AF807325

New Directions in Welfare History

Series Editors
Julia Moses, Department of History, University of Sheffield, Sheffield, UK
Martin Lengwiler, Department of History, University of Basel, Basel, Switzerland
Emma Hunter, School of History, Classics and Archaeology, University of Edinburgh, Edinburgh, UK

This series offers a unique perspective on the history of the welfare state, social policy and related social questions. It brings together research from around the world on a broad spectrum of related issues, from poverty and related questions of social justice and inequality to labour rights, family policy, social security legislation, connections between international development and social policy, and beyond. Books within it seek to highlight broader global, international, transnational and comparative aspects of these issues, while at the same time remaining sensitive to local and national histories. Moreover, they cut across traditional disciplinary boundaries, drawing on history, sociology, politics and law, as well as different theoretical and methodological approaches – from institutionalist perspectives to social history, gender history, economic history and beyond – in order to shed new light on these areas. In this way, the series problematises the nature of 'the social' and related questions of social rights, as well as the role of the state, civic organisations and international bodies in addressing these.

Andy Holroyde

Sheltered Employment and Disability in the British Welfare State

Remploy, 1944–1979

palgrave
macmillan

Andy Holroyde
Decent Work and Productivity
Research Centre
Manchester Metropolitan University
Manchester, UK

ISSN 2730-7662 ISSN 2730-7670 (electronic)
New Directions in Welfare History
ISBN 978-3-031-87875-6 ISBN 978-3-031-87876-3 (eBook)
https://doi.org/10.1007/978-3-031-87876-3

© The Editor(s) (if applicable) and The Author(s), under exclusive license to Springer Nature Switzerland AG 2025

This work is subject to copyright. All rights are solely and exclusively licensed by the Publisher, whether the whole or part of the material is concerned, specifically the rights of translation, reprinting, reuse of illustrations, recitation, broadcasting, reproduction on microfilms or in any other physical way, and transmission or information storage and retrieval, electronic adaptation, computer software, or by similar or dissimilar methodology now known or hereafter developed.
The use of general descriptive names, registered names, trademarks, service marks, etc. in this publication does not imply, even in the absence of a specific statement, that such names are exempt from the relevant protective laws and regulations and therefore free for general use.
The publisher, the authors and the editors are safe to assume that the advice and information in this book are believed to be true and accurate at the date of publication. Neither the publisher nor the authors or the editors give a warranty, expressed or implied, with respect to the material contained herein or for any errors or omissions that may have been made. The publisher remains neutral with regard to jurisdictional claims in published maps and institutional affiliations.

Cover illustration: Amy Shore/Getty Images

This Palgrave Macmillan imprint is published by the registered company Springer Nature Switzerland AG
The registered company address is: Gewerbestrasse 11, 6330 Cham, Switzerland

If disposing of this product, please recycle the paper.

For Archer

Series' Foreword

Amidst the remarkable global socio-economic developments of the twenty-first century, the history of the welfare state, social policy and related social questions warrants sustained reflection more than ever before. From the economic downturn and austerity politics since the early 2000s to the Covid-19 pandemic and its long-lasting public health drama, recent history has encouraged historians to ask new questions—and revisit longstanding ones—about the role of the state and international organisations in handling 'social problems', as well as what exactly constitutes societal rather than individual concerns and who is deemed 'deserving' in these considerations. *New Directions in Welfare History* brings together first-class research from around the world in the form of full-length and shorter monographs as well as edited collections to address these kinds of questions.

This volume speaks to several issues that this series seeks to highlight. It focuses on the creation of new opportunities to employ disabled people in postwar Britain, starting with the introduction of the Disabled Persons (Employment) Act 1944 and its creation of the Remploy programme, which ran until 2013. The topic itself has not received due attention in literature on the history of welfare and social policy, for Britain or elsewhere. Yet, this book goes further by showing how these programmes demonstrated the specificity and expansive reach of the new post-1945 British welfare state, even if the thinking behind them—including concepts of disability and welfare—in certain ways predated 1945 and emerged out of experiences with disability in the aftermath of the First World War. In this way, the volume builds on others in this series, for example, by Michele Mioni and collaborators, who have sought to probe and push the boundaries of historical periodizations of European social policies, let alone their geographical coverage in historical scholarship. Through detailed analysis going into the late twentieth century, Holroyde shows that Britain's experience with the employment of the disabled was subject to a surprising degree of cross-party consensus lasting decades in postwar Britain, extending over time despite the introduction of new governments, social programmes, understandings of health and disability, and assistive technologies. He also suggests Remploy's international impact, as it stood at the forefront of postwar rehabilitative employment programmes and therefore offered an example abroad.

By focusing on the purposeful employment of disabled and injured workers, Holroyde sheds novel light on a subject examined in detail elsewhere in this series: ideas about the relationship between leisure, work, and periods of not working. In his contribution to *New Directions in Welfare History*, Robert Snape shows how leisure was discussed in nineteenth- and twentieth-century Britain as an essential counter to work, and was enshrined in legislation reducing working hours as well as in everyday practices like setting up allotments or social clubs. By contrast, this volume shows how disabled workers were actively integrated into the workplace so that they would neither be relegated to a life of poverty from lack of earnings, or to a life where their social contributions sat (willingly or not) outside the realm of labour. As Holroyde shows, in the second half of the twentieth century, and indeed into the present, these issues were of course not without controversy. Did programmes offering sheltered employment best serve disabled people? What is the relationship between welfare, work and disability? Writing in spring 2025, these issues remain at the forefront of political and popular debate in the UK, as the current government considers ways to encourage workers on various kinds of social benefits—including those receiving different strands of disability benefits—to go to work. At the same time, the UK is considering a new Employment Bill of Rights that enshrines, for example, the right to sick leave for workers from their first day of illness. In this context, Holryode's book offers a pressing reminder that these issues have a long and fraught history in Britain, as elsewhere, that continues to shape the concepts and social programmes related to disability today.

Manchester, UK

Julia Moses
Martin Lengwiler
Emma Hunter

Acknowledgements I owe an enormous debt to the many academics who taught me at the University of Huddersfield over the years. In particular, I would like to express my gratitude to Barry Doyle, Tim Thornton, Katherine Lewis, Pat Cullum, Rebecca Gill and Paul Ward for all their help and support. My thanks also to Alice Brumby who has provided helpful advice and a friendly ear throughout the writing of this book. Most importantly I want to thank Rob Ellis, without whom the thesis upon which this book is based would not have been completed. I would also like to thank all the staff and fellow students in the Heritage Consortium, and I remain very grateful to the Arts and Humanities Research Council for funding the Ph.D., as well as to The Economic History Society, The Royal Historical Society, The Society for the Social History of Medicine, The Society for the Study of Labour History, The University of Huddersfield and the Crossley Heath Careers Fund for providing additional grants.

My love of history was kindled during my time at the Crossley Heath School, where I benefited from the inspirational teaching of Steve Donlan and Jonathan Davies. I would also like to extend my gratitude to Tom Hicks and David Felton, who welcomed me to Remploy when I began the Ph.D., and who supported the project throughout. I am also grateful for the help I have received from the staff at The National Archives on several research trips.

I have benefitted enormously from the support of many friends and colleagues throughout my studies and during the completion of this book. There are too many to mention here by name, but I would like to say a huge thank you to you all. I am particularly grateful to Peter Connor for his constant encouragement and friendship. I would like to especially thank my parents, Christina and Paul Holroyde, as well as Lauretta Langham-Lopez and Peter Holroyde, for all their love and support.

Finally, and most importantly, I want to express my love and eternal gratitude to Angie Fryers, who was utterly instrumental in allowing me to complete this book, and to Archer, who made it all worthwhile.

Competing Interests The author is currently employed by Maximus, which Remploy joined in 2015. The research which forms the basis of this book was undertaken prior to this appointment.

Contents

Abbreviations

ALO	Area Liaison Officer
BEC	British Employers' Confederation
BLESMA	British Limbless Ex-Service Men's Association
DA	Disability Alliance
DE	Department of Employment
DIG	Disablement Income Group
DPEA	Disabled Persons (Employment) Act
DRO	Disablement Resettlement Officer
ESA	Employment Services Agency
LA	Local Authority
MOL	Ministry of Labour
MP	Member of Parliament
MSC	Manpower Services Commission
NACED	National Advisory Council on the Employment of the Disabled
NAIBD	National Association of Industries for the Blind and Disabled
NHS	National Health Service
NLBD	National League of the Blind and Disabled
SEC	Sheltered Employment Committee
TB	Tuberculosis
TNA	The National Archives
TUC	Trades Union Congress

List of Tables

CHAPTER 1

Introduction

In October 2013, the few remaining Remploy factories closed their doors for the final time. The decision taken by the then Coalition Government to close these factories was controversial, attracting widespread media attention, and effectively marked the end of a long history of a particular form of employment and welfare provision. The factories provided sheltered employment, a term used to denote workplaces dedicated to employing disabled people in a supposedly safe and supportive environment protected, or 'sheltered', from the competitive pressures of the'open' or 'mainstream' labour market. Remploy was established by the British Government as part of the Disabled Persons (Employment) Act 1944 (DPEA), with the aim of providing sheltered employment on a national scale for those severely disabled people who were considered unable to gain work otherwise. Funded by the Treasury, Remploy grew rapidly to become the dominant provider of sheltered employment in the postwar period. In terms of its workforce, the scheme reached its height in the late 1980s when it employed over 9000 disabled people in 94 factories across Great Britain. As the inclusion of disabled people in mainstream employment became an ever-greater priority, Remploy adapted over time to reflect this aim. Remploy factories began to be closed down and replaced by offices on the high street, which focused on providing employment services to support jobseekers with disabilities

© The Author(s), under exclusive license to Springer Nature Switzerland AG 2025

A. Holroyde, *Sheltered Employment and Disability in the British Welfare State*, New Directions in Welfare History,
https://doi.org/10.1007/978-3-031-87876-3_1

or health conditions into work. Following the closure of the final factories in 2013, further change occurred when, in April 2015, Remploy left government ownership and joined Maximus, an international provider of health and employment services.

Despite its place as the key provider of sheltered employment in Britain, and a pioneering attempt by any government to provide this kind of national scheme, a detailed analysis of Remploy by historians has been a stark omission. Similarly, the historiography regarding sheltered employment more generally is incomplete, comprising of brief mentions and small-scale case studies. The objective of this book is therefore to provide the first detailed examination of Remploy in the period 1944–1979, over the course of which the company provided work in its factories for more than 40,000 disabled people.[1] In so doing, it seeks to develop a fuller understanding of Remploy and sheltered employment, focusing on some fundamental aspects of function and administration. The second aim is to position Remploy within some of the key debates concerning the British welfare state in this period, deepening our understanding of a key policy area for disabled people, and contributing to the wider aim of adding the experience of disability to more established areas of historical research.

From Disability Studies to Disability History

Given the occasionally blurred lines between disability history and disability studies, it is first necessary to properly position the aims and scope of this book. Until relatively recently, historians have shown little interest in disability as a category of analysis. As a result of this neglect, considerations of disability in the past were provided primarily by those working in the fields of sociology, anthropology, literature and most notably, disability studies.[2] Sometimes referred to as 'emancipatory disability studies', this field emerged in Britain during the 1970s as disability activists sought to 'rescue' disabled people from the perceived overarching dominance of what was termed the 'medical model' of

[1] 'World Interest', *Remploy News*, 124 (November, 1978).

[2] H. Stiker, *A History of Disability* (Ann Arbor, University of Michigan Press, 1999); S. Burch, 'Disability History: Suggested Readings—An Annotated Bibliography', *The Public Historian*, vol. 27, no. 2 (2005), pp. 63–74; C. Kudlick, 'Disability History: Why We Need Another "Other"', *The American Historical Review*, vol. 108, no. 3 (2003), pp. 763–93.

disability.[3] In this 'medical model', disability is defined in medical terms, with the focus on the 'dysfunctional individual body' which establishes 'physical, social and economic parameters' for disabled people.[4] Disability is therefore a physical fault with the individual, alleviated only, if at all, through the intervention of medical professionals.

The 'social model' was developed to directly challenge this perception, stemming from the activist work of the Union of the Physically Impaired Against Segregation, which came to lead the disability movement in Britain, and its proponents, such as Vic Finkelstein and Michael Oliver, who would establish its outlook in the academic field—the latter coining the term 'social model of disability' in 1983.[5] The model defines disability in social terms 'as the barriers erected, attitudes toward, and exclusion of disabled people by society'.[6] Thus it is not individual impairment that makes someone disabled, it is the constraints placed upon such individuals by wider society.[7] While it has not gone unchallenged itself, the social model has since become the dominant 'structural analysis of disabled people's social exclusion' in Britain.[8]

Although primarily concerned with contemporary issues, proponents of the social model such as Oliver and Colin Barnes have outlined the history of disabled people in their work, presenting a narrative of increasing marginalisation, exclusion and isolation with the growth of industrial capitalism.[9] Employment is therefore a central theme in such

[3] J. Anderson and A. Carden-Coyne, 'Enabling the Past: New Perspectives in the History of Disability', *European Review of History*, vol. 14, no. 4 (2007), pp. 447–57; J. Anderson, *War, Disability and Rehabilitation in Britain: 'Soul of a Nation'* (Manchester, Manchester University Press, 2011), pp. 4–7.

[4] Andersonand Carden-Coyne, 'Enabling the Past'; J. Anderson, 'Review Article: Voices in the Dark: Representations of Disability in Historical Research', *Journal of Contemporary History*, vol. 44, no. 1 (2009), pp. 107–16.

[5] T. Shakespeare, 'The Social Model of Disability', in L.J. Davies (ed.) *The Disability Studies Reader*, 4th Edition (Abingdon, Routledge, 2013), p. 215.

[6] Anderson, *War, Disability and Rehabilitation in Britain*, pp. 4–7.

[7] Shakespeare, 'The Social Model of Disability', pp. 214–7.

[8] Ibid., p. 214; J. Morris, *Pride Against Prejudice: A Personal Politics of Disability* (London, The Women's Press, 1991).

[9] M. Oliver, *The Politics of Disablement* (Basingstoke, Macmillan, 1990), pp. 25–42; M. Oliver and C. Barnes, *Disabled People and Social Policy: From Exclusion to Inclusion* (London, Longman, 1998), pp. 25–35.

work, yet these interpretations of historical developments rest upon generalised assumptions, rather than close investigation, and reflect the purpose of the social model as a contemporary activist tool.[10] Such histories are therefore problematic for historians and do not represent what would be considered robust analysis in the discipline of history.[11]

In response to these limitations, historians have brought greater attention to bear on disability as an area of analysis. The field of disability history has seen enormous growth over the last twenty or so years, becoming an established area of research.[12] This growth was initially confined largely to the United States with the dawn of 'new disability history', a term used to distinguish it from 'disability studies history'.[13] In one of the key works bearing this term as its title, Paul K. Longmore and Lauri Umansky argued that 'disability belongs with race, class, and gender as a "standard analytical tool" of historical analysis'.[14] Catherine J. Kudlick elaborated on this in 2003, suggesting that disability allowed a new perspective on all aspects of history, allowing historians 'to reconsider virtually every concept, every event, every "given" we have taken for granted'.[15] With a number of published works across a wide range of themes and periods, dedicated academic conferences and the formation of societies and associations devoted to the field, Beth Linker was able to claim in 2013 that disability history had truly 'arrived' in the United States.[16]

[10] E. Hall, 'Workspaces: Refiguring the Disability—Employment Debate', in R. Butler and H. Parr (eds.) *Mind and Body Space: geographies of illness, impairment and disability* (Abingdon, Routledge, 1999), pp. 138–54.

[11] For criticisms see B.J. Gleeson, 'Disability Studies: A historical materialist view', *Disability & Society*, vol. 12, no. 2 (1997), pp. 179–202; B. Gleeson, *Geographies of Disability* (London, Routledge, 1999) pp. 22–3; Anderson and Carden-Coyne, 'Enabling the Past'; Anderson, 'Voices in the Dark'; J. Hampton, 'Discovering Disability: The General Classes of Disabled People and the Classic Welfare State, 1948–1964', *The Historian*, vol. 75, no. 1 (2013), p. 72.

[12] Anderson, *War, Disability and Rehabilitation in Britain*, pp. 4–7.

[13] P. K. Longmore and L. Umansky, 'Disability History: From the Margins to the Mainstream', in P.K. Longmore and L. Umansky (eds.) *The New Disability History: American Perspectives* (New York, New York University Press, 2001), pp. 15–7.

[14] Longmore and Umansky, 'Disability History', p.15; S. Burch, 'Disability History'.

[15] Kudlick, 'Disability History', p. 767.

[16] B. Linker, 'On the Borderlands of Medical and Disability History: A Survey of the Fields', *Bulletin of the History of Medicine*, vol. 87, no. 4 (2013), p. 499. See also R.

The development of disability history in the United Kingdom was initially slower, but has since gathered pace. The first comprehensive historical study was Anne Borsay's *Disability and Social Policy in Britain since 1750: A History of Exclusion*.[17] While it is rightly held up as an important work and instigator for subsequent disability history, it is limited for historians by the fact that Borsay, as the title of her study suggests, was focused on supporting the notion of the assumed exclusion of disabled people propounded by the social model of disability. The primary purpose of the work was to 'raise personal and political consciousness' as a reflection of the aims of 'emancipatory disability studies'.[18] The field has since moved away from such links with disability studies to instead reflect something more of the 'new disability history', in terms of considering disability in historical contexts in the same way as with any other area of enquiry.

A key UK disability history conference took place in 2005, followed by the publication of three major volumes considering disability across a range of themes, periods and locations.[19] A further conference took place in 2010, and the following year saw the publication of a major study from Julie Anderson, *War, Disability and Rehabilitation in Britain: 'Soul of a Nation'*.[20] While noting that some progress had been made in the field, Anderson called in this work for further effort by historians to consider disability, using a range of historical sources and methodologies, in a variety of periods and locations, in order to provide a more

Garland-Thomson, (ed.) *Freakery: Cultural Spectacles of the Extraordinary Body* (New York, New York University Press, 1996); D.Z. Fleischer and F. Zames, *The Disability Rights Movement: From Charity to Confrontation* (Philadelphia, Temple University Press, 2011); K. Ott, D. Serlin, and S. Mihm, (eds.) *Artificial Parts, Practical Lives: Modern Histories of Prosthetics* (New York, New York University Press, 2002); S. Burch and M. Rembis, *Disability Histories* (Urbana, University of Illinois Press, 2014).

[17] A. Borsay, *Disability and Social Policy in Britain Since 1750: A History of Exclusion* (Basingstoke, Palgrave Macmillan, 2005).

[18] Borsay, *Disability and Social Policy in Britain Since 1750*, p. 207.

[19] N. Pemberton, 'Enabling the Past: New Perspectives in the History of Disability', *History Workshop Journal*, no. 61 (2006), pp. 292–5; D.M. Turner and K. Stagg (eds.) *Social Histories of Disability and Deformity* (Abingdon, Routledge, 2006); W. Ernst (ed.) *Histories of the Normal and the Abnormal* (Abingdon, Routledge, 2006); P. Dale and J. Melling (eds.) *Mental Illness and Learning Disability since 1850: Finding a Place for Mental Disorder in the United Kingdom* (Oxon, Routledge, 2006).

[20] D.M. Turner, 'Disability History: Looking Forward to a Better Past?', *History Workshop Journal*, no.71 (2011), pp. 283–7.

balanced, contextual picture of disability in history.[21] The call appears to have been heeded with an increasing major engagement with disability by historians now apparent.[22] Recent years have witnessed a steady stream of journal articles in the field, as well as the publication of important works including Matthias Reiss' *Blind Workers Against Charity*, Jameel Hampton's *Disability and the Welfare State in Britain* and David M. Turner and Daniel Blackie's *Disability in the Industrial Revolution*.[23] A dedicated *Disability History* series by Manchester University Press has released several volumes exploring a range of periods and contexts.[24]

[21] Anderson, *War, Disability and Rehabilitation in Britain*, pp. 1–11, 215–6.

[22] B. Curtis and S. Thompson, "A plentiful crop of cripples made by all this progress': Disability, Artificial Limbs and Working-Class Mutualism in the South Wales Coalfield, 1890–1948', *Social History of Medicine*, vol. 27, no. 4 (2014), pp. 708–27; Hampton, 'Discovering Disability', pp. 69–93; M. Mantin, 'Educational Experiences of Deaf Children in Wales: The Cambrian Institution for the Deaf and Dumb, 1847–1914', unpublished PhD Thesis, Swansea University (2010); J. Hampton, 'Disabled People and the Classic Welfare State, 1948–1975: Changes in Perception, Developments in Policy', unpublished PhD Thesis, University of Bristol (2012); G. Millward, 'Invalid Definitions, Invalid Responses: Disability and the Welfare State, 1965–1995', unpublished PhD Thesis, London School of Hygiene and Tropical Medicine (2013).

[23] M. Reiss, *Blind Workers Against Charity: The National League of the Blind of Great Britain and Ireland, 1893–1970* (London, Palgrave Macmillan, 2015); J. Hampton, *Disability and the Welfare State in Britain: Changes in perception and policy 1948–79* (Bristol, Policy Press, 2016); D. M. Turner and D. Blackie, *Disability in the Industrial Revolution: Physical impairment in British coalmining, 1780–1880* (Manchester, Manchester University Press, 2018); J. Gulland, *Gender, Work and Social Control: A Century of Disability Benefits* (Palgrave Macmillan, 2019); J. Anderson, "Jumpy Stump': Amputation and trauma in the first world war', *First World War Studies*, vol. 6, no. 1, (2015), pp. 9–19; G. Millward, 'Social Security Policy and the Early Disability Movement—Expertise, Disability, and the Government, 1965–77', *Twentieth Century British History*, vol. 26, no. 2 (2015), pp. 274–97; M. Mantin, 'Coalmining and the National Scheme for Disabled Ex-Servicemen after the First World War', *Social History*, vol. 41, no. 2 (2016), pp. 155–70; G. Millward, 'A Disability Act? The Vaccine Damage Payments Act 1979 and the British Government's Response to the Pertussis Vaccine Scare', *Social History of Medicine*, vol. 30, no. 2 (2017), pp. 429–47; A. Turner and A. McIvor, "Bottom Dog Men': Disability, Social Welfare and Advocacy in the Scottish Coalfields in the Interwar Years, 1918–1939', *Scottish Historical Review*, vol. 96, no. 2 (2017), pp. 187–213; B. Curtis and S. Thompson, 'Disability and the Family in South Wales Coalfield Society, c.1920–1939', *Family and Community History*, vol. 20, no. 1, (2017), pp. 25–44.

[24] This includes K. Bohata et al., *Disability in Industrial Britain: A Cultural and Literary History of Impairment in the Coal Industry, 1880–1948* (Manchester, Manchester University Press, 2020); M. Robinson, *Shell-shocked British Army Veterans in Ireland, 1918–39: A Difficult Homecoming* (Manchester, Manchester University Press, 2022);

The intention of this book is to contribute to this recent engagement with disability within the discipline of history, through detailed research and analysis, divorced from the activist position associated with 'emancipatory disability studies', and thereby add to our understanding of disability within historical contexts. This book aims therefore to provide the first detailed examination of Remploy and to add this to the current understanding of disability and the British welfare state.

Remploy and Sheltered Employment

That an examination of Remploy has not been undertaken until now has not meant that the company has gone unmentioned. Remploy is typically referenced as *the* example of postwar sheltered employment, yet it is evoked uncritically. This is the case across academic disciplines, and in wider public discourse. The result is that Remploy has tended to appear in scholarly works as a monolithic scheme with a predetermined and usually uncomplicated agenda. The company and from this, sheltered employment more generally, are then appropriated in various ways to support wider conclusions.

This begins with Remploy's inception and creation as part of the DPEA. Occasional references have been made to the birth of Remploy, but few attempts have been made to explain its formation.[25] An enduring popular viewpoint is that it was created as a direct result of the Second World War and this simplistic reference remained the long-held view of Remploy themselves and a common focus in media reports on the

I. Hutchinson, M. Atherton, & J. Virdi (eds.) *Disability and the Victorians: Attitudes, Interventions, Legacies* (Manchester, Manchester University Press, 2022).

[25] Borsay, *Disability and Social Policy in Britain Since* 1750, p. 135; S. Wheatcroft, *Worth Saving: Disabled Children During the Second World War* (Manchester, Manchester University Press, 2013), p. 168; S. Humphries and P. Gordon, *Out of Sight: The Experience of Disability 1900–1950* (Plymouth, Northcote House, 1992), p. 138. Further brief references are made in, L. Bryder, *Below the Magic Mountain: A Social History of Tuberculosis in Twentieth-Century Britain* (Oxford, Clarendon Press, 1988), p. 237; A. Land, R. Lowe and N. Whiteside, *The Development of the Welfare State 1939–1951: A Guide to Documents in the Public Record Office* (London, HMSO, 1992), pp. 203–4; P. Bridgen and R. Lowe, *Welfare Policy Under the Conservatives 1951–1964* (London, PRO, 1998), p. 262. Also in the field of Social Policy in S. Shah and M. Priestley, *Disability and Social Change: Private Lives and Public Policies* (Bristol, Policy Press, 2011), p. 139; E. Topliss, *Provision for the Disabled* (Oxford, Basil Blackwell, 1979), pp. 55–6.

company.[26] Some academic works have also tended to simply identify Remploy as an element of wartime legislation.[27] In other cases this has been made more explicit, with both Reiss and Anderson, for example, suggesting that Remploy came about as a direct result of the experiences of the war.[28] Perhaps the most influential academic interpretation of Remploy's creation was provided by Helen Bolderson, who viewed it as a result of a bargain with industry to segregate 'non-productive' workers away from the labour market.[29] This view was then repeated in Steve Humphries and Pamela Gordon's *Out of Sight*, and subsequently adopted by Borsay in her influential study, to reinforce the notion of Remploy as an element in the perpetual discrimination of disabled people.[30] In other cases too, Remploy's formation has been invoked in support of overarching statements about employment provision in the postwar period.[31]

There have been differing views on the primary function of Remploy and sheltered employment in this period, presented by academics across fields. One narrative, espoused by disability studies scholars such as Barnes, Sonali Shah and Mark Priestley, suggests that 'until the late

[26] T. Jeffries, 'The Remploy Resource', *Industrial Management & Data Systems*, vol. 86, no. 1/2 (1986), p. 7; A. Kochan, 'Remploy: disabled and thriving', *Assembly Automation*, vol. 16, no. 1 (1996), p. 40; BBC News 'What are Remploy workers doing now?', (31.11.2014). http://www.bbc.co.uk/news/uk-29843567. Accessed 16 August 2024.

[27] J. Anderson, "Turned into Taxpayers': Paraplegia, Rehabilitation and Sport at Stoke Mandeville, 1944-56', *Journal of Contemporary History*, vol. 38, no. 3 (2003), p. 469; E. Elsey, 'The Rehabilitation and Employment of Disabled Ex-Servicemen after the Two World Wars', unpublished PhD Thesis, University of Teesside (1994), pp. 276–7; Oliver, *The Politics of Disablement*, pp. 88–9; Wheatcroft, *Worth Saving*, p. 168; M. Hyde, 'Sheltered and Supported Employment in the 1990s: The experiences of disabled workers in the UK', *Disability & Society*, vol. 13, no. 2 (1998), pp. 199–215; Bryder, *Below the Magic Mountain*, p. 237.

[28] Reiss, *Blind Workers Against Charity,* p. 140; Anderson, *War, Disability and Rehabilitation in Britain,* pp. 183–5.

[29] H. Bolderson, *Social Security, Disability and Rehabilitation: Conflicts in the Development of Social Policy 1914–1946* (London, Jessica Kingsley Publishers, 1991), pp. 109–110.

[30] Humphries and Gordon, *Out of Sight*, p. 138; Borsay, *Disability and Social Policy in Britain Since* 1750. This was also highlighted by Wheatcroft, *Worth Saving*, pp. 168–70.

[31] Hampton, 'Discovering Disability', p. 77; Anderson, *War, Disability and Rehabilitation in Britain,* pp. 183–5.

1970s the role of sheltered workshops was widely regarded as humanitarian rather than economic'.[32] In this view, Remploy operated primarily as a social service, with welfare prioritised over commercial efficiency. This function was then transformed following the election of Margaret Thatcher in 1979 to one in which commercial principles became paramount.[33] A similar notion was put forward by the historian Gareth Millward, who highlighted the 1980s as the period in which Remploy underwent economic rationalisation, something he viewed as a significant change from previous policy.[34] The perception here is of something akin to a 'golden age' of Remploy during the period of the classic welfare state, before the Thatcher governments fundamentally changed its primary focus from providing a social service to maximising its commercial efficiency. An alternative view, proposed by social policy scholars Susan Lonsdale and Eda Topliss, suggests instead that there was always something of an 'uneasy compromise' in Remploy and sheltered employment between humanitarian and economic considerations.[35]

A similar situation arises in terms of who was being employed by Remploy and upon what basis. The composition of Remploy's workforce has largely been taken for granted. In many cases, mentions of Remploy have, with a variety of phrasing, simply referenced that it was for disabled people,[36] or for severely disabled people.[37] Other descriptions of Remploy, such as those of Borsay, Bolderson and Pat Thane

[32] C. Barnes, *Disabled People in Britain and Discrimination* (London, C. Hurst & Co., 2000), p. 73; Shah and Priestley, *Disability and Social Change,* pp. 138–40.

[33] Barnes, *Disabled People in Britain and Discrimination,* p. 73.

[34] Millward, 'Invalid definitions, invalid responses', pp. 184–5.

[35] S. Lonsdale, *Work and Inequality* (Harlow, Longman, 1985), p. 138; Topliss, *Provision for the Disabled,* pp. 55–7.

[36] Hampton, 'Discovering Disability', p. 80; Bryder, *Below the Magic Mountain,* p. 237; Wheatcroft, *Worth Saving,* p. 168; Hyde, 'Sheltered and Supported Employment in the 1990s', p. 200; Bridgen and Lowe, *Welfare Policy Under the Conservatives 1951–1964,* pp. 262–3.

[37] Bolderson, *Social Security, Disability and Rehabilitation,* p. 109; Topliss, *Provision for the Disabled,* p. 56; Reiss, *Blind Workers Against Charity,* p. 139; Elsey, 'The Rehabilitation and Employment of Disabled Ex-Servicemen after the Two World Wars', pp. 276–7; Anderson, 'Turned into Taxpayers', p. 469 refers to 'seriously disabled'; Barnes, *Disabled People in Britain and Discrimination,* p. 71; Land, Lowe and Whiteside, *The Development of the Welfare State 1939–1951,* p. 204; Mantin, 'Coalmining and the National Scheme for Disabled Ex-Servicemen after the First World War', p. 170.

have suggested it was reserved for those disabled people deemed to be ineffective or non-productive workers.[38] The common assumption here has been that in forming its workforce, Remploy simply met the requirements outlined in the DPEA, and provided employment for those too severely disabled to be considered able to gain employment in the open job market, officially designated by the Act as 'Section II' disabled people. Similarly, with a single exception, all descriptions of the Remploy workforce make no mention of any gender distinction. Consideration of the place of women in Remploy specifically has only been given brief consideration by Anderson, who suggested that women were excluded from Remploy due to its nature as an industrial enterprise, as well as issues of accommodation and transport.[39] Other descriptions of Remploy's workforce have highlighted specific groups of disabled people. One enduring view, which framed Remploy's own explanation of its origins, held that the company was created specifically for disabled ex-service personnel.[40] Most recently, Roddy Slorach in his socialist interpretation of disability history echoed this view.[41] Historians considering disability have often tended to focus on those disabled during war.[42] Disabled ex-service

[38] Borsay, *Disability and Social Policy in Britain Since 1750*, p. 135; Bolderson, *Social Security, Disability and Rehabilitation*, p. 109; H. Bolderson, 'The Origins of the Disabled Persons Employment Quota and its Symbolic Significance', *Journal of Social Policy*, vol. 9, no. 2 (1980), p. 178; P. Thane, *Foundations of the Welfare State, 2nd Edition* (London, Longman, 1996), p. 225, who does not mention Remploy by name but refers to the sheltered workshops provided by the DPEA.

[39] Anderson, *War, Disability and Rehabilitation in Britain*, p. 170; J. Anderson, 'British Women, Disability and the Second World War', *Contemporary British History*, vol. 20, no. 1 (2006), p. 49.

[40] Ex-Servicemen have typically been highlighted, sometimes alongside 'miners', for example, BBC News 'What are Remploy workers doing now?', (31.11.2014). http://www.bbc.co.uk/news/uk-29843567. Accessed 16 August 2024.

[41] R. Slorach, *A Very Capitalist Condition: A History and Politics of Disability* (London, Bookmarks, 2016), p. 141.

[42] Anderson, *War, Disability and Rehabilitation in Britain*; J. Anderson, "Jumpy Stump': Amputation and trauma in the first world war', pp. 9–19; Anderson, 'Turned into Taxpayers'; J. Anderson and N. Pemberton, 'Walking Alone: Aiding the War and Civilian Blind in the Inter-war Period', *European Review of History*, vol. 14, no. 4 (2007), pp. 459–79; J. Meyer, "Not Septimus Now': wives of disabled veterans and cultural memory of the First World War in Britain', *Women's History Review*, vol. 13, no. 1 (2004), pp. 117–138; M. Kowalsky, "This Honourable Obligation": The King's National Roll Scheme for Disabled Ex-servicemen, 1915–1944', *European Review of History*, vol. 14, no. 4 (2007), pp. 567–84; A. Borsay, 'Disability in British Poetry of the First World

personnel have been considered as a distinct group who received preferential treatment in welfare and employment provision owing to the origin of their disability.[43] Such work has tended to focus on the durations of the two World Wars themselves or the interwar period, with very little consideration of the place of disabled ex-service personnel post-1945.[44] The exception is Anderson who, in considering the immediate aftermath of the Second World War, highlighted Remploy as part of the continued 'special treatment' this group received.[45] In addition to this focus on ex-service personnel, Anderson further suggested that Remploy concentrated its provision upon people with certain disabilities or conditions.[46]

In all these descriptions of Remploy, the workforce consists entirely of disabled people. This is also implicit in descriptions of sheltered employment as 'segregated employment', with the absolute separation of

War', *Disability & Society*, vol. 30, no. 4 (2015), pp. 499–512; J. Bourke, *Dismembering the Male: Men's Bodies, Britain and the Great War* (London, Reaktion Books, 1996); D. Cohen, *The War Come Home: Disabled Veterans in Britain and Germany 1914–1939* (Los Angeles, University of California Press, 2001); D. A. Gerber (ed.) *Disabled Veterans in History* (Ann Arbor, University of Michigan Press, 2012); F.L. Bernstein, 'Rehabilitation Staged: How Soviet Doctors "Cured" Disability in the Second World War', in S. Burch and M. Rembis (eds.) *Disability History* (Urbana, University of Illinois Press, 2014), pp. 218–236; J.M. Kinder, "Lest We Forget': Disabled Veterans and the Politics of War Remembrance in the United States' in S. Burch and M. Rembis (eds.) *Disability History* (Urbana, University of Illinois Press, 2014), pp. 163–182; K. Muir, "That bastard's following me!' Mentally Ill Australian Veterans Struggling to Maintain Control', in D.M. Turner, and K. Stagg, (eds.) *Social Histories of Disability and Deformity* (Abingdon, Routledge, 2006), pp. 161–174; J. Reznick, 'Work-Therapy and the Disabled British Soldier in Great Britain in the First World War: The Case of Shepherd's Bush Military Hospital, London', in D. A. Gerber (ed.) *Disabled Veterans in History* (Ann Arbor, University of Michigan Press, 2012), pp. 185–203.

43 W. Gagen, 'Remastering the Body, Renegotiating Gender: Physical Disability and Masculinity during the First World War, the Case of J.B. Middlebrook', *European Review of History*, vol. 14, no. 4, pp. 536–7; Bourke, *Dismembering the Male,* pp. 37–9; Hampton, *Disability and the Welfare State in Britain,* pp. 53–4.

44 M. Kowalsky, 'Enabling the Great War: ex-servicemen, the mixed economy of welfare and the social construction of disability, 1899–1930', unpublished PhD Thesis, University of Leeds (2007), p. 236.

45 Anderson, 'Turned into Taxpayers', pp. 469–70; Anderson, *War, Disability and Rehabilitation in Britain,* p. 211.

46 Anderson, *War, Disability and Rehabilitation in Britain,* p. 183.

disabled people in such places.[47] That the company only ever employed disabled people in its production workforce was also the belief of Remploy themselves, expressed in conversations with senior management undertaken through this research, and this was understood to be a key difference between Remploy and sheltered employment programmes in other countries, in which the inclusion of a proportion of non-disabled workers to boost productivity was the norm. It was suggested that this had often been cited in discussions with policy-makers and disability employment providers around the world, as one of the reasons why Remploy's factories ultimately proved uneconomical—in that they had lacked the 'advantage' of a non-disabled element in their workforce. Such views run contrary to the claim made by Topliss in the 1970s, that the inclusion of a proportion of non-disabled workers was 'always envisaged' for Remploy 'in order to ensure the efficiency of organisation and running of production'.[48]

Furthermore, with any mention or consideration of postwar sheltered employment focusing almost exclusively upon Remploy, there has been an assumption that it became the only meaningful provider. The impression is that the voluntary sheltered workshops which existed prior to the Second World War, which themselves have received only very limited attention from historians, were made largely redundant following the establishment of Remploy.[49] Only Anderson has suggested that voluntary sheltered employment survived in the immediate postwar period, though to what extent is unclear.[50] It is also the case that wherever Remploy is referenced, it is presented as a coherent, monolithic scheme, with no sense of any discrepancy between policy and how it functioned in reality. This is largely because any considerations of Remploy have relied on very limited sources, if any, which invariably reflect only central policy. How Remploy and sheltered employment operated at the local factory level, and how far

47 Millward, 'Invalid Definitions, Invalid Responses', pp. 184–5; Humphries and Gordon, *Out of Sight*, p. 138; Wheatcroft, *Worth Saving*, p. 168; Slorach, *A Very Capitalist Condition*, p. 141; Hyde, 'Sheltered and Supported Employment in the 1990s', p. 200; Barnes, *Disabled People in Britain and Discrimination*, p. 74.

48 Topliss, *Provision for the Disabled*, pp. 55–6.

49 Anderson, *War, Disability and Rehabilitation in Britain;* Cohen, *The War Come Home*; Bolderson, *Social Security, Disability and Rehabilitation.*

50 Anderson, *War, Disability and Rehabilitation in Britain*, p. 184.

this reflected the aims of the legislation and the policies espoused, has not yet been explored.

There has been, therefore, no comprehensive account of Remploy in terms of how and why it was created, how it functioned, who it was for and how far it dominated the provision of sheltered employment. With the company commonly used across disciplines as *the* example of sheltered employment, it is important these foundational areas are clarified. Furthermore, as the accepted chief provider of sheltered employment in the period, it is the key to understanding how this form of employment and welfare was understood and functioned for severely disabled people. Our understanding of disability in postwar Britain is not complete without Remploy, and as the first attempt to provide sheltered employment on this scale, it has also served as an international exemplar. Although sheltered employment has largely been phased out in Britain, it is still relatively common across the world, and has also remained controversial with ongoing debates about its validity in serving disabled people.[51] An understanding of how Remploy functioned is not therefore solely a question of academic interest, but also of relevance in informing such debates. This book therefore provides this first detailed examination of Remploy in the period 1944–1979, in order to address these fundamental issues.

The 'Classic' Welfare State

The further aim of this study is to add the case of Remploy and sheltered employment to our understanding of postwar disability and the welfare state. There can be few aspects of modern British history which capture the public imagination and receive as much comment as the welfare state,

[51] See for example, E.W. Carter, S. Bendetson and C.H. Guiden, 'Family Perspectives on the Appeals of and Alternatives to Sheltered Employment for Individuals with Severe Disabilities', *Research and Practice for Persons with Severe Disabilities*, vol. 43, no. 3 (2018), pp. 145–164; E. Hemphill and C.T. Kulik, 'The Tyranny of Fit: Yet another Barrier to Mainstream Employment for Disabled People in Sheltered Employment', *Social Policy & Administration*, vol. 51, no. 7 (2017), pp. 1119–1134; L. Visier, 'Sheltered Employment for Persons with Disabilities', *International Labour Review*, vol. 137, no. 3 (1998), pp. 347–65; M.S. Soeker et al., 'The Experiences and Perceptions of Persons with Disabilities Regarding Work Skills Development in Sheltered and Protective Workshops', *Work*, vol. 59, no. 2 (2018), pp. 303–14; L. Van Der Torre and M. Fenger, 'Policy Innovations for Including Disabled People in the Labour Market: A study of Innovative Practices of Dutch Sheltered Work Companies', *International Social Security Review*, vol. 67, no. 2 (2014), pp. 67–84.

examination of which is not work confined to historians, with a whole range of disciplines bringing along their own terms of reference, areas of focus and theoretical frameworks.[52] Yet an immediate issue is the definition of the term itself.[53] As Derek Fraser expressed, the concept is difficult to define as 'it has meant different things to different people'.[54] Many scholars have traced the origins of the term in various contexts and periods and called into question how viable a term it is to describe the postwar programme of social welfare in Britain.[55] To this we can layer further complexity by recognising that this was not a solely British phenomenon, with a range of welfare states, incorporating differing aspects of economic and social policies, developing in diverse forms around the world in the second half of the twentieth century.[56] Constraining this to a Western welfare state or even a British welfare state still brings many conceptual challenges.[57] Despite these musings, the fact is that the term continues to be used and as such requires a usable definition. One oft-cited definition was provided by Asa Briggs in 1961, who described a welfare state as one in which market forces were modified to guarantee a minimum income, reduce insecurity and provide citizens with an agreed range of

[52] D. Gladstone, *The Twentieth-Century Welfare State* (Basingstoke, Palgrave Macmillan, 1999), p. 4; G. Esping-Anderson, *The Three Worlds of Welfare Capitalism* (Princeton, Princeton University Press, 1990); C. Pierson, *Beyond the Welfare State? The New Political Economy of Welfare* (Cambridge, Polity Press, 1991), chapters 1–3; M. Hill, *The Welfare State in Britain: A Political History since 1945* (Aldershot, Edward Elgar Publishing, 1993), pp. 3–10; R. Lowe, *The Welfare State in Britain Since 1945* (Basingstoke, Palgrave Macmillan, 2005) pp. 23–48; H. Glennerster, *British Social Policy: 1945 to the Present*, 3rd Edition (Oxford, Blackwell Publishing, 2007), pp. 8–19; D. Fraser, *The Evolution of the British Welfare State*, 4th Edition (Basingstoke, Palgrave Macmillan, 2009), p. 2; K. Laybourn, *The Evolution of British Social Policy and the Welfare State, c.1800–1993* (Keele, Keele University Press, 1995), p.10.

[53] Lowe, *The Welfare State in Britain Since 1945*, p. 12; Pierson, *Beyond the Welfare State?*, pp. 6–7.

[54] Fraser, *The Evolution of the British Welfare State*, p. 1. See also N. Timmins, *The Five Giants: A Biography of the Welfare State*, New Edition (London, Harper Collins, 2001), pp. 6–7; D. E. Ashford, 'The Whig Interpretation of the Welfare State', *Journal of Policy History*, vol. 1, no. 1 (1989), pp. 24–25.

[55] Lowe, *The Welfare State in Britain Since 1945*, pp. 12–16; Glennerster, *British Social Policy*, p. 1.

[56] D. Béland, et al., 'Introduction', in D. Béland, et al., (eds.) *The Oxford Handbook of the Welfare State: Second Edition* (Oxford, Oxford University Press, 2021), pp. 1–19.

[57] Ibid.

social services.[58] Rodney Lowe took a pragmatic approach and defined a welfare state as one born from the 1940s, with a government which 'actively accepts responsibility' for the welfare of all citizens, and which supplies those citizens with 'an inalienable core of universal services'.[59] For Keith Laybourn, the welfare state could be characterised through the government interruption of the free market to protect vulnerable groups, to offer social services, and to safeguard the general population from the 'exigencies of working life'.[60]

The issue of precisely defining a welfare state is perhaps of greater importance for comparative studies or those which consider the extent to which Britain has indeed been a welfare state at various times. The more practical definitions suffice here for describing the programme of social provision enacted in Britain following the Second World War.[61] The focus here is upon the period often referred to as the 'classic welfare state' in Britain, which provides both the timeframe and the key areas of analysis. This term is used to distinguish the welfare provision in Britain which emerged after the war and existed until either 1976, with the imposition of cash limits on spending and the abandonment of the policy of full employment, or 1979, with the election of the Thatcher Government, at which points fundamental changes in the welfare state are seen to have occurred.[62] The period is characterised as one of faith in increased statutory welfare, and the central importance of the maintenance of full,

[58] A. Briggs, 'The Welfare State in Historical Perspective', *European Journal of Sociology*, vol. 2, no. 2 (1961), p. 228; J. Brown, *The British Welfare State: A Critical History* (Oxford, Blackwell, 1995), p. 5.

[59] Ibid., pp. 16–17.

[60] Laybourn, *The Evolution of British Social Policy and the Welfare State*, p. 9.

[61] Fraser, *The Evolution of the British Welfare State*, p. 1.

[62] A. Digby, *British Welfare Policy: Workhouse to Workfare* (London, Faber and Faber, 1989); Fraser, *The Evolution of the British Welfare State*, p. 287; Lowe, *The Welfare State in Britain Since 1945*, p. 77; Glennerster, *British Social Policy*, pp. 8–9; B. Harris, *The Origins of the British Welfare State* (Basingstoke, Palgrave Macmillan, 2004), p. 301; Gladstone, *The Twentieth-Century Welfare State*, pp. 7, 32, 73; D. Gladstone, 'The Welfare State and the State of Welfare', in D. Gladstone, (ed.) *British Social Welfare: Past, Present and Future* (London, UCL Press, 1995), p. 2; Laybourn, *The Evolution of British Social Policy and the Welfare State*, pp. 221–237; R. Page, *Revisiting the Welfare State* (Maidenhead, Open University Press, 2007), p. 47; Hampton, *Disability and the Welfare State in Britain*; B. Coxall and L. Robins, *British Politics Since the War* (Basingstoke, Macmillan, 1998), p. 49.

or near-full, employment.[63] As such, the perception is of the period as something of a 'golden age' in terms of both welfare and work.[64] This has not gone unchallenged in terms of other provisions of the welfare state, though in terms of Remploy, a degree of this perception remains, with something of a 'golden age' until the economic rationalisation that supposedly followed in the 1980s.[65] With no detailed consideration of Remploy having taken place, the company has been entirely absent from the major examinations of this period. Yet Remploy was an important part of the postwar welfare settlement for disabled people, and is unusual in that it straddles the boundaries between the two key aspects—welfare and employment. It therefore provides a pertinent case study to consider these aspects of the welfare state for disabled people.

Disability in the Welfare State

As Hampton remarked, disability has been largely absent from work considering the welfare state, both in the twentieth century and in the *longue durée*, with a tendency for historians to focus on areas 'with more contemporary, historical, and popular esteem', such as the National Health Service (NHS).[66] In terms of the period under consideration here, disability has indeed been a stark omission, with the major works in the field including only occasional and brief mentions of disability legislation and issues.[67] With such neglect it was, until recently, left for

[63] Hampton, 'Disabled People and the Classic Welfare State', p. 1.

[64] Lowe, *The Welfare State in Britain Since 1945*, p. 84; Thane, *Foundations of the Welfare State*, p. 277; K.O. Morgan, *Britain Since 1945: The People's Peace, 3rd Edition* (Oxford, Oxford University Press, 2001).

[65] Glennerster, *British Social Policy*, pp. 8–9; Lowe, *The Welfare State in Britain Since 1945*, pp. 139–172; Laybourn, *The Evolution of British Social Policy and the Welfare State*, p. 214; I. Gough, *The Political Economy of the Welfare State, Critical Texts in Social Work and the Welfare State* (London, Palgrave Macmillan, 1979); C. Barnett, *The Audit of War: The Illusion and Reality of Britain as a Great Nation* (London, Macmillan, 1986), p. 26.

[66] Hampton, 'Discovering Disability', pp. 71–2.

[67] Fraser, *The Evolution of the British Welfare State*, pp. 258, 271–2; Lowe, *The Welfare State in Britain Since 1945*, pp. 146, 166, 277–8, 283, 346; K. Jones, *The Making of Social Policy in Britain 1830–1990*, 2nd Edition (London, Athlone Press, 1996), pp. 125–7, 153–5, 174, 191; Glennerster, *British Social Policy*, pp. 46, 118, 237–8; Thane, *Foundations of the Welfare State*, pp. 224–5; Harris, *The Origins of the British Welfare State*; Hill, *The Welfare State in Britain*, pp. 14, 92, 116–7; G. Finlayson, *Citizen, State,*

those working in other disciplines, such as social and political scientists, to consider the place of disabled people. The most notable example was Deborah Stone's *The Disabled State,* which proposed the existence of a 'distributive dilemma' in disability policy, with society having to balance the need to promote the impetus to work with provision for those unable to do so.[68] Despite its influence, Stone's study has similar limitations to 'disability studies history', with its wide focus in term of place and chronology, and its proposition of an overarching theory without empirical evidence.[69] A more focused contribution was made by Sally Sainsbury, who outlined some aspects of disability legislation in the postwar period through the development of the Personal Social Services.[70] Though offering greater historical context, this still provided only a brief survey over the period in order to consider more recent developments which reflected the true focus of the work.[71] Borsay's major study of disability, though including the period considered here as part of her broad timeframe from 1750, similarly remains limited in its application. This is particularly true in terms of the postwar period, elements of which are included in the thematic chapters into which the study is structured but which lack substantive detail. The key issue, as stated, is with the study's very nature and purpose to support a predetermined conclusion. The argument in relation to disabled people was that the measures of the welfare state 'failed to guarantee them against poverty and financial exclusion', but this conclusion was never in doubt.[72] Despite these

and Social Welfare in Britain 1830–1990 (Oxford, Clarendon Press, 1994), pp. 220–6, 316–7, 327–9; Timmins, *The Five Giants*, pp. 19, 55–6, 227–8, 274, 285–7, 342–3; A. Deacon, 'Spending More to Achieve less? Social Security Since 1945' in D. Gladstone, (ed.) *British Social Welfare: Past, Present and Future* (London, UCL Press, 1995), p. 86; Laybourn, *The Evolution of British Social Policy and the Welfare State*, p. 251; Gladstone, *The Twentieth-Century Welfare State*, p. 67; Brown, *The British Welfare State,* pp. 39–41; Digby, *British Welfare Policy*, pp. 91–3.

[68] D. Stone, *The Disabled State* (Philadelphia, Temple University Press, 1984).

[69] For criticisms see B.J. Gleeson, 'Disability Studies: A Historical Materialist View', *Disability & Society*, vol. 12, no. 2 (1997), pp. 179–202.

[70] S. Sainsbury, 'Disabled People and the Personal Social Services', in D. Gladstone, (ed.) *British Social Welfare: Past, Present and Future* (London, UCL Press, 1995), pp. 183–195.

[71] Ibid.

[72] Borsay, *Disability and Social Policy in Britain Since 1750*, p. 168.

limitations, the work does serve to highlight many of the key areas of the welfare state which were relevant to disabled people.

As part of the growing interest in disability history, work which considers disability and the welfare state firmly within the discipline of history has recently begun to appear, with the first major study produced by Hampton in 2016.[73] Focusing on those disabled people described as the 'general classes' (those whose disability was not the result of injury received in war or from industrial accident), Hampton addressed how welfare policy for, and perceptions of, disabled people changed over the period 1948–1979.[74] The overall argument was that these general classes of disabled people were failed by the initial elements which established the welfare state, and though they were gradually recognised as a group in need of further provision, statutory measures remained limited both in terms of their aims and impact.[75] Hampton concluded that the general classes were largely excluded from statutory welfare provision, and thus remained 'the wretched' of the welfare state.[76]

Similar studies on disability have also tended to focus on social services and welfare for those disabled people consider unable to work.[77] Yet employment is an important area when we consider that securing 'full employment' among the general population was a key element in the classic welfare state settlement, and has been seen as a genuine and major achievement by scholars such as Lowe, Howard Glennerster and Robert Page.[78] For Sainsbury, this concept of full employment was also supposed to extend to disabled people—with work both a *right*, and an *obligation*, for anyone capable.[79] There has been some consideration of disability employment in the twentieth century.[80] The Second World War is seen

[73] Hampton, *Disability and the Welfare State in Britain.*

[74] Ibid.

[75] Ibid.

[76] Ibid.

[77] Gulland, *Gender, Work and Social Control.*

[78] Lowe, *The Welfare State in Britain Since 1945*, pp. 80–1, 115–9; Page, *Revisiting the Welfare State*, p. 38; Fraser, *The Evolution of the British Welfare State*, pp. 267–8; Glennerster, *British Social Policy*, p. 5; Laybourn, *The Evolution of British Social Policy and the Welfare State*, p. 241.

[79] Sainsbury, 'Disabled People and the Personal Social Services', p. 184.

[80] Anderson, *War, Disability and Rehabilitation in Britain,* pp. 88–92; Borsay, *Disability and Social Policy in Britain Since 1750*, pp. 119–139; Bolderson, 'The Origins

as a watershed moment, with Anderson and Borsay arguing that the manpower shortage caused by the war led to the inclusion of disabled people in significant numbers in the workforce for the first time.[81] The DPEA itself included a range of provision alongside Remploy. The Act divided disabled people into two groups, those designated 'Section I', who were considered able to access open employment in some way (representing the majority of disabled people), and those designated 'Section II', who, owing to the severity of their disability, were considered unable to do so, and therefore as requiring sheltered employment. Most of the measures in the DPEA were focused on those designated Section I, including a list of reserved occupations, a mandatory quota system requiring that 3% of an employer's workforce, if they employed 20 or more people, be made up of disabled people, and the creation of a number of training and resettlement schemes.[82]

Opinions have differed on the impact of the DPEA. Anderson described is as a 'breakthrough' moment for disabled people, and argued that it 'undoubtedly had the best interests of disabled people at its core'.[83] For Bolderson, however, the negotiations which formed the Act had become informed by 'sectional interests', which were 'detrimental to the interests of disabled people'.[84] Chiefly this was the input from employers and trade unions, who sought to ensure that the Act did not 'upset their own interests in the labour market'.[85] A similar view was echoed by Thane, Borsay and Hampton.[86] The measures of the DPEA remained

of the Disabled Persons employment Quota and its Symbolic Significance'; Meyer, 'Not Septimus Now'; Kowalsky, '"This Honourable Obligation"'; Mantin, 'Coalmining and the National Scheme for Disabled Ex-Servicemen after the First World War'.

81 Anderson, 'Turned into Taxpayers', p. 468; Anderson, *War, Disability and Rehabilitation in Britain,* pp. 8–11, 91; J. Anderson, 'British Women, Disability and the Second World War', *Contemporary British History*, vol. 20, no. 1 (2006), pp. 39–42; Borsay, *Disability and Social Policy in Britain Since 1750*, pp. 58–9, 133; Bolderson, 'The Origins of the Disabled Persons employment Quota and its Symbolic Significance'.

82 Borsay, *Disability and Social Policy in Britain Since 1750*, p. 135.

83 Anderson, 'British Women, Disability and the Second World War', p. 48; Anderson, 'Turned into Taxpayers', p. 470.

84 Bolderson, 'The Origins of the Disabled Persons Employment Quota and its Symbolic Significance', pp. 169–70.

85 Ibid., pp. 172, 181.

86 Thane, *Foundations of the Welfare State*, pp. 224–5; Borsay, *Disability and Social Policy in Britain Since 1750,* pp. 135–6; Hampton, 'Discovering Disability', p. 77.

in place throughout the period considered here, and their long-term success, with the exception of Remploy, has been seriously questioned.[87] Bolderson, considering the employment quota in 1980, judged that it had been largely unsuccessful in placing disabled people in open employment.[88] She suggested that this failure had been widely recognised for years, but that the principles enshrined in the Act were 'difficult to discard'.[89] Borsay likewise argued that the measures had largely failed disabled people.[90] As such, these other measures of the DPEA are seen to have met with little real success. The common view is therefore that disabled people were largely excluded from the welfare state, and did not reap the benefits of the 'golden age' of welfare and employment. With Remploy representing one of the few examples of statutory provision for disabled people at this time, the extent to which it conforms to this narrative is a central element in this study. Beyond this, the case of Remploy can further be marshalled to shed new light on some of the key areas of debate and analysis concerning the welfare state, which will be outlined here in turn.

The Creation of the Welfare State

Significant attention has been placed on the creation of the British welfare state, and the extent to which it was brought about directly by the Second World War.[91] This debate was sparked by the influential work of R. M. Titmuss, who argued that it was the unique and specific experience of the war which turned welfare from the selectivity of the prewar years to the statist universalism of the late 1940s.[92] This view has been subject to a range of criticism, with scholars such as Kenneth O. Morgan, Anne Digby,

[87] Borsay, *Disability and Social Policy in Britain Since 1750*, p. 135; Bolderson, 'The Origins of the Disabled Persons Employment Quota and its Symbolic Significance', pp. 171, 184; A. Roulstone and S. Prideaux, *Understanding Disability Policy* (Bristol, Policy Press, 2012), pp. 26–32.

[88] Bolderson, 'The Origins of the Disabled Persons Employment Quota and its Symbolic Significance', pp. 170–2.

[89] Ibid., pp. 171, 184.

[90] Borsay, *Disability and Social Policy in Britain Since 1750*, pp. 135–9.

[91] Laybourn, The *Evolution of British Social Policy and the Welfare State*, p. 222.

[92] R.M. Titmuss, *Problems of Social Policy* (London, HMSO and Longmans, 1950), p. 508.

David Gladstone and Angus Calder questioning the social unity espoused by Titmuss.[93] The notion of the war instigating a popular will to create a welfare state has also been challenged by Lowe, Kathleen Jones, Steven Fielding, Peter Thompson and Nick Tiratsoo.[94] A number of historians have stressed the importance of longer term prewar developments. For Henry Pelling, while the war did spur improvements in several areas, social and political developments leading to the welfare state would likely have occurred without it.[95] Similarly for Calder, the war acted to move Britain along an already determined course, albeit slightly faster, rather than initiating a fundamental change.[96] More recently, historians have highlighted areas of continuity between pre- and postwar social provision, calling into question any discourse which suggests the Second World War represented a clean break in the history of welfare provision.[97]

Generally however, the debate reflects a range of variations rather than an entrenched dialectic. There is recognition that it was not only Britain that saw expansion in welfare following the war, with the impact of the conflict resulting in a need for economic reconstruction internationally and leading to a common commitment to improving social outcomes.[98] Titmuss' view represents therefore an extreme side of the scale, with historians taking positions along it, in which the war has differing degrees of impact alongside other factors—such as the role of the postwar Labour

[93] Morgan, *The People's Peace*, p. 18; Digby, *British Welfare Policy*, pp. 54–55; Gladstone, 'The Welfare state and the State of Welfare', p. 3; A. Calder, *The Myth of the Blitz* (London, Pimlico, 1991); S. O. Rose, *Which People's War? National Identity and Citizenship in Wartime Britain 1939–1945* (Oxford, Oxford University Press, 2003), p. 3.

[94] R. Lowe, 'The Second World War, Consensus, and the Foundation of the Welfare State', *Twentieth Century British History*, 1 (1990) quoted in Rose, *Which People's War?* p. 23; Jones, *The Making of Social Policy in Britain*, p. 122; S. Fielding, Peter Thompson, and N. Tiratsoo, *'England Arise!': The Labour Party and Popular Politics in 1940s Britain* (Manchester, 1995) in Rose, *Which People's War?* p. 23.

[95] H. Pelling, *Britain and the Second World War* (London, Collins, 1970).

[96] A. Calder, *The People's War: Britain 1939–1945* (London, Pimlico, 1969).

[97] F. K. Prochaska, *The Voluntary Impulse: Philanthropy in Modern Britain*, (London, Faber, 1988); P. Thane, 'Voluntary Action in Britain Since Beveridge', in M. Oppenheimer and N. Deakin (eds.) *Beveridge and Voluntary Action in Britain and the Wider British World* (Manchester: Manchester University Press, 2011), pp. 121–34; Millward, 'Invalid Definitions, Invalid Responses', p. 23; T. Alborn, 'Senses of Belonging: The Politics of Working-class Insurance in Britain, 1880–1914', *Journal of Modern History*, vol. 73, no.3 (2001), p. 567.

[98] Béland, et al., 'Introduction'.

Government.[99] Most historians therefore, see the war as having had an impact, but not one divorced from traditional social and political division, pre-1939 developments and continuing trends.[100]

Work in the field of disability history has tended to focus on the impact of war on disability and the two World Wars in the twentieth century have provided a common focus. In most cases this has been the First World War,[101] though the Second World War[102] has also received some attention. Both are viewed as watershed moments in the history of disability.[103] That war is seen to be important in the development of disability policy

[99] Laybourn, *The Evolution of British Social Policy and the Welfare State*, pp. 209–18; A. Marwick, *Britain in the Century of Total War: War, Peace and Social Change 1900–1967* (Middlesex, Penguin, 1970); Harris, *The Origins of the British Welfare State*, p. 289; G. Wright, *The Ordeal of Total War, 1939–1945* (London, Harper & Row, 1968); Fraser, *The Evolution of the British Welfare State*, chapter 9; P. Addison, *The Road to 1945: British Politics and the Second World War, Revised Edition* (London, Pimlico, 1994), pp. 13–14, 118; H.L. Smith, (ed.), *War and Social Change: British Society in the Second World War*, New Edition (Manchester, Manchester University Press, 1990); Glennerster, *British Social Policy*, p. 4; K.O. Morgan, *Labour in Power 1945–51* (Oxford, Oxford University Press, 1984); Jones, *The Making of Social Policy in Britain 1830–1990*, p. 122.

[100] T.H. Marshall, *Social Policy in the Twentieth Century* (London, Hutchinson, 1975), pp. 84, 99; Lowe, *The Welfare State in Britain Since 1945*, pp. 16–17; Gladstone, *The Twentieth-Century Welfare State*, p. 51.

[101] See for example, Gerber, (ed.) *Disabled Veterans in History*. A. Carden-Coyne, *Reconstructing the Body: Classicism, Modernism, and the First World War* (Oxford, Oxford University Press, 2009); A. Carden-Coyne, 'Ungrateful Bodies: Rehabilitation, Resistance and Disabled American Veterans of the First World War', *European Review of History*, vol. 14, no. 4 (2007), pp. 543–65; Cohen, *The War Come Home*; S. Koven, 'Remembering and Dismemberment: Crippled Children, Wounded Soldiers and the Great War in Great Britain', *American Historical Review*, vol. 99, no. 4, (1994), pp. 1167–202; Kowalsky, "This Honourable Obligation'; Kowalsky, 'Enabling the Great War'; Meyer, 'Not Septimus now'; J. Reznick, *Healing the Nation: Soldiers and the Culture of Caregiving in Britain During the Great War* (Manchester, Manchester University Press, 2005); E. Elsey, 'Disabled Ex-servicemen's Experiences of Rehabilitation and Employment After the First World War', *Oral History*, vol. 25, no. 2 (1997), pp. 49–58; W. J. Gagen, 'Remastering the Body, Renegotiating Gender: Physical Disability and Masculinity during the First World War, the case of J.B. Middlebrook', *European Review of History*, vol. 14, no. 4 (2007), pp. 525–41; Bourke, *Dismembering the Male*.

[102] Anderson, 'Turned into Taxpayers'; Anderson, *Disability and Rehabilitation in Britain*; Anderson, 'British Women, Disability and the Second World War'; Wheatcroft, *Worth Saving*; Bernstein, 'Rehabilitation Staged'; Kinder, "Lest We Forget'; Muir, "That bastard's following me!'.

[103] Anderson, 'British Women, Disability and the Second World War'; Anderson, *Disability and Rehabilitation in Britain*.

rests on the increase in the disabled population that results from conflict, and in the political profile afforded those who become disabled in service to the nation.[104] Wars in general, and the two World Wars in particular, are therefore highlighted as important catalysts for developments in disability policy. Considering the case of Remploy here will further expand our understanding of the impact of the Second World War on the creation of the welfare state.

The Postwar Consensus

A further area of long-standing debate is the notion of a consensus in welfare and employment policy across the governments of the period, which suggests that there was little real difference between Labour and Conservative governments until the election of Margaret Thatcher in 1979.[105] Historians and political scientists have subjected this notion to review and a number of debates have arisen around the existence and nature of the so-called 'postwar consensus'. The debate is generally considered to have commenced with Addison's assertion that the experience of the Second World War gave rise to a centre-left consensus in politics and resulted in a postwar settlement centred on commitment to the welfare state, full employment, and Keynesian economics.[106] Support for this view has come from David Dutton, Anthony Seldon, Dennis Kavanagh, Peter Morris, Bill Coxall and Lynton Robins.[107] Jones also

[104] D. A. Gerber, 'Introduction: Finding Disabled Veterans in History', in D.A. Gerber (ed.) *Disabled Veterans in History* (Ann Arbor, University of Michigan Press, 2012), pp. 1–51.

[105] H. Jones, 'Introduction', in H. Jones and M. Kandiah (eds.), *The Myth of Consensus: New Views on British History, 1945–64* (Basingstoke, Macmillan, 1996), p. xiii.

[106] P. Addison, *The Road to 1945: British Politics and the Second World War,* (London, Cape, 1975); Addison later refined his interpretation of consensus as a 'Whitehall consensus', *The Road to 1945: British Politics and the Second World War, Revised Edition* (London, Pimlico, 1994), p. 281; D. Fraser, 'The Postwar Consensus: A Debate Not Long Enough?', *Parliamentary Affairs*, vol. 53, no. 2 (2000), p. 347; A. Marwick, 'Middle Opinion in the Thirties: Planning, Progress and Political 'Agreement'', *English Historical Review*, vol. 79, no. 311 (1964), pp. 285–98; Calder, *The People's War*; R. Toye, 'From "Consensus" to "Common Ground": The Rhetoric of the Postwar Settlement and its Collapse', *Journal of Contemporary History*, vol. 48, no. 1 (2012), p. 5.

[107] D. Dutton, *British Politics Since 1945, 2nd Edition* (Oxford, Blackwell, 1997); D. Kavanagh and P. Morris, *Consensus Politics from Attlee to Major,* 2nd Edition (Oxford, Blackwell, 1994); A. Seldon, 'Consensus: A Debate Too Long?', *Parliamentary Affairs*,

embraced this view, suggesting that for both Labour and Conservatives it was then taken for granted that governments should provide welfare services consisting of both universal services and special services for those who could not be self-supporting.[108]

Other scholars have criticised the very existence of such a consensus. Most notably, Ben Pimlott argued that 'consensus is a mirage, an illusion that rapidly fades the closer one gets to it'.[109] Similar views were expressed by Nicholas Deakin, Harriet Jones, Michael Kandiah and Neil Rollings among others.[110] For these scholars, the traditional adversarial party system continued unabated, with Labour and Conservatives representing ideological opposed positions and maintaining numerous differences on policy.[111] Further areas of debate have arisen around the correct terminology relating to consensus, the precise time when consensus ended, and the influence of factors beyond Whitehall.[112]

vol. 47, no. 4 (1994), pp. 501–514; Coxall and Robins, *British Politics Since the War*, p. 49.

108 Jones, *The Making of Social Policy in Britain 1830–1990,* pp. ix–x.

109 B. Pimlott, 'The Myth of Consensus', in L.M. Smith (ed.), *The Making of Britain: Echoes of Greatness,* (Basingstoke, Macmillan, 1988), p. 136.

110 Jones and Kandiah, *The Myth of Consensus*, contains chapters from a range of historians which question the notion of consensus; N. Deakin, quoted in Fraser, 'The Postwar Consensus', p. 347; N. Rollings, 'Poor Mr Butskell: A Short Life, Wrecked by Schizophrenia"? *Twentieth Century British History*, vol. 5, no. 2 (1994), pp. 183–205. Other works taking a sceptical line towards consensus include: K. Jefferys, *The Churchill Coalition and Wartime Politics, 1940–1945* (Manchester, Manchester University Press, 1991); S. Kelly, *The Myth of Mr. Butskell: The Politics of British Economic Policy, 1950–55* (Aldershot, Ashgate, 2002).

111 Fraser, 'The Postwar Consensus', p. 348.

112 For considerations of terminology see Seldon, 'Consensus', p. 508; Kavanagh and Morris, *Consensus Politics from Attlee to Major,* p. 13; Pimlott, 'Myth of Consensus', p. 130; Fraser, 'The Postwar Consensus', p. 349. For debate over when consensus ended see, B. Harrison, 'The Rise, Fall and Rise of Political Consensus in Britain since 1940', *History,* vol. 84, no. 274 (1999), pp. 301–24; Laybourn, *The Evolution of British Social Policy and the Welfare State*, p. 237; Jones, *The Making of Social Policy in Britain 1830–1990*, pp. ix–x, 164–5; Fraser, 'The Postwar Consensus', pp. 355–6. For wider factors see, P. Dorey, *British Politics Since 1945* (Oxford, Blackwell, 1995), pp. 59–65; Fraser, 'The Postwar Consensus', pp. 59–61, 351–4; P. Dunleavy and C.T. Husbands, *British Democracy at the Crossroads: Voting and Party Competition in the 1980s* (London, Allen & Unwin, 1985); P. Dunleavy and B. O'Leary, *Theories of the State: The Politics of Liberal Democracy,* (Basingstoke, Macmillan, 1987); D. Bell, *The End of Ideology: On the Exhaustion of Political Ideas in the Fifties*, (London, Collier-Macmillan, 1962); S.M.

The crucial aspect considered here, however, is the fundamental notion of a consensus in the case of policy. Here, Richard Toye has recently suggested that historians would do well to move away from the traditional focus in this debate upon major policies such as housing, education and the NHS, and consider neglected areas which have not yet been examined.[113] The case of Remploy is one such example. The traditional view has been that 'disability' was not 'discovered' as a political issue until the 1960s.[114] Considerations of disability policy in this debate have therefore been few and have focused exclusively on aspects of welfare. For Millward, although a true ideological consensus did not exist, there was a 'common response' to disability welfare policy during the period prior to Thatcher's Government and therefore a 'consensus in action'.[115] Hampton, similarly saw consensus in government response, if not in ideological position, suggesting both main parties saw welfare provision for disabled people as an expense 'and subject to a minimum standard of provision'.[116] As one of the few examples of statutory provision for disabled people, and as the central government sheltered employment scheme, Remploy represents a pertinent new case to consider.

Welfare and Employment for Women

It is not only disabled people who have been seen as having been largely excluded from the provisions of the welfare state.[117] The postwar settlement received serious criticism almost immediately for its differential treatment of men and women, and this grew in the wake of 'second wave' feminism in the 1960s, until the gender analysis of the welfare state became a major focus of the academic study of social policy in

Lipset, *Political Man*, (London, Mercury Books, 1963); K. Jefferys, *Retreat from the New Jerusalem, British Politics 1951–64* (London, Palgrave, 1997).

113 Toye, 'From "Consensus" to "Common Ground"', p. 23.

114 Hampton, 'Discovering Disability', pp. 70–1; Hampton, *Disability and the Welfare State in Britain*, pp. 8, 50; Sainsbury, 'Disabled People and the Personal Social Services', pp. 183–88; E. Younghusband, *Social Work in Britain: 1950–1975* (London, Allen and Unwin, 1978), pp. 210–11.

115 Millward, 'Invalid Definitions, Invalid Responses', pp. 165, 284.

116 Hampton, *Disability and the Welfare State in Britain*, p. 244.

117 Laybourn, *The Evolution of British Social Policy and the Welfare State*, pp. 254–6; Lowe, *The Welfare State in Britain Since 1945*, pp. 40–3.

the 1980s.[118] By the mid-1990s, Gladstone noted it was 'impossible to evaluate the welfare state without understanding how it deals with women'.[119] The primary criticism of the welfare state itself has been that the measures failed to emancipate women, and instead tended to reinforce their traditional role in society, with an underlying assumption that women should remain primarily care-givers to the family and economically reliant on a husband.[120] This has been referred to as the 'male breadwinner logic', reflecting a male responsibility to provide for the family.[121] There has since been some counter-balance to this, with recognition that the postwar settlement did confer some benefits to women, both directly (such as family allowances), and indirectly (such as measures relating to housing and health).[122] The fundamental view

118 Lowe, *The Welfare State in Britain Since 1945*, p. 40; Gladstone, 'The Welfare State and the State of Welfare', p. 23; C. Pierson 'Theory in British Social Policy', in N. Ellison & C. Pierson (eds.) *Developments in British Social Policy* (London, Macmillan, 1998), p. 21; E. Wilson, *Women and the Welfare State* (London, Tavistock Publications, 1977), p. 170.

119 Gladstone, *The Twentieth-Century Welfare State*, pp. 6–7.

120 Lowe, *The Welfare State in Britain Since 1945*, pp. 40–3; Pierson 'Theory in British Social Policy', pp. 21–3; J. Stewart, 'The Twentieth Century: an Overview', in R. Page and R. Silburn (eds.) *British Social Welfare in the Twentieth Century* (London, Macmillan, 1999), pp. 19–21; Glennerster, *British Social Policy,* pp. 35–6; Brown, *The British Welfare State*, p. 53; P. Thane, 'Visions of Gender in the Making of the British Welfare State' in G. Bock and P. Thane (eds.), *Maternity and Gender Policies: Women and the Rise of the European Welfare States, 1880s–1950s* (London, Routledge, 1991), p. 93; C. Pierson, *Beyond the Welfare State?* (Cambridge, Polity Press, 1991), pp. 69–79; R. Crompton and K. Sanderson, *Gendered Jobs & Social Change* (London, Unwin Hyman, 1990), pp. 49–50; D.S. Wilson, 'Gender, Race and Ideal Labour Force' in L. Ryan and W. Webster (eds.), *Gendering Migration: Masculinity, Femininity and Ethnicity in Post-War Britain* (Aldershot, Ashgate, 2008), p. 89.

121 Stewart, 'The Twentieth Century'; L. King, *Family Men: Fatherhood and Masculinity in Britain, 1914–1960* (Oxford, Oxford University Press, 2015), pp. 29–30; Gulland, *Gender, Work and Social Control*, p. 9.

122 H. Jones 'The State and Social Policy', in I. Zweiniger-Bargielowska (ed.), *Women in Twentieth-Century Britain* (London, Routledge, 2014), pp. 329–330; Lowe, *The Welfare State in Britain Since 1945*, pp. 40–3; R. Lowe, 'Introduction: The Road from 1945', in H. Fawcett and R. Lowe (eds.) *Welfare Policy in Britain: The Road from 1945* (Basingstoke, Macmillan, 1999), pp. 10–11; Gladstone, *The Twentieth-Century Welfare State*, p. 6; P. Thane, 'Women in the British Labour Party and the Construction of State welfare, 1906–39' in S. Koven and S. Michel (eds.), *Mothers of a new world: maternalist politics and the origins of welfare states* (London, Routledge, 1993), pp. 343–77; J. Lewis, 'Gender, the Family and Women's Agency in the Building of States: the British Case',

remains however, that the welfare state did not treat men and women equally, with women neglected in its provision.[123]

Changes in employment for women in the postwar period has also proved a ripe area for study. The traditional view held that the Second World War instigated fundamental change, largely based on the expansion in the number of women in work, which, as Harold Smith illustrated, saw an increase of almost 50% between 1939 and 1943.[124] This narrative has since been complicated with historians such as Penny Summerfield, Sue Bruley, Hugh Pemberton and Gerry Holloway, highlighting how the increased role of women in work during the war was largely considered a temporary situation.[125] Examinations of the postwar period considered here have revealed a mixed picture. On the one hand, there was an increasing number of women entering into employment, driven by the huge increase in numbers of married women (including mothers) working, which could not but lead to change.[126] On the other hand, true

Social History, vol. 19, no. 1 (1994), pp 37–55; T. Skocpol and G. Ritter, 'Gender and the Origins of Modern Social Policies in Britain and the United States', *Studies in American Political Development*, vol. 5, no. 1 (1991), pp. 36–93; S. Koven and S. Michel, 'Womanly Duties: Maternalist Politics and the Origins of Welfare States in France, Germany, Great Britain and the United States, 1880–1920', *American Historical Review*, vol. 95, no. 4 (1990), pp. 1076–1108; J. Misra and F. Akins, 'The Welfare State and Women: Structure, Agency, and Diversity', *Social Politics*, vol. 5, no. 3 (1998), pp. 260–78.

[123] Page, *Revisiting the Welfare State*, p 40; Gladstone, 'The Welfare State and the State of Welfare', p. 23; N. Deakin, *The Politics of Welfare: Continuities and Change* (London, Harvester Wheatsheaf, 1994), p. 4; Gladstone, *The Twentieth Century Welfare State*, pp. 6–7; Digby, *British Welfare Policy*, pp. 62–3; Pierson, *Beyond the Welfare State?*, pp. 69–79.

[124] H. L Smith, 'The Effect of the War on the Status of Women', in H.L.Smith (ed.), *War and Social Change: British Society in the Second World War* (Manchester, Manchester University Press, 1986), p. 211; A. Marwick, *War and Social Change in the Twentieth Century: a Comparative Study of Britain, France, Germany, Russia and the US* (London, Macmillan, 1974).

[125] P. Summerfield, *Women Workers in the Second World War: Production and Patriarchy in Conflict* (London, Routledge, 1984); G. Braybon and P. Summerfield, *Out of the Cage: Women's Experiences in Two World Wars* (Abingdon, Routledge, 2013); S. Bruley, *Women in Britain Since 1900* (Basingstoke, Palgrave, 1999); G. Holloway, *Women and Work in Britain Since 1840* (London, Routledge, 2005), pp. 162–78; H. Pemberton, 'The Transformation of the Economy', in P. Addison and H. Jones (eds.) *A Companion to Contemporary Britain 1939–2000* (Oxford, Blackwell, 2005), pp. 190–1.

[126] Summerfield, *Women Workers in the Second World War;* M. Pugh, *Women and the Women's movement in Britain 1914–1959* (London, Macmillan, 1992); H. McCarthy,

equality in employment remained largely out of reach. There is agreement among a wide range of scholars that women's employment in the period was typified by gender segregation, low pay, inferior status and a lack of opportunity for advancement.[127] Such studies did not consider whether this was the case for disabled women as well. This is important, for as Bruley has noted, women are not a 'homogenous group', and it is crucial that historians examine the various factors which 'mediated their experiences'.[128] Disability is clearly one such factor.

Though gender has long been a central element in the field of disability studies, there has been relatively little consideration of women in disability history.[129] What research has been done with regards to the welfare state, suggests that disabled women were also neglected compared to disabled men. Anderson asserted that disabled women faced a more difficult postwar climate than disabled men generally, with areas such as transport, accommodation and welfare payments favouring the latter.[130] Millward similarly argued that women were discriminated against in

Double Lives: A History of Working Motherhood (London, Bloomsbury, 2020); Gladstone, *The Twentieth-Century Welfare State*, p. 119; Bruley, *Women in Britain Since 1900*, pp. 99–119; Wilson, 'Gender, Race the Ideal Labour Force', pp. 89–91; D.S. Wilson, 'A New Look at the Affluent Worker: The Good Working Mother in Post-War Britain', *Twentieth Century British History*, vol. 17, no. 2 (2006), pp. 206–29; L. King, 'How Men Valued Women's Work: Labour In and Outside the Home in Post-War Britain', *Contemporary European History*, 28 (2019), p. 455.

[127] Lowe, *The Welfare State in Britain Since 1945*, pp. 42–3; K. Laybourn, *Unemployment and Employment Policies Concerning Women in Britain, 1900–1951* (Lampeter, Edwin Mellen Press, 2002), p. 187; Bruley, *Women in Britain Since 1900*, pp. 99–119; Summerfield, *Women Workers in the Second World War;* M. Glucksmann, *Women Assemble: Women Workers and the New Industries in Inter-War Britain* (London, Routledge, 1990), p. 281; Gladstone, *The Twentieth-Century Welfare State*, pp. 119–122; Holloway, *Women and Work in Britain Since 1840*, p. 186; P. Thane, 'Towards Equal Opportunities? Women in Britain since 1945', in T. Gourvish and A. O'Day (eds.), *Britain Since 1945* (Basingstoke, Macmillan, 1991), pp. 183–208; J. Lewis, *Women in Britain Since 1945: Women, Family, Work and the State in the Post-War Years* (Oxford, Blackwell, 1992), pp. 78–91; J. Lewis, *Women in England 1870–1950: Sexual Divisions and Social Change* (Brighton, Wheatsheaf Books Ltd, 1984); H. Bradley, *Men's Work, Women's Work* (Cambridge, Polity Press, 1989), p. 116; Wilson, 'Gender, Race the Ideal Labour Force'.

[128] Bruley, *Women in Britain Since 1900*, p. 93.

[129] Gleeson, *Geographies of Disability*, p. 17.

[130] Anderson, *War, Disability and Rehabilitation in Britain*, p. 168; Anderson, 'British Women, Disability and the Second World War'.

disability welfare.[131] Hampton also suggested that welfare provision differed 'according to sex', with women suffering an 'absence of provision in cash and services under the postwar settlement'.[132] Jackie Gulland further noted the extension of the breadwinner logic to disabled women in assumptions underpinning incapacity benefits.[133] The result is that in the area of welfare, disabled women are seen as a group who experienced a particular neglect, as both women and disabled people, or what Oliver termed a 'double disability'.[134]

In terms of work, Borsay suggested that the suspension of gender roles during the Second World War, which allowed an increase in the number of women entering the labour market generally, did not necessarily extend to disabled women.[135] The chief work in this area was done by Anderson, who focused on disabled women during the Second World War and into its immediate aftermath.[136] For Anderson, while the wartime labour shortage had allowed some disabled women to enter the labour market and gain a measure of 'personal independence', this was neither universal nor permanent.[137] Disabled women in the postwar period were thus left struggling to find employment and experienced a training and work environment which was 'gendered and segregated'.[138] Thane also suggested that the DPEA itself overlooked the needs of disabled women.[139] Both Hampton and Sainsbury likewise argued that disability services associated with employment 'were allocated overwhelmingly to men'.[140] A study of Remploy is therefore a valuable opportunity to consider the experiences

[131] Millward, 'Social Security Policy and the Early Disability Movement', pp. 281–2.

[132] Hampton, *Disability and the Welfare State in Britain*, p. 119.

[133] Gulland, Gender, *Work and Social Control*, p. 127.

[134] Oliver, *The Politics of Disablement*, p. 70.

[135] Borsay, *Disability and Social Policy in Britain Since 1750*, p. 134.

[136] Anderson, *War, Disability and Rehabilitation in Britain*, pp. 152–175; Anderson, 'British Women, Disability and the Second World War', pp. 37–53.

[137] Anderson, *War, Disability and Rehabilitation in Britain*, pp. 158–9, 154–5, 168–9, 170–1.

[138] Ibid., pp. 169–70; Anderson, 'British Women, Disability and the Second World War', p. 50.

[139] Thane, *Foundations of the Welfare State*, pp. 224–5.

[140] Sainsbury, 'Disabled People and the Personal Social Services', p. 188; Hampton, *Disability and the Welfare State in Britain*, p. 119.

of disabled women, both in terms of their relative exclusion from the welfare state and the conditions they faced in sheltered employment.

The Mixed Economy and Moving Frontier of the State

The extent of the expanding state in postwar Britain and its effect on the traditional provision of welfare by voluntary organisations has remained an important focus for scholars.[141] The traditional view was that the expansion of statutory welfare in the 1940s left voluntarism redundant until it experienced something of a resurgence in the mid-to-late-1960s.[142] Thus the Wolfenden Report on voluntary organisations in 1978 described the intervening period as one in which the sector was left 'marking time'.[143] Barry Knight went further and suggested that voluntarism was effectively 'moribund'.[144] This was occasionally highlighted in contemporary opinion as a 'welfare state escalator', with the inexorable rise of state responsibility culminating in the creation of the welfare state.[145] This 'whiggish' view of the steady evolution of statutory welfare in Britain has since been forcefully challenged, with scholars such as Geoffrey Finlayson, Eileen Younghusband, Marilyn Taylor, Frank Prochaska, Pat Thane, Jeremy Kendall and Martin Knapp, all revealing the survival of the voluntary sector.[146] The result is a concept of a 'mixed economy of welfare', with a combination of statutory and voluntary provision during the period of the classic welfare state, followed by a radical

[141] The terms 'charitable' and 'voluntary' are used here interchangeably to reflect the overall non-statutory sector and range of organisations providing sheltered employment.

[142] Gladstone, *The Twentieth-Century Welfare State*, p. 66.

[143] *The Future of Voluntary Organisations: Report of the Wolfenden Committee* (London, Croom Helm, 1978).

[144] B. Knight, *Voluntary Action (*London, Centris 1993).

[145] Hampton, *Disability and the Welfare State in Britain;* M. Bruce, *The Coming of the Welfare State* (London, Harper Collins, 1971); G Kitson-Clark, *An Expanding Society: Britain 1830–1900* (Cambridge, Cambridge University Press, 1967).

[146] Finlayson, *Citizen, State and Social Welfare in Britain 1830–1990*; Younghusband, *Social Work in Britain;* M. Taylor, 'Voluntary Action and the State', in D. Gladstone, (ed.) *British Social Welfare: Past, Present and Future* (London, UCL Press, 1995), p. 215; Prochaska, *The Voluntary Impulse*; Thane, *Foundations of the Welfare State*, p. 277; J. Kendall and M. Knapp, *The Voluntary Sector in the United Kingdom* (Manchester, Manchester University Press, 1996), pp. 51–57.

shift in the climate under the subsequent Thatcher Government.[147] This is not to suggest that the increase in statutory provision had no effect on the charitable sector and it is widely accepted that voluntary provision became a 'junior partner in the welfare firm'.[148]

This expansion of the state was neither complete nor steady, however, and it has been suggested that state involvement represented a 'moving frontier', with a changing relationship with non-statutory providers over the period.[149] Finlayson explained that there was a 'constant interrelationship between voluntarism, in its various guises, and the state'.[150] This was also noted by Kendall and Knapp, who considered that the state continuously looked for 'new ways of working with the voluntary sector'.[151] Alongside this, was the expansion of the role of local authorities (LAs) in delivering welfare, which moved into increasing partnership with voluntary organisations to provide services.[152] Examination of this moving frontier has been noted as requiring further work, with both Julie Grier and Hampton calling for a more nuanced analysis of the mixed economy, exploring the complex and changing relationships between the various parties involved.[153]

The non-statutory sector has been considered particularly important for the study of disability.[154] As Younghusband illustrated, hundreds of voluntary organisations, large and small, national and local, contributed

[147] Kendall and Knapp, *The Voluntary Sector in the United Kingdom*, pp. 133–9.

[148] D. Owen, *English Philanthropy: 1660–1960* (London, Belknap Press, 1964), p. 527; Digby, *British Welfare Policy*, p. 89; Kendall and Knapp, *The Voluntary Sector in the United Kingdom*, pp. 51–57, 133–9.

[149] G. Finlayson, 'A Moving Frontier: Voluntarism and the State in British Social Welfare 1911–1949', *Twentieth Century British History*, vol. 1, no. 2 (1990), pp. 183–206.

[150] Finlayson, *Citizen, State and Social Welfare in Britain 1830–1990*, pp. 11–12.

[151] Kendall and Knapp, *The Voluntary Sector in the United Kingdom*, pp. 51–57.

[152] Ibid.

[153] J. Grier, 'Voluntary Rights and Statutory Wrongs: The Case of Child Migration, 1948–67', *History of Education*, vol. 31 no. 3 (2002), pp. 263–4; Hampton, *Disability and the Welfare State in Britain*, p. 8.

[154] Hampton, *Disability and the Welfare State in Britain*, p. 8; Gladstone, *The Twentieth-Century Welfare State*, p. 66.

welfare services for disabled men, women and children, including accommodation, medical support, holidays and education.[155] The importance placed upon the voluntary sector in disability history stems from an understanding that the state made only limited attempts to expand into the provision of statutory welfare for disabled people.[156] Hampton, for example, concluded that the period saw 'a major change in opinion about the appropriate place of disabled people within the mixed economy', with the view developing that the state should provide 'a significant portion of their welfare' developing only in the mid-1970s.[157] Such research has focused on out-of-work welfare and on the creation of campaigning groups for various causes around disability in the 1960s, such as the Disablement Income Group (DIG), the Disability Alliance (DA), the Spastics Society and the National Association for Mental Health (MIND).[158] Given that so much of the welfare provision for disabled people was of the non-statutory kind, it is important to consider what this position was for sheltered employment.[159] This book will therefore illuminate the wider field, to consider whether a mixed economy existed. Furthermore, given Remploy's place as the central government scheme, representing the 'frontier of the state', it is possible to examine a previously unexplored set of relationships between the various providers across the period.

[155] Younghusband, *Social Work in Britain*, pp. 261–3.

[156] Digby, *British Welfare Policy*, p. 91; Kendall and Knapp, *The Voluntary Sector in the United Kingdom*, pp. 51–7; Hampton, *Disability and the Welfare State in Britain*; M. Brenton, *The Voluntary Sector in British Social Services* (Harlow, Prentice Hall Press, 1985).

[157] Hampton, *Disability and the Welfare State in Britain*, pp. 240–1.

[158] Millward, 'Invalid Definitions, Invalid Responses', p. 22; Hampton, *Disability and the Welfare State in Britain*.

[159] Hampton, *Disability and the Welfare State in Britain*, p. 56.

Timeframe and Terminology

The precise point the classic welfare state began has variously been stated as 1944,[160] with the passing of social service legislation such as the Education Act; 1945,[161] with the close of the war in Europe and the election of the Labour Government; or 1948,[162] as major provision such as the NHS became operative. In this study, the start of the classic welfare state is taken as 1944, the year Remploy was created as part of the DPEA and in order to encapsulate all potential aspects, it takes the period through to 1979. Though this is the timeframe which focuses the analysis, in consideration of the origins of Remploy in Chapter 2, some attention is given to pre-1944 developments.

Definitions of 'disability' can be problematic, both in terms of accuracy and suitability—reflecting the shifting contexts, cultures and models in which the term has been applied. This book adopts the approach of Millward in taking a 'bureaucratic' definition of disability.[163] As such, the use of terms such as 'disability', 'disabled people', 'severely disabled people', 'Section I and II disabled people', 'fit people', 'mentally disabled people' and 'sighted people', solely reflect the precise bureaucratic categories applied during the period in determining eligibility for sheltered employment and are not intended to reflect lived experience nor personal or group identity.[164] Chapter 4 considers this further in relation to the eligibility criteria which defined disability in the context of accessing Remploy. Similarly, the use of 'sheltered employment', as opposed to 'segregated employment', reflects the term given to this form of provision within the period. There are also occasional uses of what is now considered derogatory language in direct quotation from primary sources. This

[160] Gladstone, *The Twentieth-Century Welfare State*, pp. 32, 73; Gladstone 'The Welfare State and the State of Welfare', p. 2.

[161] Lowe, *The Welfare State in Britain Since 1945*, p. 77; Hill, *The Welfare State in Britain*, p. 11.

[162] N. Johnson, *The Welfare State in Transition: The Theory and Practice of Welfare Pluralism* (Amherst, The University of Massachusetts Press, 1987), p. 4; M. Jones and R. Lowe, *From Beveridge to Blair: The First Fifty Years of Britain's Welfare State, 1948–98* (Manchester, Manchester University Press, 2002), p. 3.

[163] Millward, 'Invalid Definitions, Invalid Responses', pp. 43–9.

[164] Ibid.

is done purely in the interests of historical accuracy and is not intended to condone any subsequent use of such terms.

Remploy itself was initially called ‘The Disabled Persons Employment Corporation’, with its factories referred to as ‘British Factories’. The name Remploy was in use from 1946 and officially adopted in 1949, though reference to the ‘Corporation’ continued for some years. In the interests of clarity, the term ‘Remploy’ is used throughout, with the exception of direct quotation. In terms of government departments, the key reference here is to the Ministry of Labour and National Service, which became the Ministry of Labour in 1959, the Department of Employment and Productivity in 1968 and the Department of Employment in 1970. Again, in the interests of clarity, the terms used to refer to this department are the Ministry of Labour (MOL) until 1968, and the Department of Employment (DE) thereafter.

Sources and Approach

This study takes a historical and empirical approach using archival material to consider the development of Remploy and sheltered employment. The focus on Remploy was determined by its position as the key provider of sheltered employment and, more practically, by the availability of archival source material. Contrary to the traditional belief that disability is absent from the archives, there exists an abundance of source material concerning disabled people.[165] In the case of Remploy, official material is held by The National Archives, Kew. This includes a wide range of records from the company itself, such as annual accounts, internal reports, correspondence, minutes and papers of the Board of Directors, and copies of *Remploy News* (a regular newsletter produced by the company from 1952). Statistics included here, especially those presented in tables, are often compiled from a range of these sources, and there can be numerous discrepancies across documents reflecting purpose, scope and date. In addition to these, are records compiled in relation to Remploy by various government departments, most notably the MOL. Such sources are particularly abundant for the period considered here, and there is certainly ample material for further consideration by historians. This book also makes use

[165] J. Campbell and M. Oliver, *Disability Politics: Understanding Our Past, Changing Our Future* (London, Routledge, 1996), p. 17; Anderson, *War, Disability and Rehabilitation in Britain*, p. 6.

of a range of other sources including legislation, parliamentary committee reports and papers and local and national press coverage. Remploy was also one of the chief topics of discussion concerning disability in the House of Commons during the period and extensive use is made of *Hansard* to understand policy and areas of political debate.

Though this study is focused primarily on Remploy, there is consideration, particularly in Chapter 6, of the alternative providers. Unfortunately, sheltered employment beyond Remploy, such as that provided by voluntary organisations, has much less presence in the archive, reflecting the disparate nature of such provision. This is not an issue unique to sheltered employment as the study of any non-statutory group is particularly challenging for historians. As Thane stated, voluntarism 'does not survive in official records as state action does'.[166] Finlayson likewise noted that attempting to provide a comprehensive account of the extent of voluntarism 'is impossible', suggesting 'all that can be done is to provide exemplar material'.[167] This is equally the case here. There are few records from the sheltered workshops themselves; the reliance is instead on government records, particularly those of the MOL, the National Advisory Council on the Employment of the Disabled (NACED), which was established to oversee the enacting of the provisions of the DPEA, and of Remploy. It is apparent when examining these records that contradictory evidence abounds, even in some cases within one document, which reflects the diverse and fragmentary nature of voluntary provision. Such information can usually only indicate the 'approved' sheltered employment schemes and how many were operating informally cannot be known.

This study is also limited to exploring what was accepted at the time by governments and officials as constituting 'sheltered employment' comparable with Remploy. This did not include some cases where disabled people were incorporated into enclaves in open industry. Perhaps the most notable example of such schemes were the Grenfell Factories in Wales, which were offered some financial incentives, such as a reduction in rent, for employing a proportion of disabled people in their workforce.[168]

[166] Thane, *Foundations of the Welfare State*, p. 277.

[167] Finlayson, *Citizen, State and Social Welfare in Britain 1830–1990*, p. 327.

[168] The National Archives (TNA) BD 40, Welsh Office: Economic Planning Division, 'Note on Matters arising out of Welsh Debate' (23.10.1962).

These were still considered competitive 'open employment' factories, however, and not as sheltered employment in the same vein as Remploy and other workshops.[169] Similarly, there is only limited reference to sheltered employment for the blind. Consideration of the experiences of blind people has formed its own field in disability history, reflecting the distinct development of exclusive welfare services for this group.[170] Sheltered employment was one such service and was similarly demarcated by officials at the time from the general provision. There was some overlap in this area, however, which is referenced where relevant. This is similarly the case for work, training and occupational therapy which took place within the wider context of medical rehabilitation. Furthermore, while recognising that sheltered employment developed in other countries and welfare states in various forms after the Second World War, this study is confined to the British context. Inevitably with sheltered employment having received such limited attention there is much yet to be uncovered and explored. These aspects—among many others—all merit further attention, but this is beyond the scope of this book. The focus here is on examination of core aspects of Remploy and the field of comparable sheltered employment as it was understood and referred to during the period, and in relation to key aspects of the classic welfare state in Britain which have been outlined. It is hoped this will provide a foundation upon which further research can continue to build.[171]

Finally, this study is firmly in the discipline of history, and seeks to understand Remploy and sheltered employment in its historical context. In doing so, it makes no judgement on sheltered employment as a concept. Sheltered employment has long been controversial, and remains so in many parts of the world where it is still widespread. For some, it is inherently about segregation and is inferior to the attainment of work in an inclusive mainstream employment environment. For others, it represents a better prospect for work and fulfilment than the possibility of unemployment in a competitive labour market. It is not my intention to enter into this debate by suggesting sheltered employment was either

[169] TNA BD 40, Welsh Office: Economic Planning Division, 'Note on MOL' (03.04.1963); MOL, 'Note to Welsh Office' (15.02.1963).

[170] Reiss, *Blind Workers against Charity*, pp. 152–6.

[171] Further research which involved a deeper exploration of those disabled workers who accessed sheltered employment, as well as broader considerations of gender, concepts of disability, and medical discourse would be particularly beneficial.

'good' or 'bad'. Any contribution to this debate is in terms of correcting misconceptions about the past and providing a better understanding of historical developments in disability policy within their own context.

Chapter Themes and Structure

This book is structured thematically, with each chapter considering a fundamental element of understanding Remploy and the corresponding aspect of the welfare state. Chapter 2 considers the formation of Remploy in the DPEA alongside the wider debate about the creation of the welfare state. Remploy's origins have rarely been considered beyond it being among the measures contained within the Act, but this chapter shows that it had its own distinct formation. Longer term policy developments during the interwar period are considered alongside the impact of the Second World War itself, and close examination is made of the short-term political processes which led to the DPEA. Existing explanations for the creation of Remploy are explored, with particular attention paid to the influential interpretation that it was done to placate industry. The chapter shows that Remploy, while owing something to prewar developments and ideas, and the impetus of the Second World War, was driven through primarily by the efforts of the wartime Minister of Labour, Ernest Bevin. Importantly, however, it demonstrates that Remploy was not created with a predetermined *modus operandi*, leaving fundamental aspects unresolved as it began to operate in 1945.

Chapter 3 takes up this final point to consider the prime purpose of Remploy across the period, exploring the central policy negotiated between successive governments and the Remploy Board of Directors. The implications of this for the debate over the existence of a postwar consensus are then explored, by considering the extent to which the two main political parties shared a common understanding and approach to Remploy. The chapter demonstrates that Remploy's function was initially contested, but a consensus eventually formed through a common approach based on economics and commercial performance, and a shared conception of the benefits of providing work. The chapter then expands this analysis to consider the extent to which overall policy was reflected at the local factory level.

The book then moves on to explore Remploy's disabled workforce across two chapters. Chapter 4 focuses upon recruitment and retention, considering who was employed by Remploy and the basis upon which this occurred. It highlights the various barriers which prevented many disabled people from gaining work with Remploy and argues that the key factor in securing and maintaining employment with the company was perceived individual productivity. This chapter highlights both central recruitment policy over the period and the local variations in practice. In so doing, it adds Remploy to the current understanding of the exclusion of disabled people from the measures of the welfare state, and demonstrates that the achievement of full employment in the period was not extended to severely disabled people through sheltered employment.

Chapter 5 then explores the place of women in Remploy, in relation to the wider understanding of women's experiences of welfare and employment during the period. In terms of the former, it considers the number of disabled women employed by the company and the factors which may have prevented them from joining, to determine if the relative exclusion of women from the provisions of the welfare state also extended to Remploy. It then considers the current understanding of women's employment in the period, as one characterised by segregation, low pay, low status, and limited advancement, exploring the experiences of disabled women in Remploy to determine the extent to which this was also reflected in sheltered employment.

Finally, Chapter 6 considers the wider field beyond Remploy. By examining a previously unexplored set of relationships, it explores the existence and extent of a mixed economy in sheltered employment. The analysis is framed around Remploy's place as the 'frontier of the state', with the chapter examining the movement of this frontier across three distinct periods. Demonstrating that Remploy operated as the core element in a tripartite mixed economy, alongside both voluntary providers and LAs, it shows how this approach ultimately failed to deliver a cohesive overall system.

CHAPTER 2

'When the War-Drums Cease to Roll', Creating the Postwar Scheme

Introduction

Remploy was created as one element of the Disabled Persons (Employment) Act (DPEA) in 1944. A landmark piece of legislation, the Act set out a range of measures for the training and employment of disabled people. The majority of these were aimed at those designated as 'Section I', who were considered able to access 'open' or 'mainstream' employment in some way. Remploy was then to provide sheltered employment for those considered too severely disabled to do so, designated as 'Section II'. Typically, considerations of the creation of the DPEA have tended to focus on the Section I measures, with sheltered employment simply identified as a further aspect of the Act.[1] By focusing on the creation of

[1] A. Borsay, *Disability and Social Policy in Britain Since 1750: A History of Exclusion* (Basingstoke, Palgrave Macmillan, 2005); H. Bolderson, *Social Security, Disability and Rehabilitation: Conflicts in the Development of Social Policy 1914–1946* (London, Jessica Kingsley Publishers, 1991); S. Wheatcroft, *Worth Saving: Disabled Children During the Second World War* (Manchester, Manchester University Press, 2013), p. 168; M. Reiss, *Blind Workers Against Charity: The National League of the Blind of Great Britain and Ireland, 1893–1970* (London, Palgrave Macmillan, 2015), pp. 138–41; J. Anderson, *War, Disability and Rehabilitation in Britain: 'Soul of a Nation'* (Manchester, Manchester University Press, 2011), pp. 183–5; P. Thane, *Foundations of the Welfare State, 2nd Edition* (London, Longman, 1996), pp. 224–5; L. Bryder, *Below the Magic Mountain: A Social History of Tuberculosis in Twentieth-Century Britain* (Oxford, Clarendon Press,

© The Author(s), under exclusive license to Springer Nature Switzerland AG 2025

A. Holroyde, *Sheltered Employment and Disability in the British Welfare State*, New Directions in Welfare History,
https://doi.org/10.1007/978-3-031-87876-3_2

Remploy specifically, this chapter will chart its own distinct journey into being.

A popular viewpoint has held that Remploy was created as a direct consequence of the Second World War.[2] This has also been suggested by a number of academics, including historians such as Reiss and Anderson.[3] Wars in general, and the two World Wars of the twentieth century in particular, have provided a common focus for studies in disability history and are thereby considered important drivers of disability policy. The Second World War has been described as a watershed moment for disabled people, particularly in terms of employment owing to the manpower shortage it created and evidenced by the passing of the DPEA itself.[4] More broadly, the impact of the conflict on the establishment of the welfare state represents an aspect of long-standing debate, in which Remploy might appear to support Titmuss' overall view of the primacy of the unique and specific experience of the Second World War.[5]

1988), p. 237; S. Lonsdale, *Work and Inequality* (Harlow, Longman, 1985), p. 120; S. Shah and M. Priestley, *Disability and Social Change: Private Lives and Public Policies* (Bristol, Policy Press, 2011), pp. 121–2; C. Barnes, *Disabled People in Britain and Discrimination* (London, C. Hurst & Co., 2000), pp. 71–2; E. Topliss, *Provision for the Disabled* (Oxford, Basil Blackwell, 1979), p. 55; M. Hyde, 'Sheltered and Supported Employment in the 1990s: The Experiences of Disabled Workers in the UK', *Disability & Society*, vol. 13, no. 2 (1998), p. 200.

[2] See for example, BBC News 'What are Remploy workers doing now?', (31.11.2014). http://www.bbc.co.uk/news/uk-29843567. Accessed 16 August 2024.

[3] Reiss, *Blind Workers Against Charity,* p. 140; Anderson, *War, Disability and Rehabilitation in Britain,* pp. 183–5; J. Anderson, "Turned into Taxpayers': Paraplegia, Rehabilitation and Sport at Stoke Mandeville, 1944–56', *Journal of Contemporary History*, vol. 38, no. 3 (2003), p. 469; E. Elsey, 'The Rehabilitation and Employment of Disabled Ex-Servicemen after the Two World Wars', unpublished PhD Thesis, University of Teesside (1994), pp. 276–7; M. Oliver, *The Politics of Disablement* (Basingstoke, Macmillan, 1990), pp. 88–9; Wheatcroft, *Worth Saving*, p. 168; Hyde, 'Sheltered and Supported Employment in the 1990s', pp. 199–215; Bryder, *Below the Magic Mountain*, p. 237; T. Jeffries, 'The Remploy Resource', *Industrial Management & Data Systems*, vol. 86, no. 1/2 (1986), p. 7; A. Kochan, 'Remploy: Disabled and Thriving', *Assembly Automation*, vol. 16, no. 1 (1996), p. 40.

[4] Borsay, *Disability and Social Policy in Britain Since 1750*, p. 135; J. Anderson, 'British Women, Disability and the Second World War', *Contemporary British History*, vol. 20, no. 1 (2006), p. 48; Anderson, 'Turned into Taxpayers', p. 470; Anderson, *Disability and Rehabilitation in Britain.*

[5] R.M. Titmuss, *Problems of Social Policy* (London, HMSO and Longmans, 1950), p. 508.

The majority of historians, however, have highlighted the importance of considering the war alongside longer term developments in policy and the role of Labour politicians in both coalition and majority governments.[6] The Minister of Labour in Winston Churchill's wartime Coalition Government, Ernest Bevin, universally recognised by both contemporaries and later scholars as having played a central role in the formation and passing of the DPEA, was himself adamant that it was not the war which was responsible for the measures contained in the Act, but long experience of the employment problems faced by disabled people.[7] This chapter will therefore explore the factors which led to the creation of Remploy, through consideration of the state of sheltered employment prior to the Second World War, the impact of the war itself and a close examination of its development through the formation of the DPEA.

The most detailed interpretation of Remploy's creation remains that proposed by Bolderson, subsequently adopted by Borsay, Humphries and Gordon, which sees the creation of the company as being a result of a bargain with industry to gain approval for the other measures of the DPEA, by segregating those non-productive disabled workers within the

[6] H. Pelling, *Britain and the Second World War* (London, Collins, 1970); A. Calder, *The People's War: Britain 1939–1945* (London, Pimlico, 1969); F. K. Prochaska, *The Voluntary Impulse: Philanthropy in Modern Britain*, (London, Faber, 1988); P. Thane, 'Voluntary Action in Britain Since Beveridge', in M. Oppenheimer and N. Deakin (eds.) *Beveridge and Voluntary Action in Britain and the Wider British World* (Manchester: Manchester University Press, 2011), pp. 121–34; G. Millward, 'Invalid Definitions, Invalid Responses: Disability and the Welfare State, 1965–1995', unpublished PhD Thesis, London11 School of Hygiene and Tropical Medicine (2013), p. 23; T. Alborn, 'Senses of Belonging: The Politics of Working-class Insurance in Britain, 1880–1914', *Journal of Modern History*, vol. 73, no.3 (2001), p. 567; K. Laybourn, *The Evolution of British Social Policy and the Welfare State, c.1800–1993* (Keele, Keele University Press, 1995), pp. 209–10; B. Harris, *The Origins of the British Welfare State* (Basingstoke, Palgrave Macmillan, 2004), p. 289; G. Wright, *The Ordeal of Total War, 1939–1945* (London, Harper & Row, 1968); D. Fraser, *The Evolution of the British Welfare State*, 4th Edition (Basingstoke, Palgrave Macmillan, 2009); P. Addison, *The Road to 1945: British Politics and the Second World War, Revised Edition* (London, Pimlico, 1994), pp. 13–4; H. Glennerster, *British Social Policy: 1945 to the Present*, 3rd Edition (Oxford, Blackwell Publishing, 2007), p. 4; K.O. Morgan, *Labour in Power 1945–51* (Oxford, Oxford University Press, 1984); K. Jones, *The Making of Social Policy in Britain 1830–1990*, 2nd Edition (London, Athlone Press, 1996), p. 122; R. Lowe, *The Welfare State in Britain Since 1945* (Basingstoke, Palgrave Macmillan, 2005) pp. 16–17; D. Gladstone, *The Twentieth-Century Welfare State* (Basingstoke, Palgrave Macmillan, 1999), p. 51.

[7] Mr. Ernest Bevin, *Hansard*, 395, col. 1349 (10.12.1943).

scheme.[8] This influential interpretation merits close attention and this chapter will explore it in detail. A common assumption across many references to the creation of Remploy is that it appeared as a fully formed, coherent company, with a determined objective and *modus operandi* as it began to operate.[9] By examining the development of the company prior to the first meeting of the Board of Directors on 30 May 1945, this chapter will further consider whether this was indeed the case and the degree to which Remploy was established with a predetermined agenda.

To explore these areas, this chapter will initially expand the chronological focus to consider the provision of sheltered employment in the interwar period, in order to determine the existence of any notion of such a scheme prior to the Second World War. Following this, the impact of the war itself will be considered. The chapter will then turn to a close examination of the development of what would become Remploy through the formation and passage of the DPEA. This will be followed by a detailed analysis of the case made by Bolderson, and will conclude with consideration of the particular role of Bevin himself. The final section will then consider the extent to which Remploy began to operate with a defined purpose already in place. The chapter will thereby shed new light on the specific developments which led to Remploy, and consider this within the wider context of the creation of the welfare state.

[8] Bolderson, *Social Security, Disability and Rehabilitation*, pp. 109–110; S. Humphries and P. Gordon, *Out of Sight: The Experience of Disability 1900–1950* (Plymouth, Northcote House, 1992), p. 138; Borsay, *Disability and Social Policy in Britain Since 1750*.

[9] See for example, J. Hampton, 'Discovering Disability: The General Classes of Disabled People and the Classic Welfare State, 1948–1964', *The Historian*, vol. 75, no. 1 (2013), p. 77; Anderson, *War, Disability and Rehabilitation in Britain*, pp. 183–5; Topliss, *Provision for the Disabled*, pp. 55–6; Barnes, *Disabled People in Britain and Discrimination*, p. 71; Shah and Priestley, *Disability and Social Change*, pp. 139–40; Lonsdale, *Work and Inequality*, p. 137; H. Bolderson, 'The Origins of the Disabled Persons Employment Quota and its Symbolic Significance', *Journal of Social Policy*, vol. 9, no. 2 (1980), p. 178.

Interwar Developments in Sheltered Employment, 1918–1939

Prior to the First World War, scant provision for disabled people was made through a combination of outdoor and indoor relief, with employment reliant on very limited philanthropic endeavours.[10] Following the end of the war, with some 20 million men wounded, and 8 million permanently disabled, the question of how to reintegrate these people back into society was a challenge for states throughout Europe.[11] Thus in Britain, disability employment became a pressing issue, though this was focused almost entirely upon ex-servicemen, who received unique consideration in welfare owing to their having become disabled in service to the nation.[12] The dominant view of this period, espoused by Cohen and Bolderson, is that interwar governments wished to limit their responsibility for providing employment for disabled ex-servicemen, preferring instead to rely on the awarding of pensions, the goodwill of employers, and the efforts of the voluntary sector wherever possible.[13] This appears

[10] J. Hampton, *Disability and the Welfare State in Britain: Changes in Perception and Policy 1948–79* (Bristol, Policy Press, 2016), pp. 21–33; J. Reznick, 'Work-Therapy and the Disabled British Soldier in Great Britain in the First World War: The Case of Shepherd's Bush Military Hospital, London', in D. A. Gerber (ed.) *Disabled Veterans in History* (Ann Arbor, University of Michigan Press, 2012), pp. 187–9; Borsay, *Disability and Social Policy in Britain Since 1750*, pp. 119–39; D. Cohen, *The War Come Home: Disabled Veterans in Britain and Germany 1914–1939* (Los Angeles, University of California Press, 2001); pp. 18–9; J. Bourke, *Dismembering the Male: Men's Bodies, Britain and the Great War* (London, Reaktion Books, 1996); pp. 44–5; M. Kowalsky, "This Honourable Obligation": The King's National Roll Scheme for Disabled Ex-servicemen, 1915–1944', *European Review of History*, vol. 14, no. 4 (2007), pp. 576–7.

[11] D. Cohen, 'Will to Work: Disabled Veterans in Britain and Germany after the First World War', in D. A. Gerber (ed.) *Disabled Veterans in History* (Ann Arbor, University of Michigan Press, 2012), p. 295.

[12] The National Archives (TNA) LAB 20/3, MOL, 'Memorandum on Scheme Adopted for Training Persons Disabled in the Last War'. For overview of special provisions for ex-servicemen see, Hampton, *Disability and the Welfare State in Britain*, pp. 37–40. See also G. L. Hudson, 'Disabled Veterans and the State in Early Modern England', in D. A. Gerber (ed.) *Disabled Veterans in History* (Ann Arbor, University of Michigan Press, 2012), pp. 117–44.

[13] Cohen, 'Will to Work', pp. 297–300; Cohen, *The War Come Home*, pp. 16–7; Bolderson, *Social Security, Disability and Rehabilitation*, pp. 36–45, 56–7, 160–61; See also Reznick, 'Work-Therapy and the Disabled British Soldier in Great Britain in the First World War', p. 198; Anderson, *War, Disability and Rehabilitation in Britain*, pp. 15, 46–8; Kowalsky, 'This Honourable Obligation', pp. 570–1, 568–9; J. Meyer, "Not Septimus

to have been a result of both a common and persistent ideological resistance to state involvement in such issues, and the problems of industrial unrest, economic depression and mass unemployment faced by successive interwar governments, which are seen as having limited the initial commitment to reconstruction and social welfare measures more generally.[14]

In terms of disability employment, several measures were put in place, perhaps the most important being the establishment of the King's National Roll in 1919.[15] This was a voluntary scheme intended to evoke employers' patriotic sense of duty with a royal appeal for them to ensure at least 5% of their workers were disabled ex-servicemen.[16] In addition to this, were numerous schemes for training and instruction, in which the government was involved to varying degrees.[17] While indicating the beginning of a gradual movement towards state responsibility for the employment of disabled ex-servicemen, these steps were inadequate. Faith in industry absorbing disabled ex-servicemen proved to be misplaced.[18] Pensions, upon which such emphasis was placed, were

Now': Wives of Disabled Veterans and Cultural Memory of the First World War in Britain', *Women's History Review*, vol. 13, no. 1 (2004), p. 122. TNA CAB 27/49, 'Demobilisation Committee: DM-57' (15.1.1919).

[14] Cohen, 'Will to Work', pp. 297–300; Cohen, *The War Come Home*, pp. 16–7; Bolderson, *Social Security, Disability and Rehabilitation*, p. 161; Gladstone, *The Twentieth-Century Welfare State*, pp. 21–31; Laybourn, *The Evolution of British Social Policy and the Welfare State*, pp. 188–206; Thane, *Foundations of the Welfare State*, pp. 153–206; A. Digby, *British Welfare Policy: Workhouse to Workfare* (London, Faber and Faber, 1989), pp. 49–51; Hampton, *Disability and the Welfare State in Britain*, pp. 38–9.

[15] TNA LAB 20/56, Inter-Departmental Committee on the Rehabilitation and Resettlement of Disabled Persons, 'Note by the Ministry of Pensions'.

[16] Ibid. For details of the scheme see Kowalksy, 'This Honourable Obligation'; M. Mantin, 'Coalmining and the National Scheme for Disabled Ex-Servicemen after the First World War', *Social History*, vol. 41, no. 2 (2016), p. 170.

[17] TNA LAB 20/56, 'Memorandum on Training of Disabled Ex Service Men After the Great War: R.D.4'. Anderson, *War, Disability and Rehabilitation in Britain*, pp. 46–8; Kowalsky, 'This Honourable Obligation', p. 570.

[18] TNA PIN 15/35, Bedford and District Employment Committee, 'Employment Sub Committee for Disabled Sailors and Soldiers' (1920). Cohen, 'Will to Work', pp. 302-3; Bolderson, *Social Security, Disability and Rehabilitation*, pp. 56-7; Wheatcroft, *Worth Saving*, pp. 96-8.

insufficient and often subject to dispute.[19] The King's Roll and the government's training programmes could also claim only partial success.[20] Collectively these efforts, while generally well intentioned, proved insufficient to provide a definitive solution to the problem of unemployment for disabled ex-servicemen.[21]

This was particularly the case for those who were severely disabled. These men were referred to as the 'unemployables', who, because of the severity of their disability, found securing work virtually impossible.[22] Estimates differed on how many such cases there were, but it could have been as many as 25,000.[23] For these men there was little option for work beyond that provided by sheltered employment schemes run by charitable organisations. Some of these provided training or limited employment in residential settings, such as the Star and Garter Home for Disabled Soldiers and Sailors, opened in 1916.[24] More ambitious schemes, such as the Enham Village Centre involved whole sheltered communities.[25] The

[19] Cohen, *The War Come Home*, p. 4; Meyer, 'Not Septimus Now', p. 122; Bolderson, *Social Security, Disability and Rehabilitation*, pp. 46–7.

[20] TNA CAB 24/106/55, 'Report from the Ministry of Labour' (26.05.1920); TNA LAB 20/416, 'Extract from Select Committee Report on Training and Employment of Disabled Ex-Service Men', p. vi; 'Note by Mr. R. Gomme to Mr. Glen' (26.02.1941); 'Disabled Men's Workshops', *The Times* (19.05.1921); TNA CAB 24/84/92, 'Cabinet Memorandum: The Labour Situation. Report from the Ministry of Labour' (23.7.1919). *Report from the Select Committee on Pensions,* 185 (1920), p. iv. Kowalsky, 'This Honourable Obligation', p. 573; Reznick, 'Work-Therapy and the Disabled British Soldier in Great Britain in the First World War', p. 198; Anderson, *War, Disability and Rehabilitation in Britain*, p. 47; Bolderson, *Social Security, Disability and Rehabilitation*, pp. 36–41; Cohen, *The War Come Home*, pp. 39–40; Cohen 'Will to Work', pp. 302–3; Mantin, 'Coalmining and the National Scheme for Disabled Ex-Servicemen after the First World War', p. 170.

[21] Meyer, 'Not Septimus Now', pp. 117–38; Cohen, *The War Come Home*, pp. 104–14; Hampton, *Disability and the Welfare State in Britain*, p. 39.

[22] TNA PIN 15/35, Bedford and District Employment Committee, 'Employment Sub-Committee for Disabled Sailors and Soldiers' (1920).

[23] TNA PIN 15/34, 'The Return of the Disabled Solider to Civil Life', *The Lancet* (04.09.1920); TNA PIN 15/35, Committee on Employment of Severely Disabled Ex-Service Men, 'Minutes of the First Meeting' (30.09.1920).

[24] Anderson, *War, Disability and Rehabilitation in Britain*, pp. 49–55; J. Anderson and N. Pemberton, 'Walking Alone: Aiding the War and Civilian Blind in the Inter-war Period', *European Review of History*, vol. 14, no. 4 (2007), pp. 459–79.

[25] TNA PIN 15/34, 'Village Settlements for Disabled Ex-Service Men Scheme' (November. 1917); 'Village Settlements for the Disabled', *The Lancet*, (03.11.1917);

majority, however, offered employment in non-residential settings, the most prominent of which were the Lord Roberts Memorial Workshops. Operated by the Soldiers and Sailors Help Society following the Boer War, these were renamed in honour of Field Marshall Lord Roberts, a trustee of the workshops and recipient of the Victoria Cross, who had passed away during a visit to the front in 1914.[26] The Lord Roberts Workshops expanded during the First World War, and at the end of 1919 employed over 600 men in several locations around the country.[27] Charitable workshops such as these continually faced financial and operational challenges, being run on very slight budgets reliant on public generosity.[28]

There was some consideration of a government scheme of sheltered employment in the aftermath of the First World War under David Lloyd George's Coalition Government—with a proposal for 'state factories' for severely disabled ex-servicemen raised during a meeting of the War Cabinet Demobilisation Committee in January 1919.[29] The Committee concluded that the Government should indeed 'provide a certain number of factories solely for the employment of certain classes of disabled men who, on account of special disability, may be found to be unable to engage in ordinary industrial occupations'.[30] Within just a few months, however, the MOL determined that such a scheme was not 'practicable'.[31] The idea would be raised again the same year in a cabinet report explaining that 'the Government have already anticipated that it may be necessary for them to create direct employment for very badly disfigured men', with

'Reconstruction: Village Settlements for Disabled Ex-Service Men', *Westminster Gazette*, (09.11.1917); TNA PIN 15/37, Village Centres Council, 'First Annual Report' (1919); TNA PIN 15/36, Committee on Employment of Severely Disabled Ex-Service Men, 'Minutes of the Third Meeting' (20.10.1920). Cohen, *The War Come Home*, p. 35.

[26] TNA LAB 20/78, 'The Incorporated Soldiers, Sailors and Airmen's Help Society and Lord Roberts Memorial Fund and Workshops Annual Report for 1944' (1944), pp. 28–9.

[27] Ibid.; TNA LAB 20/56, Inter-departmental Committee on the Rehabilitation and Resettlement of Disabled Persons, 'Note by the Ministry of Pensions: R.D.9'.

[28] See Cohen, *The War Come Home*, pp. 112–4; Anderson, *War, Disability and Rehabilitation in Britain*, pp. 27–8; M. Kowalsky, 'Enabling the Great War: Ex-servicemen, the Mixed Economy of Welfare and the Social Construction of Disability, 1899–1930', unpublished PhD Thesis, University of Leeds (2007), pp. 102–3.

[29] TNA CAB 27/49, 'War Cabinet Demobilisation Committee: DM -57' (15.01.1919).

[30] Ibid.

[31] TNA CAB 24/80/62, 'Cabinet Memorandum: The Labour Situation. Report from the Ministry of Labour' (28.05.1919).

the responsibility sitting with the Ministry of Pensions.[32] The Ministry, however, claimed there was no justification 'for putting up factories for employment'.[33]

The issue was resurrected the following year by the cross-party Select Committee on Pensions, which recognised that there was a significant number of severely disabled men who could not find ordinary employment and for whom no government provision was being made.[34] As part of its proceedings, the Committee took evidence from the Minister of Labour, Thomas Macnamara, a Coalition Liberal and close associate of Lloyd George, who admitted the need for sheltered workshops, but not necessarily for state involvement.[35] Referencing charitable schemes such as the Lord Roberts Workshops, he concluded that 'provision of this kind is necessary for men who cannot hope to compete in the industrial world'.[36] However, despite noting that existing voluntary schemes were not sufficient, and under repeated questioning from the Committee on government involvement, Macnamara would admit no more than it being a matter 'which we are seriously considering'.[37] Thus the attitude of the MOL was non-committal, while the attitude of the Ministry of Pensions appears to have been that such individuals would have to rely solely on their pension.[38] Despite this, in its report produced in August 1920, the Committee recommended that arrangements including 'special workshops' be made for those who 'possess some potential earning capacity, but could only exercise it if some special arrangements were made for enabling them to do so'.[39]

[32] TNA CAB 24/87/60, 'Cabinet Memorandum: The Labour Situation. Report from the Ministry of Labour' (27.08.1919).

[33] See evidence given by Colonel J.S. Bostock, Director of the Treatment-Training Branch of the Medical Services Division of the Ministry of Pensions, *Report from the Select Committee on Pensions,* 185 (1920), p. 110.

[34] Ibid., p. iv; *Ministry of Labour, Committee on Re-Employment of Ex-Servicemen, Interim Report,* 951 (1920).

[35] R. Betts, 'Macnamara, Thomas James (1861–1931), educationist and politician', *Oxford Dictionary of National Biography* (03.01.2008). https://www.oxforddnb.com/. Accessed 8 July 2018; *Report from the Select Committee on Pensions,* 185 (1920), p. 184.

[36] *Report from the Select Committee on Pensions,* 185 (1920), p. 184.

[37] Ibid., pp. 185–7.

[38] Ibid., p. 110.

[39] Ibid., pp. ix-xii.

The idea of state-run sheltered employment was given its full and final consideration later in the year. In response to demand 'from all sides', the MOL led formation of the inter-departmental Committee on the Employment of Severely Disabled Ex-Servicemen in September 1920.[40] Part of this demand came from the Lord Roberts Workshops themselves, which were specifically referenced in the terms of the Committee. The Comptroller of the workshops, Sir Algernon Tudor-Craig, had approached the Minister of Labour the previous year to inform him that the workshops were on the brink of ruin and to propose either that the Government gave financial assistance or took control entirely.[41] The Committee heard evidence from a wide range of interested parties including representatives of charitable sheltered employment schemes, trade unions, ex-serviceman organisations, employers and local employment committees.[42] There was a great deal of support for the idea of state factories, with arguments highlighting the national debt owed to these ex-servicemen and that only a large government-backed network of sheltered employment could provide adequate, and equal, provision.[43] There was, however, significant opposition to the idea from a number of local employment committees, and from within the Committee itself, centred on the Ministry of Pensions' Adair Hore.[44] Described by Cohen as being

[40] TNA PIN 15/35, Committee on Employment of Severely Disabled Ex-Service Men, 'Minutes of the First Meeting' (30.09.1920).

[41] TNA PIN 15/34, 'Proposals Made by the Comptroller of the Lord Roberts' Memorial Workshops for Assistance by the Government'.

[42] For a list see TNA PIN 15/37, 'Provisional Interim Report of the Committee Appointed to Consider the Employment of Severely Disabled Ex-Service Men' (18.01.1921).

[43] TNA PIN 15/37, 'Summary of Replies of Local Employment Committees to Questionnaire, Memo 60' (1921); 'The Employment of Severely Disabled Men, Memo no. 37' (27.11.1920); Committee on Employment of Severely Disabled Ex-Service Men, 'Minutes of the Sixth Meeting' (11.11.1920); 'Minutes of the Tenth Meeting' (26.11.1920); 'Minutes of the Twelfth Meeting' (09.12.1920); 'Provisional Interim Report of the Committee Appointed to Consider the Employment of Severely Disabled Ex-Service Men' (18.01.1921).

[44] TNA PIN 15/37, Committee on Employment of Severely Disabled Ex-Service Men, 'Minutes of the Seventh Meeting' (17.11.1920); 'G. Crosfield reply to questionnaire, Memo no. 35' (26.11.1920); TNA PIN 15/36, 'Note from A. Hore' (08.10.1920); TNA PIN 15/37, 'Provisional Interim Report of the Committee Appointed to Consider the Employment of Severely Disabled Ex-Service Men' (18.01.1921). Bolderson, *Social Security, Disability and Rehabilitation*, pp. 41–3; Cohen, *The War Come Home*, pp. 40–5.

'among the most powerful officials' in the Ministry and as someone particularly resistant to state involvement in the issue of employment provision for disabled people, Hore seems to have been against the idea from the beginning.[45] Collectively, a number of objections were raised, including: that the factories would run at a loss; that they would not gain the approval of industry;that they would involve moving disabled ex-servicemen away from their homes and families; that the factories would be unable to sell their products; that employed disabled ex-servicemen would abandon their work to join the scheme; that state involvement would lead to demands for higher wages; and that a national scheme would not be flexible enough to deal with local issues.[46] Hore circulated a memorandum outlining his own objections to the idea to members of the Committee, suggesting such a scheme was beyond the responsibility of the state and, contrary to the general opinion of the Committee, that pensions were an adequate substitute.[47]

The result was a recommendation that state factories should not be established and instead the best solution was 'to be along the lines of voluntary effort locally organised and administered but with a certain amount of central guidance and central assistance'.[48] The burden of administration and finance would fall to LAs working with charitable enterprise.[49] Government was to provide financial assistance only, through the awarding of grants set at £25 per capita, per annum—only a quarter of the average loss per worker in the Lord Roberts Workshops.[50]

[45] Cohen, *The War Come Home*, p. 42.

[46] TNA PIN 15/35, 'Memorandum by Training Department on the employment of men whose disabilities preclude their absorption into industry'; TNA PIN 15/36, 'Note from A. Hore' (08.10.1920); TNA PIN 15/36, Committee on Employment of Severely Disabled Ex-Servicemen, 'Minutes of Second Meeting' (07.10.1920); TNA PIN 15/37, 'Provisional Interim Report of the Committee Appointed to Consider the Employment of Severely Disabled Ex-Service Men' (18.01.1921).

[47] TNA PIN 15/33, C.F.A. Hore, 'Memorandum, Committee on the Employment of Severely Disabled Men' (16.12.1920); TNA PIN 15/37, 'Provisional Interim Report of the Committee Appointed to Consider the Employment of Severely Disabled Ex-Service Men' (18.01.1921).

[48] TNA PIN 15/37, 'Provisional Interim Report of the Committee Appointed to Consider the Employment of Severely Disabled Ex-Service Men' (18.01.1921).

[49] Ibid.

[50] TNA CAB 24/123/79, 'Cabinet Summary of the Report of the Committee Appointed to Consider the Employment of Severely Disabled Ex-Service Men'.

Even this limited proposal received opposition, chiefly from the Treasury, with the Chancellor of the Exchequer, Sir Robert Horne, a Conservative in the Coalition Government, writing a memorandum for the Cabinet in June 1921 registering his opposition.[51] By the time of Horne's appointment in April, a severe economic downturn had led to calls from industry and from within his own party for reductions in government expenditure.[52] His memorandum reflected this overall agenda as he explained that 'the state of national finance makes it impossible to contemplate any further increase of expenditure'.[53] Noting the rising levels of unemployment generally, he also evoked the argument that pensions were an adequate provision, explaining that in his view 'so far as the grievance of these men is that they cannot find employment, their case is not different at the present time from that of an unprecedented number of other men and women, who do not draw pensions from the state'.[54] Horne's interjection succeeded with the Committee's proposals initially rejected by the Cabinet.[55] They were eventually accepted, albeit in weakened form, with grants awarded to support charitable employment schemes when, and only when, public funding through charitable donations proved insufficient.[56] Even with the small amounts involved it is apparent that the Treasury would do all it could to limit their award, much to the dismay of the sheltered workshops and sympathetic members of government.[57]

There was to be no change to this approach. A prevalent economic understanding that 'good governance' involved balancing the budget

(25.05.1921); TNA PIN 15/34, 'Memo by Finance Department as to the Financial Position of the Lord Roberts Memorial Workshops'. Bolderson, *Social Security, Disability and Rehabilitation*, p. 42.

51 TNA CAB 24/125/13, 'Cabinet Memorandum by the Chancellor of the Exchequer, The Employment of Severely Disabled Ex-Servicemen' (03.06.1921).

52 P. Williamson, 'Horne, Robert Stevenson, Viscount Horne of Slamannan (1871–1940), politician and businessman', *Oxford Dictionary of National Biography (06.01.2011)*. https://www.oxforddnb.com/. Accessed 14 July 2018.

53 TNA CAB 24/125/13, 'Cabinet Memorandum by the Chancellor of the Exchequer, The Employment of Severely Disabled Ex-Servicemen' (03.06.1921).

54 Ibid.

55 Ibid; TNA PIN 15/33, 'Note from C.F.A Hore' (16.08.1921).

56 TNA PIN 15/38, MOL, 'Scheme of Grants to Undertakings Formed for the Employment of Severely Disabled Ex-Service Men' (06.12.1923). Cohen, *The War Come Home*, p. 45.

57 Cohen, *The War Come Home*, p. 45.

brought wider and sustained expenditure cuts, beginning with the so-called 'Geddes Axe' of 1922, named after the Secretary to the Treasury, Sir Eric Geddes, who chaired the committee which recommended the policy of economic retrenchment and the abandonment of many reconstruction promises.[58] During the interwar period, the MOL made grants to 'thirty separate enterprises' providing sheltered employment, which Cohen suggests probably employed around 2000 workers, 'only a fraction of those who according to the Government's figures needed work'.[59] This appears to have been the pattern of support, or lack thereof, for sheltered workshops throughout the interwar period, regardless of which political party was in power.[60] Continuing high unemployment and economic difficulties punctuated by crises such as the General Strike in 1926 and the Wall Street Crash in 1931, limited advances in statutory welfare and perpetuated a reliance on the voluntary sector to deal with disabled people.[61] The Conservative Government's reply to a parliamentary question on sheltered employment provision in 1938 confirmed that the awarding of grants to voluntary workshops was still considered 'the most practicable' system.[62]

The decision not to provide a state sheltered employment scheme did not put an end to the concept, with continued calls for government to reconsider voiced throughout the interwar period. Those charged with attempting to assist severely disabled ex-servicemen into employment clearly recognised a need, as the MOL continued to receive requests for state sheltered employment from a number of its local employment committees.[63] Such sentiments were shared by administrators of the

[58] Jones, *The Making of Social Policy in Britain*, pp. 104–5; Hampton, *Disability and the Welfare State in Britain*, pp. 38–9, 57; Lowe, *The Welfare State in Britain Since 1945*, p. 92.

[59] Cohen, *The War Come Home*, pp. 45–6.

[60] Ibid., pp. 44–6.

[61] Jones, *The Making of Social Policy in Britain*, pp. 104–5; Hampton, *Disability and the Welfare State in Britain*, pp. 38–9, 57; Lowe, *The Welfare State in Britain Since 1945*, p. 92.

[62] Sir Smedley Crooke to Mr E.Brown, *Hansard* (22.12.1938), vol. 342 cc. 3101-3w.

[63] TNA CAB 24/80/62, 'Cabinet Memorandum: The Labour Situation. Report from the Ministry of Labour for the week ending 28th May 1919' (28.05.1919); TNA CAB 24/73/30, 'Cabinet Memorandum: The Labour Situation. Report from the Ministry of Labour for the week ending 1st January 1919' (01.01.1919); TNA PIN 15/35,

King's Roll, who noted the increasing difficulty of placing such men into work.[64] There was also sustained discussion of the issue in both the national and local press.[65]

A testament to the continued demand for sheltered employment from disabled people themselves was indicated by a report in *The Times*, which noted that a short paragraph in a previous issue on the opening of a workshop by the Disabled Soldiers' and Sailors' Workshops Association, had resulted in over 2000 applications from disabled ex-servicemen.[66] The issue thus became a key area of campaigning for organisations representing disabled people. As Hampton has noted, a political profile in the interwar period was reserved for disabled ex-servicemen, the industrially injured and the blind, who were each represented by advocate groups.[67] As part of the wider welfare measures contained in the 1920 Blind Persons Act, LAs had already been made responsible for providing some sheltered employment exclusively for the blind, though as Reiss has noted, the creation of a coherent national state network of sheltered employment remained a 'core goal' and a continued focus of campaigning for the National League of the Blind.[68] In the case of ex-servicemen, two of the most important groups, the British Legion and the British Limbless Ex-Service Men's Association (BLESMA), the latter of which grew out of the 'grassroots working class movement' Limbless Ex-Servicemen's Association, were both actively campaigning for further sheltered employment provision in the years preceding the Second World War.[69] A report in *The Times* from 1932 detailed the evidence given by the Chairman of

'Extract from the Minutes of the Meeting of the Northampton Employment Committee' (30.08.1920); 'Disabled Men's Future', *The Times* (11.02.1919); TNA PIN 15/34, 'Letter from Chester, Harwich and District Local Committee' (02.09.1920); TNA PIN 15/36, 'Resolution RE. Employment of Disabled Men Passed by the DundeeLocal War Pensions Committee' (October, 1920).

64 TNA CAB 24/121/7, 'Cabinet Memorandum: The Labour Situation. Report from the Ministry of Labour for the week ending 12 March 1921' (12.03.1921).

65 See numerous examples in TNA PIN 15/34.

66 'Disabled Men's Workshops', *The Times* (19.05.1921).

67 Hampton, *Disability and the Welfare State in Britain*, pp. 53–4.

68 Reis, *Blind Workers against Charity*, p. 140; TNA LAB 20/1429, DE, 'Sheltered Employment: A Draft Consultative Document' (October, 1973), p. 5.

69 P. Ryde, *Out on a Limb* (British Limbless Ex-Service Men's Association, 1982); Kowalsky, 'Enabling the Great War', pp. 182–9.

the British Legion, Colonel John Brown, to the Royal Commission on Unemployment Insurance, in which the Colonel explained that it had always been the policy of the British Legion that sheltered employment was necessary for 'the severely disabled ex-Service man', and he called on government involvement in providing this.[70] In 1938, a series of press articles followed a petition sent to the then Prime Minister, Neville Chamberlain, from BLESMA, calling for government provision of sheltered employment.[71] Following the petitions refusal, a BLESMA representative was reported as saying that 'the association would persist in its request'.[72] In addition to this campaigning, awareness of existing charitable workshops, such as those provided by the British Legion and the Lord Roberts Workshops, was maintained through charitable appeals in the press and fundraising activities.[73] Though no government was to acquiesce, both the demand and desire for a state-run sheltered employment scheme from those groups representing disabled people was clearly evident.

It is important to note that interwar developments were not unique to the question of sheltered employment, with two of the other key measures of the DPEA also receiving consideration at this time. The idea of a compulsory quota of disabled workers for industry was raised frequently by the Committee on the Employment of Severely Disabled Men, but was rejected in favour of the voluntary King's Roll.[74] Similarly, the idea of reserved trades for disabled people was put to the Cabinet by the Minister of Labour and the Minister of Pensions in 1918, but was not to survive the following general election.[75] Employment prospects for disabled ex-servicemen more generally have also been shown by historians such as

[70] 'Unemployment Insurance', *The Times* (05.03.1932).

[71] 'Ex-Service Men's Request Refused', *The Times* (10.09.1938); 'War-Disabled Men's Pensions', *The Manchester Guardian* (04.04.1938); 'Premier's Reply to Ex-Servicemen', *The Manchester Guardian* (09.07.1938); 'Ex-Servicemen and their widows', *The Manchester Guardian* (10.09.1938).

[72] 'Ex-Servicemen and their widows', *The Manchester Guardian* (10.09.1938).

[73] See for example, 'National Tribute Fund', *The Times* (20.05.1918); 'Lord Roberts', *The Times* (22.05.1918); 'Christmas Appeals', *The Times* (24.12.1929); 'Occupational Therapy', *The Times* (06.09.1937); 'Men with nerves wrecked by the war', *The Times* (04.08.1939); 'This week is National Tribute Week', *Daily Mail* (20.05.1918); Kowalsky, 'Enabling the Great War', p. 189.

[74] Kowalsky, 'This Honourable Obligation', p. 573.

[75] Bolderson, *Social Security, Disability and Rehabilitation*, pp. 38–9, Kowalsky, 'This Honourable Obligation', pp. 577–8.

Cohen, Anderson and Kowalksy, to have enjoyed sustained interest from both politicians and the public throughout the interwar period.[76] The question of sheltered employment was therefore part of a growing wider discourse on employment provision for disabled ex-servicemen.

In the case of sheltered employment, it is clear that there were significant developments in the interwar period which appear to follow the same broad process as disability employment provision more generally. We see increased, though strictly limited, government measures focused on ex-servicemen, which proved insufficient, and thereby resulted in sustained, though unsuccessful, campaigning for further support. Crucially, the idea of state-run sheltered employment and the demand for it, did not suddenly appear during the Second World War. The idea of a government scheme in the vein of what would become Remploy, was raised and seriously considered in the aftermath of the First World War, and though it was ultimately abandoned by Lloyd George's Coalition Government, further demand and campaigning efforts ensured that the notion did not disappear from public and political discourse.

The Impact of the Second World War

While the idea of a state scheme of sheltered employment was not a new one, it was finally enacted during the Second World War. The outbreak of war certainly placed the issue of support for disabled people on the agenda with an urgency which would have been unlikely otherwise, particularly in relation to those disabled by the war itself, which for the first time included significant numbers of women and civilians. Concern for the treatment, both in the long- and short-term, of disabled people was

[76] TNA CAB 24/88/84, 'Cabinet Memorandum: The Labour Situation. Report from the Ministry of Labour' (17.09.1919); TNA CAB 24/118/79, 'Cabinet Memorandum: The Labour Situation. Report from the Ministry of Labour' (22.01.1921); TNA PIN 15/33, which contains numerous press cuttings throughout the period containing articles, news and correspondence on the issue. *Report of the Committee appointed by the President of the Local Government Board upon the Provision and Employment of Sailors and Soldiers Disabled in the War*, 7915 (1915); Bolderson, *Social Security, Disability and Rehabilitation*, pp. 38–9; Cohen, *The War Come Home*, pp. 22–5, 45–6; Wheatcroft, *Worth Saving*, pp. 24–5; Reznick, 'Work-Therapy and the Disabled British Soldier in Great Britain in the First World War', p. 198; Anderson, *War, Disability and Rehabilitation in Britain*, pp. 46–8; Borsay, *Disability and Social Policy in Britain Since 1750*, p. 130; Kowalsky, 'This Honourable Obligation', pp. 567–78.

evident in both the public and political spheres throughout.[77] This also encapsulated the related issue of medical rehabilitation for those injured, with the need to preserve manpower, both in terms of the armed forces and the civilian population, necessitating rapid improvements in such provision.[78]

The manpower shortage caused by the Second World War has often been seen as having had a significant impact on the position of disabled people.[79] Historians such as Anderson and Borsay have suggested that the shortage of labour allowed disabled people to enter into a diminished workforce and prove their ability to be productive.[80] Disabled people thus became an important source of manpower for British industry.[81] This entry into the workforce occurred both naturally, as existing workers left for military service, and as the result of government intervention through the 'Interim Scheme' which provided training and employment advice.[82] Access to mainstream employment extended to some severely disabled people as well, which meant they could rely less on charitable sheltered employment schemes. Thus, the sheltered settlement established by The Derwen Cripples' Training College saw its number of workers decline from 45 in July 1939, to just 13 in May 1940; while the Queen Elizabeth

[77] TNA LAB 20/3, 'Report of the Inter-Departmental Committee on the Vocational Training of War Casualties' (1940); TNA LAB 20/2, 'Note from J.M. Glen' (22.10.1940). 'Work for disabled Service men', *The Times* (08.12.1943); 'Workshop for casualties', *The Daily Herald* (09.12.1943); TNA LAB 20/108, 'Town has jobs for them', *The Daily Dispatch*, (06.10.1944); 'Adjusting Conditions of Work', *The Manchester Guardian* (04.04.1945).

[78] Bolderson, *Social Security, Disability and Rehabilitation*, pp. 97–9; Wheatcroft, *Worth Saving*, pp. 167–70; TNA LAB 20/84, H. Balme, 'Britain Advances: The Unfit made Fit' (1943).

[79] Wheatcroft, *Worth Saving*, pp. 167–70; Hampton, *Disability and the Welfare State in Britain*, p. 53; Anderson, *War, Disability and Rehabilitation in Britain*, p. 212; Borsay, *Disability and Social Policy in Britain Since 1750*, pp. 133–4; Hampton, 'Discovering Disability', p. 77.

[80] Anderson, *War, Disability and Rehabilitation in Britain*, p. 212; Borsay, *Disability and Social Policy in Britain Since 1750*, pp. 133–4.

[81] Bolderson, *Social Security, Disability and Rehabilitation*, pp. 7–8.

[82] Ibid., pp. 104–5.

Training College for the Disabled could claim that by 1941, nearly 350 of its trainees had entered munitions work.[83]

While there can be little doubt that this inclusion was beneficial, there was no guarantee that it would itself lead to permanent change. At the end of the war the munitions industries which had employed so many disabled people would be scaled-back for peacetime and those disabled people employed in other industries would be unlikely to keep any job in competition with a returning soldier or other non-disabled person. The anomaly of the wartime situation was recognised at the time, as policy-makers attempted 'to visualise the peace-time position'.[84] Similarly, Bevin himself emphasised the longer term manpower requirements for the task of reconstruction following the war in justification for the measures contained in the DPEA.[85] The Act would therefore function to maximise 'the productive capacity of every human being we have at our disposal'.[86] The most important impact of the manpower shortage caused by the Second World War in terms of the creation of Remploy, and of the other measures of the DPEA, was therefore to assist in the recognition of the ability of disabled people to be productive and contribute both to the war effort and to the task of reconstruction that would follow.

For Bolderson, a further key impact of the Second World War was to add a sense of urgency in the political psyche for the proposals put forward regarding rehabilitation and disabled people.[87] While Bevin may have insisted that the DPEA was not the result of the war, this does not seem to have been the opinion of other Members of Parliament (MPs).[88] The impact of the war on the DPEA was addressed directly in the House of Commons during its reading at Bill stage. The Conservative MP, Rear-Admiral Beamish, whose own son was twice wounded during the Second World War, remarked that 'I maintain that the Bill was produced…solely

[83] TNA LAB 20/56, Inter-departmental Committee on the Rehabilitation and Resettlement of Disabled Persons, 'Memorandum by the Board of Education on the Vocational Training of Cripples: R.D.17'. Wheatcroft, *Worth Saving*, p. 102.

[84] TNA LAB 14/429, 'George Tomlinson to the Factory and Welfare Advisory Board' (09.03.1943).

[85] Mr. Ernest Bevin, *Hansard* (10.12.1943), vol. 395, cc. 1349.

[86] Ibid.

[87] Bolderson, *Social Security, Disability and Rehabilitation*, p. 106.

[88] Mr. Ernest Bevin, *Hansard* (10.12.1943), vol. 395, cc. 1345; Mr. Ernest Bevin, *Hansard* (18.01.1944), vol. 396, cc. 106.

and wholly because we are at war...I repeat again that the Bill would never have come before the House if it had not been for the war'.[89] The war was frequently referenced in these deliberations in emotive terms. The Labour MP, Tom Brown, who had campaigned for years on behalf of miners, foundry and textile workers suffering from respiratory diseases, remarked:

> If by keeping them in suitable employment, we can prevent men who have served on the field of battle or men who have served in industry from becoming degraded, we shall have gone a long way towards bringing about that new world that has been promised us often in days gone by.[90]

A desire to avoid the perceived failures of the last war was also evoked. The Labour MP, Ellis Smith, who was on the committee of the Trades Union Congress (TUC) looking into rehabilitation, had remarked in 1942: 'I intend to do all I can to prevent this and future generations being treated as my generation was treated. We came home after the last war and scarcely anyone bothered with us'.[91] He went on to express the hope that 'all public-spirited men and women in this House will join in seeing that we shall not after this war allow human suffering and tragedies to exist as they did for 20 years—the best part of my life—after the [last] war'.[92] Similar sentiments were expressed during the readings of the DPEA, with the widely-respected Labour MP Jack Lawson asserting that 'there is no subject which has caused the people of this country more heart-searching than the way in which the soldier was treated after the last war'.[93] The Labour MP, and former Trade Union organiser, Evelyn Walkden, also warned that 'the tide of patriotism in war-time recedes quickly when the

[89] Rear-Admiral Beamish, *Hansard* (18.01.1944), vol. 396, cc. 109; P. Cosgrave, 'Beamish, Tufton Victor Hamilton, Baron Chelwood (1917–1989), army officer and politician', *Oxford Dictionary of National Biography* (08.01.2015). https://www.oxforddnb.com/. Accessed 26 August 2019.

[90] Mr. Tom Brown, *Hansard* (10.12.1943), vol. 395, cc. 1299–1302; 'Obituary: Mr Tom Brown', *The Times* (11.11.1970).

[91] Mr. Ellis Smith, *Hansard* (22.07.1942), vol. 382, cc. 50–126.

[92] Ibid.

[93] Mr. Lawson, *Hansard* (10.12.1943), vol. 395, cc. 1283; D. Bythell, 'Lawson, John James [Jack], Baron Lawson (1881–1965), coalminer and politician', *Oxford Dictionary of National Biography* (23.09.2004). https://www.oxforddnb.com/. Accessed 6 February 2018.

war-drums cease to roll'.[94] This attitude is perhaps best exemplified by the Conservative MP, Sir Ian Fraser, who had long campaigned on behalf of fellow blind ex-servicemen, and who noted that 'good sometimes comes out of evil…the tragic consequences of war have stirred the imagination and accelerated tendencies, which have already been in people's minds, to action'.[95] With the level of praise heaped upon the Bill, the Labour MP George Isaacs was able to claim, with perhaps only some exaggeration, that 'the whole House seems to be rejoicing that a Bill of this kind has come before it'.[96] Thus the war certainly appears to have ensured general support for the DPEA and its swift movement through Parliament.

The DPEA did not, of course, appear in isolation, as there were other welfare measures being considered during the course of the war which would form the subsequent welfare state, such as the Education Act 1944, and some preliminary discussions on health reform which would eventually lead to the formation of the NHS.[97] While the famous Beveridge Report produced in 1942 did not make mention of the specifics of provision for disabled people such as sheltered employment, the system of social security advocated was predicated on employment contributions to social insurance and, as such, emphasised the obligation for the Government to support employment for all those capable of undertaking it.[98] So while the Report was non-specific, the idea of sheltered employment was entirely compatible with its overall aims. Indeed, the notion of the maintenance of 'full employment' was a central aspect of postwar social policy aims outlined in the Report and in the wartime Coalition Government's 1944 White Paper on Employment Policy.[99] The provision of employment for the disabled in the DPEA was therefore part of this overall vision

[94] Mr. Evelyn Walkden, *Hansard* (10.12.1943), vol. 395, cc. 1340; Lord Robens of Woldingham, 'Obituary: Mr Evelyn Walkden', *The Times* (17.09.1970).

[95] Sir Ian Fraser, *Hansard* (10.12.1943), vol. 395, cc. 1311.

[96] Mr. George Isaacs, *Hansard* (10.12.1943), vol. 395, cc. 1307.

[97] M. Hill, *The Welfare State in Britain: A Political History since 1945* (Aldershot, Edward Elgar Publishing, 1993), pp. 11–24.

[98] *Social Insurance and Allied Services*, 6404 (1942), para. 22, p. 12; para. 130, p. 58.

[99] D. Gladstone, 'The Welfare State and the State of Welfare', in D. Gladstone, (ed.) *British Social Welfare: Past, Present and Future* (London, UCL Press, 1995), p. 2; Gladstone, *The Twentieth-Century Welfare State*, p. 33.

for welfare and employment which would then create the welfare state.[100] Furthermore, the war necessitated unprecedented levels of centralised government control and planning over areas of civilian life and in the tackling of social problems.[101] In this context, government ownership of a scheme of sheltered employment was perhaps not as radical a step as it was once considered. This was also reflected at a practical level, with the general disruption and wartime control over industry providing an opportune moment in which to begin to apply state-control to a large-scale sheltered employment scheme.[102] We can see, therefore, something of the displacement effect and concentration process outlined by Alan Peacock and Jack Wiseman across public expenditure more widely, with the war laying a fertile ground for expenditure and central planning directed at a nationalised scheme to address the problem of unemployment for disabled people.[103]

While we cannot therefore see the Second World War as the sole impetus for Remploy, we cannot discount the impact of it either. The war served to demonstrate the productivity potential of disabled people, including the severely disabled; provided the impetus needed to take bold action; and aided the acceptance of state involvement in the provision of employment for the disabled. More generally, we cannot ignore that Remploy, as with the other measures of the DPEA, was formulated, discussed and created during the Second World War alongside other reforms which would create the welfare state. It is to a closer examination of the development of the sheltered employment scheme in the creation of the DPEA during this time that this chapter will now turn.

[100] S. Sainsbury, 'Disabled People and the Personal Social Services', in D. Gladstone, (ed.) *British Social Welfare: Past, Present and Future* (London, UCL Press, 1995), p. 184.

[101] B. Coxall and L. Robins, *British Politics Since the War* (Basingstoke, Macmillan, 1998), pp. 9–10; Gladstone, *The Twentieth-Century Welfare State*, pp. 36–7.

[102] *Report of Inter-departmental Committee on the Rehabilitation and Resettlement of Disabled Persons*, 6415 (1943), para. 92, p. 35.

[103] A.T. Peacock & J. Wiseman, *The Growth of Public Expenditure in the United Kingdom* (Unwin University Books, 1967).

Remploy in the Development of the DPEA: Committees and Parliament

The DPEA was formed through the deliberations of several committees, chiefly the Inter-Departmental Committee on the Rehabilitation and Resettlement of Disabled Persons (Tomlinson Committee), and the Standing Rehabilitation and Resettlement Committee (Ince Committee), as well as a subsequent series of debates in Parliament.

Attention was given to those disabled during the Second World War from its beginning, though this was chiefly focused on the area of medical rehabilitation under the Ministry of Health.[104] Following Bevin's appointment as Minister of Labour in Churchill's new Coalition Government in May 1940, numerous committees came into being and considered the issue of rehabilitation and employment for disabled people more generally.[105] The first of these, the Inter-Departmental Committee on the Vocational Training of War Casualties (Glen Committee), which deliberated in 1940, was limited to considering a scheme for vocational training for those injured as a result of the war.[106] Even within this narrow remit, it expressly did not consider those who had been injured working in industry, nor those 'persons so badly disabled that they cannot be trained for any industrial occupation'.[107] For these severely disabled people the Committee simply noted that 'special provision will no doubt be made'.[108]

Bevin had set out his own views in a memorandum for the Home Policy Committee in February 1941.[109] Though it laid out his aims of a comprehensive service inclusive of both those injured in war and in

[104] Bolderson, *Social Security, Disability and Rehabilitation*; pp. 95–9.

[105] C. Wrigley, 'Bevin, Ernest (1881–1951), trade unionist and politician', *Oxford Dictionary of National Biography* (01.03.2008). https://www.oxforddnb.com/. Accessed 7 September 2016.

[106] TNA LAB 20/3, Inter-Departmental Committee on the Vocational Training of War Casualties, 'Minutes of the Fourth Meeting' (19.09.1940); 'Minutes of the Fifth Meeting' (03.10.1940).

[107] TNA LAB 20/3, 'Report of the Inter-Departmental Committee on the Vocational Training of War Casualties' (1940).

[108] Ibid.

[109] TNA LAB 20/2, 'Draft Memorandum' (01.02.1941); the draft of this memorandum seems the only copy available; 'Note by F.N. Tribe' (04.02.1941).

industry, and referenced an expanded quota scheme on the lines of the King's Roll, it made no mention of sheltered employment.[110] Following the rejection of his plans by the Committee, Bevin and his officials in the MOL were, as one official noted, free 'to go ahead and make a start in our schemes for dealing at least with men who have been disabled by enemy action in the present war'.[111] The result of this was the so-called 'Interim Scheme', which was announced in October 1941 and through which disabled people were given advice about employment or trained for 'war work'.[112]

To fully consider the issue, the Committee on the Rehabilitation and Resettlement of Disabled Persons, was established under the chairmanship of Bevin's Parliamentary Secretary George Tomlinson and would meet for the first time on 22 January 1942.[113] Tomlinson was a former textile worker who had established himself in local politics before becoming a Labour MP in 1938.[114] Held in high regard by Bevin, he was later to serve in Attlee's Government as Minister of Works and then as Minister of Education.[115] The Tomlinson Committee was to consider both the immediate provision for those not provided for by the Interim Scheme, and for provision after the war for rehabilitation and the securing of 'satisfactory employment' for disabled people 'of all categories'.[116] This was

[110] TNA LAB 20/2, 'Draft Memorandum' (01.02.1941).

[111] TNA LAB 20/2, 'Note by F.N. Tribe' (27.02.1941); 'Note by F.N. Tribe' (12.02.1941); 'Note from J. Worsfold' (12.02.1941); Home Policy Committee, 'Memorandum by the Minister of Health on Rehabilitation' (24.02.1941); 'Memorandum by the Chancellor of the Exchequer' (22.02.1941); 'Memorandum by the Home Secretary on Rehabilitation' (25.02.1941).

[112] Bolderson, *Social Security, Disability and Rehabilitation*; pp. 104–5.

[113] TNA CAB 67/9/160, 'Rehabilitation, Training and Employment of Disabled Persons: Note by the Minister of Labour and National Service' (31.12.1941). The committee comprised members of the Ministries of Labour, Health, and Pensions as well as the Board of Education, the Scottish Office, the Treasury, and the Minister without Portfolio and, from the third meeting onwards, the Home Office, TNA LAB 20/56, Inter-departmental Committee on the Rehabilitation and Resettlement of Disabled Persons, 'Terms of Reference' (1942); 'Minutes of the Third Meeting' (26.02.1942).

[114] K. Jefferys, 'Tomlinson, George (1890–1952), politician', *Oxford Dictionary of National Biography* (06.01.2011). https://www.oxforddnb.com/. Accessed 7 September 2016.

[115] Ibid.

[116] TNA LAB 20/56, Inter-departmental Committee on the Rehabilitation and Resettlement of Disabled Persons, 'Terms of Reference' (1942).

the first time that the notion of securing satisfactory employment for all disabled persons, regardless of the cause of disability, had been considered a role for the state. While the Committee's initial focus was on aspects of the Interim Scheme, the issue of sheltered employment was briefly raised on several occasions in terms of the voluntary provision available and the decision to not enact a state scheme following the First World War.[117] The Tomlinson Committee submitted an Interim Report on 10 March 1942, focusing on additions to the existing Interim Scheme, including 'the provision of special facilities for sheltered employment for the more seriously disabled'.[118] With the emphasis on meeting immediate wartime needs, these recommendations were limited however to simply making better use of existing voluntary establishments.[119]

Following the publication of the Interim Report, the Tomlinson Committee moved onto consideration of the postwar situation.[120] This included the notion of a permanent sheltered employment scheme, though the precise nature of these discussions is not clear. References were made at the sixth and seventh meetings to a 'Memorandum R.D.14', which is unfortunately not included in the file of the Tomlinson Committee held at The National Archives.[121] There was mention at the

[117] TNA LAB 20/56, Inter-departmental Committee on the Rehabilitation and Resettlement of Disabled Persons, 'Note by the Join Secretaries on the Resettlement of Tuberculous Persons' (13.05.1942); 'Minutes of the Second Meeting' (12.02.1942); 'Memorandum of Training of Disabled Ex-Service Men After the Great War: Based on Memorandum submitted by the Ministry of Labour: R.D. 4'; Inter-Departmental Committee on the Rehabilitation and Resettlement of Disabled Persons, 'Note by the Ministry of Pensions: R.D. 9'; 'Memorandum by the Board of Education on the Vocational Training of Cripples: R.D.17'.

[118] TNA LAB 20/56, Inter-departmental Committee on the Rehabilitation and Resettlement of Disabled Persons, 'First Report to the Minister of Labour and National Service' (March, 1942); *Report of Inter-departmental Committee on the Rehabilitation and Resettlement of Disabled Persons*, 6415 (1943), para. 3, p. 3.

[119] TNA LAB 20/56, Inter-departmental Committee on the Rehabilitation and Resettlement of Disabled Persons, 'First Report to the Minister of Labour and National Service' (March, 1942); 'Minutes of the Second Meeting' (12.02.1942).

[120] TNA LAB 20/56, Inter-departmental Committee on the Rehabilitation and Resettlement of Disabled Persons, 'Minutes of the Fifth Meeting' (26.03.1942); 'Post War Scheme: Note by the Joint Secretaries'.

[121] TNA LAB 20/56, Inter-departmental Committee on the Rehabilitation and Resettlement of Disabled Persons, 'Minutes of the Sixth Meeting' (09.04.1942); 'Minutes of the Seventh Meeting' (23.04.1942).

seventh meeting of amendments to R.D.14, which included the complete substitution of the existing paragraph for a new one which dealt with the issue of sheltered employment.[122] This paragraph distinguished provision for those who may one day be able to enter into open employment and those who needed 'permanent employment under sheltered or sub-economic conditions'.[123] For the former, the use of existing voluntary institutions was advocated, while for the latter there was no indication of what provision might be made, if any, beyond this.[124]

A change appears to have taken place at the eighth meeting, which involved discussion of R.D.14 and further amendments regarding sheltered employment.[125] One such amendment was to 'paragraph 2', so that it then read:

> The Committee are of [the] opinion however that if the resources and scope of the voluntary undertakings prove insufficient to meet the requirement of a comprehensive and permanent scheme covering severe disablements from all causes, the need should be met by a system of special centres set up for the purpose.[126]

A further amendment to 'paragraphs 3 and 4' read:

> (1) the allocation to a central Government Department of general responsibility for the new service of sheltered employment, whether in voluntary undertakings or in special centres; and (2) the establishment of a public corporation for the purpose of undertaking the trading operation and the day-to-day administration of the special centres.[127]

Here we see the outline of what would become Remploy, including the first mention of a public corporation to run sheltered employment 'centres'—though it is clear that at this stage there was a preference to

[122] TNA LAB 20/56, Inter-departmental Committee on the Rehabilitation and Resettlement of Disabled Persons, 'Minutes of the Seventh Meeting' (23.04.1942).

[123] Ibid.

[124] Ibid.

[125] TNA LAB 20/56, Inter-departmental Committee on the Rehabilitation and Resettlement of Disabled Persons, 'Minutes of the Eighth Meeting' (07.05.1942).

[126] Ibid.

[127] Ibid; TNA LAB 20/56, Inter-departmental Committee on the Rehabilitation and Resettlement of Disabled Persons, 'Minutes of the Ninth Meeting' (21.05.1942).

continue to rely on voluntary undertakings if possible. These few examples are the limit of consideration and discussion of what would become Remploy by the Tomlinson Committee, whose primary focus was clearly not upon sheltered employment, but upon consideration of the other measures which would be subsequently included in the DPEA.

The Tomlinson Report was completed and presented to Parliament in January 1943, gaining widespread attention from the press.[128] The report touched on a broad range of areas including rehabilitation, resettlement and finance.[129] The emphasis of the report was on the return of disabled workers into open employment with three key recommendations; firstly, 'the introduction of a quota of disabled persons'; secondly, 'the scheduling of certain occupations for the benefit of disabled persons'; and finally, 'the creation of a Register of Persons Handicapped by Disablement'.[130] The section on 'Employment under Sheltered Conditions' came some way down the report, and noted the continued work of voluntary establishments and considered 'that the postwar scheme should include full provision for the use of facilities for sheltered employment in voluntary undertakings'.[131] However, the report continued:

> The Committee are of [the] opinion however that the resources and scope of the voluntary undertakings cannot reasonably be expected to prove sufficient to meet the requirements of a comprehensive and permanent scheme covering severe disablements from all causes, and they consider that a system of special centres under Government auspices should be set up for the purpose.[132]

The recommendations of the Committee had thus changed from the use of state centres *only* if voluntary undertakings proved insufficient, to an assumption that they would in fact be required. It is not clear why this

[128] *Report of Inter-departmental Committee on the Rehabilitation and Resettlement of Disabled Persons*, 6415 (1943); 'Work for the Disabled', *The Times* (15.01.1943); 'Reserving Jobs for the Disabled', *The Manchester Guardian* (15.01.1943); 'Charter for War Disabled', *Daily Mail* (15.01.1943).

[129] *Report of Inter-departmental Committee on the Rehabilitation and Resettlement of Disabled Persons*, 6415 (1943).

[130] Ibid, para. 72, p. 28; para. 9, p. 6.

[131] Ibid, para. 90, p. 34.

[132] Ibid, para. 91, p. 34.

occurred prior to publication, as no consideration to this was given in the minutes of the previous meetings.[133]

January 1943 also saw the establishment of the Standing Rehabilitation and Resettlement Committee, chaired by the Deputy Secretary to the Minister of Labour, Sir Godfrey Ince.[134] A civil servant in the MOL since 1919, Ince had been appointed director-general of manpower under Bevin in June 1941, with the two enjoying 'an exceptional mutual trust'.[135] The Ince Committee was to coordinate preparation of the various aspects recommended in the Tomlinson Report.[136] The issue of sheltered employment barely featured, with only three mentions of such provision in all nine committee meetings from February 1943 through to the passing of the DPEA in March 1944, and no mention afterwards.[137] Direct consideration was given only during the second meeting of the Ince Committee in which the Chairman noted that the recommendations of the Tomlinson Committee regarding sheltered employment were 'a matter for Departmental action by [the] Ministry of Labour and National Service'.[138] The Ince Committee's first report to Bevin in July 1943 simply echoed these remarks.[139]

[133] For meeting minutes see TNA LAB 20/56.

[134] TNA LAB 20/85, Standing Rehabilitation and Resettlement Committee, 'Second Report to the Minister of Labour and National Service: S.R.R.C.66'.

[135] R. Lowe, 'Ince, Sir Godfrey Herbert (1891–1960), civil servant', *Oxford Dictionary of National Biography* (03.01.2008). https://www.oxforddnb.com/. Accessed 13 July 2019.

[136] TNA LAB 20/85, Standing Rehabilitation and Resettlement Committee, 'Second Report to the Minister of Labour and National Service: S.R.R.C.66'; TNA LAB 20/87, Standing Rehabilitation and Resettlement Committee, 'Minutes of Meeting' (04.02.1943); Bolderson, *Social Security, Disability and Rehabilitation*, p. 115.

[137] See minutes of meetings in TNA LAB 20/87.

[138] TNA LAB 20/87, Standing Rehabilitation and Resettlement Committee, 'Minutes of the Second Meeting' (04.03.1943). The only other mention was in relation to the case of Thermaga Limited, a voluntary undertaking for which the Ministry of Labour was attempting to secure exclusive rights to produce materials, TNA LAB 20/84, Standing Rehabilitation and Resettlement Committee, 'Note by the Ministry of Labour and National Service, Production work for Undertakings providing sheltered employment for severely disabled persons: S.R.R.C.28'. This was mentioned again, TNA LAB 20/87 Standing Rehabilitation and Resettlement Committee, 'Minutes of the Ninth Meeting' (03.02.1944).

[139] TNA LAB 20/84, Standing Rehabilitation and Resettlement Committee, 'First Report to the Minister of Labour and National Service: S.R.R.C.19' (17.07.1943).

The Ince Committee's role in terms of sheltered employment was limited therefore to reviewing and offering amendments to the MOL's own proposals for a Bill to enact the sheltered employment scheme, presented in paper 'S.S.R.C.8'.[140] Even in this limited role, the amendments proposed by the Ince Committee reveal disagreement over the nature of the scheme. The section on sheltered employment in the original paper read:

> It is proposed that this provision should principally be made by the establishment of a public corporation under the aegis of the Minister...There are, however, a number of voluntary societies and undertakings which already provide the necessary facilities for employment under "sheltered" conditions and the Minister should therefore be empowered to provide such training and employment or to defray or contribute towards the cost of any such training or employment so provided by other persons or bodies.[141]

Another copy was amended to read, 'it is proposed that this provision should be made either through the use and development of facilities already provided by voluntary societies and undertakings or through the establishment of special centres to be set up for the purpose'.[142] A further copy had a different amendment, suggesting that 'it is proposed that this provision should be made in special centres to be set up and administered by a public corporation to be established under the aegis of the Minister'.[143] There were therefore three different versions of amendments to the MOL's proposals, either suggesting that sheltered employment should be 'principally' made through the state centres, or 'either' in these or voluntary provision, or entirely in state centres. Unlike the other measures of the DPEA, the Ince Committee had very limited input on the scheme of sheltered employment, and what input it had was inconsistent. The Ince Committee clearly did not see considerations of the sheltered

[140] TNA LAB 20/91, 'Disabled Persons Rehabilitation and Resettlement: Proposals by the Ministry of Labour and National Service for a Bill to implement the recommendations of the Tomlinson Committee: S.R.R.C.8'.

[141] Ibid.

[142] Ibid.

[143] Ibid.

employment scheme as a key part of its remit and played little part in its realisation.[144]

Finally, in terms of Parliament, as the draft Bill of the DPEA was presented to the House of Commons to consider, there was no debate on sheltered employment. Deliberation in the Commons focused on other aspects of the draft, chiefly the issue of preference for ex-servicemen across the measures, leaving no discussion of the scheme which was to become Remploy. Consideration of the proposed Bill was undertaken in the Commons on 10 December 1943. Tomlinson himself outlined the measures, including 'the creation of special facilities for the minority whose disablement prevents them permanently, or for a substantial period, obtaining employment of the ordinary kind and who require some shelter from the strain of competitive conditions'.[145] He further explained that 'the Minister may provide special facilities for this purpose in two ways. One is by the employment of a non-profit-making company, under the Companies Act, 1929, and the other is through an association or body similarly constituted and recognised for the purpose'.[146]

The Bill was debated again on 18 January 1944, with no mention of the sheltered scheme.[147] This was also the case during its reading in the House of Lords on 15 February 1944.[148] Further discussion took place in the Commons on 27 January 1944, 4 February 1944 and on 1 March 1944.[149] The sheltered employment scheme was mentioned only once in these substantial debates, with a minor amendment for clarification of the language of the relevant clause, which passed without recorded

[144] This was not due to a lack of time, as numerous meetings were postponed due to a 'lack of business', see TNA LAB 20/87.

[145] Mr. Tomlinson, *Hansard* (10.12.1943), vol. 395, cc. 1268–9.

[146] Ibid., cc. 1275.

[147] Disabled Persons (Employment) Bill, *Hansard* (18.01.1944), vol. 396, cc.67–148.

[148] Lord Snell, *Hansard* (18.01.1944), vol. 130 cc. 763–7.

[149] See *Hansard* (27.01.1944), vol. 396 cc. 877–1028; (04.02.1944), vol. 396, cc. 1546–1576; (01.03.1944), vol. 397, cc. 1427–1476.

comment.[150] There was thus no meaningful consideration of the sheltered employment scheme in Parliament prior to the DPEA gaining royal assent on 1 March 1944.[151]

Nor do we see much attention given to sheltered employment following this. The scheme was mentioned in a written question to Bevin on 24 March 1944, and when the Minister was asked about the general development of the provisions of the DPEA the following month.[152] There were several further discussions regarding the other provisions of the DPEA, but no mention of sheltered employment prior to the announcement in the Commons of the formation of the Board of Directors of Remploy on 3 May 1945.[153] This particular event has not been documented in Hansard, which has no record of the Commons sitting on this date.[154] There is only a mention of the announcement in *The Times* the following day.[155] It is not clear therefore if this drew any additional comments from MPs. In any case, these are the only mentions of the scheme prior to the first meeting of the Remploy Board later in the month.[156] It is apparent therefore, that proceedings in both Houses of Parliament provided no meaningful input.

In terms of sheltered employment, we can therefore see the extremely limited role played by the various committees and Parliament. The priority

[150] Mr. Tomlinson, *Hansard* (27.01.1944), vol. 396 cc. 969–71.

[151] See *Hansard* (27.01.1944), vol. 396 cc. 877–1028; (04.02.1944), vol. 396, cc. 1546–1576; (01.03.1944), vol. 397, cc. 1427–1476; Disabled Persons (Employment) Act, (1944). *Hansard* (01.03.1944), vol. 397, cc. 1475.

[152] Mr. R. Duckworth, *Hansard* (24.03.1944), vol. 398, cc. 1215; Mr. E. Bevin, *Hansard* (24.03.1944), vol. 398, cc. 1215; Mr. E. Bevin, *Hansard* (27.04.1944), vol. 399, cc. 906.

[153] On 14 December 1944, Bevin was asked when the Act would be brought into force, Mr. Bevin, *Hansard* (14.12.1944), vol. 406, cc. 1321; Mr Bellenger, *Hansard* (21.12.1944), vol. 406, cc. 1923–4. On 1 March 1945, Bevin responded to a question about the setting up of the register, Mr Bevin, *Hansard* (01.03.1945), vol. 408, cc. 1531; See also TNA BM 8/1.

[154] TNA LAB 20/120, 'Note from Ernest Bevin' (01.05.1945).

[155] 'Parliament', *The Times* (04.05.1945).

[156] TNA BM 8/1, Disabled Persons Employment Corporation Limited, 'First Meeting of the Board' (30.05.1945).

was the other measures of the DPEA, which would cater for a greater number of people, and on the political issue of preference for ex-service personnel. We must therefore look elsewhere for the driving force behind the creation of Remploy.

Remploy in the Development of the DPEA: Industry and Segregation

The most detailed consideration of the creation of Remploy has remained that proposed by Bolderson in her work on the DPEA.[157] It is from the need to secure the backing of industry that Bolderson saw the true origins of Remploy, as a means to allay fears that the other measures in the Act, chiefly the mandatory quota, would result in unproductive workers being forced upon them.[158] The cooperation of industry in the measures of the DPEA was therefore 'bought' at the expense of segregating 'non-productive' workers in sheltered employment. It was this view which was subsequently adopted by Borsay in her influential study on disability in Britain, and which underpinned her negative depiction of sheltered employment as one of 'segregated employment' and of the policies of the DPEA as having failed disabled people as part of the wider narrative of discrimination and marginalisation.[159]

In Bolderson's account, this bargain with industry began with the deliberations of the Tomlinson Committee, which she described as being under the influence of the TUC, as 'when opinion was divided on the committee as to the degree of fitness which a man should attain before he was placed in employment...opposition from the TUC led it to conclude that "unfit workers should not go into competition with the fit"'.[160] For this statement Bolderson cited Tomlinson 'explaining the committee's decisions to the Factory Welfare Advisory Board' on 12 January 1943, in

[157] Bolderson, 'The Origins of the Disabled Persons Employment Quota and its Symbolic Significance', pp. 169–186; Bolderson, *Social Security, Disability and Rehabilitation.*

[158] Bolderson, *Social Security, Disability and Rehabilitation*, p. 109; 'The Origins of the Disabled Persons Employment Quota and its Symbolic Significance', pp. 178–9.

[159] Borsay, *Disability and Social Policy in Britain Since 1750*, p. 135 for which she cites Bolderson, 'The Origins of the Disabled Persons Employment Quota and its Symbolic Significance', n. 86.

[160] Bolderson, *Social Security, Disability and Rehabilitation*, p. 109.

document 'FWB (43) 1', file 'LAB 14/429' at The National Archives.[161] However, 'FWB (43) 1' is a note which explains that copies of the report have been circulated to the Board and which draws attention to certain pertinent areas to focus upon.[162] The report of the committee was not discussed until the meeting on the 9 March 1943, and the statement does not appear in the minutes.[163] It is therefore unclear where this remark came from. The record of the meeting of the Factory and Welfare Advisory Board on the 9 March 1943, in which the report of the Tomlinson Committee was discussed, noted that 'the Joint Consultative Committee of the TUC and British Employers' Confederation (BEC) had set up a sub-committee to examine points raised in the Report'.[164] One member of the Board asked 'whether it was right to ask industry to engage cripples in view of their probably cramping affect on production'.[165] Tomlinson replied that 'it was the State's responsibility to see that a fair proportion of those with permanent injuries (however caused) should be absorbed into industry, and that industrial employers should take their fair share, whether the injury in the particular case was caused in industry or not'.[166] He then noted that 'some of course, could never be returned to ordinary employment and for these sheltered special occupations would have to be found'.[167] We should not, however, assume that this was considered for the benefit of industry, as subsequent comments reflected instead a concern that the pressure to compete in open employment could prove detrimental to the disabled worker. Tomlinson proceeded to mention the sheltered village settlement at Papworth, which was engaged in 'competitive' industry, which he was concerned could 'entail a dangerous over-exertion on the part of the worker'.[168] Though he did then note that 'another difficulty arising from having fit and unfit workers together was

[161] Ibid., p. 109, n. 18.

[162] TNA LAB 14/429, Factory and Welfare Advisory Board, 'Tomlinson Committee Report, F.W.B. (43)1'.

[163] TNA LAB 14/429, Factory and Welfare Advisory Board, 'Minutes of the Thirty-Seventh Meeting' (09.03.1943).

[164] Ibid.

[165] Ibid.

[166] Ibid.

[167] Ibid.

[168] Ibid.

that Union squabbles arose from the fit workers' contending that their unfit colleagues were not 100% producing agents'.[169] So while there was an awareness from Tomlinson that sheltered establishments could prevent the difficulties of having those who would not be '100%' productive from lowering production and leading to conflict with unions, there was also a clear concern of over-exertion in an attempt to remain competitive being a problem, something which was especially highlighted in cases of Tuberculosis (TB).[170] Such a view was consistent with a report the committee had considered at an earlier meeting by Dr Macauley, Medical Officer of Health to the Middlesex County Council, on the dangerous effects of over-exertion on patients in sanatoria.[171]

While it was certainly the case that the Tomlinson Committee had emphasised the importance of securing the agreement and cooperation 'of both sides of industry' in all aspects of its recommendations, there is no evidence that this was unbalanced to favour industry entirely at the expense of the severely disabled.[172] Indeed, it is notable that the final Tomlinson Report explained that the development of production in the sheltered employment scheme would undoubtedly disadvantage employers who also made those products.[173] The report demanded however, that this be recognised 'as an essential feature of any national scheme to secure satisfactory employment for disabled persons who cannot find a place in ordinary industry'.[174] In this case it was industry that would have to potentially suffer in order to provide sheltered employment for the severely disabled.

[169] Ibid.

[170] Ibid.

[171] TNA LAB 20/56, Inter-Departmental Committee on the Rehabilitation and Resettlement of Disabled People, 'Note by the Join Secretaries on the Resettlement of Tuberculous Persons: R.D.16' (13.05.1942).

[172] TNA LAB 20/56, Inter-Departmental Committee on the Rehabilitation and Resettlement of Disabled Persons, 'Draft additional paragraphs for the Report, Vocational Training, R.D.21'; 'Minutes of the Eleventh Meeting' (17.06.1942). *Report of Inter-departmental Committee on the Rehabilitation and Resettlement of Disabled Persons*, 6415 (1943), para. 89, p. 3.

[173] *Report of Inter-departmental Committee on the Rehabilitation and Resettlement of Disabled Persons*, 6415 (1943), para. 91, pp. 34–5.

[174] Ibid.

Bolderson also cited the discussion of the draft Bill of the DPEA between the TUC and BEC in support of her interpretation. Proposals for the various elements of the Bill were sent to the BEC and the TUC on 23 April 1943 for them to consider.[175] Unfortunately, the BEC was delayed in doing so and therefore a draft of the Bill was produced before the observations of industry could be given.[176] The TUC and BEC met together on the 6 July 1943 and again on the 24 August 1943, and with government representatives on 15 September 1943 and the 12 October 1943.[177] During the September meeting with government, both the TUC and the BEC agreed that those disabled people 'below a reasonable standard of employability' should not be a 'burden' for industry, but should be the responsibility of the state.[178] In earlier discussions they had noted this would be the function of the sheltered employment scheme.[179] This was confirmed to be the case by Tomlinson, who was chairing the meeting, and who 'emphasised that there was no intention to force employers to take on persons who were so incapacitated that they would be merely "passengers" in industry'.[180] Industry would be 'expected to employ those who were capable of rendering reasonably effective service'.[181] Those who were not able to do this would

[175] TNA LAB 20/91, 'Note to T.W. Phillips from TUC' (29.04.1943); 'Note to T.W. Phillips from BEC' (27.04.1943).

[176] Bolderson, *Social Security, Disability and Rehabilitation*; p. 112, suggests that this was a genuine delay due to workload. TNA LAB 20/91, 'Note to Mr. Hetherington' (26.07.1943); 'Notes from Sir. T.W.Phillips to Sir John Forbes Watson and Sir Walter Citrine' (30.07.1943); Joint Consultative Committee,'Head of Bill providing for Employment of Disabled Persons'.

[177] Bolderson, *Social Security, Disability and Rehabilitation*; p. 112.

[178] TNA LAB 20/91, 'Note of a discussion with Representatives of the British Employers' Confederation and the Trades Union Congress on 15th September 1943, on the Tomlinson Committee Report and the draft proposals for a Bill based on that Report' (15.09.1943).

[179] TNA LAB 20/91, 'Note of discussions between Representatives of the British Employers' Confederation and the TUC on the Ministry of Labour's proposals for implementing the Tomlinson Report'.

[180] TNA LAB 20/91, 'Note of a discussion with Representatives of the British Employers' Confederation and the Trades Union Congress on 15th September 1943, on the Tomlinson Committee Report and the draft proposals for a Bill based on that Report' (15.09.1943).

[181] Ibid.

be 'catered for under the sheltered employment scheme'.[182] Bolderson suggested this equated to the overall draft bill having been 'bought at the price of dividing disabled people into "effective" workers—able to take their place in open employment—and ineffective workers for whom sheltered employment would be provided'.[183] However, the idea for a scheme of sheltered employment did not come from industry, but from the MOL. The draft Bill had been produced without input from industry and the BEC and TUC had only agreed with the proposals.[184] The BEC and TUC simply recognised, correctly, that it would also mean that industry would not shoulder the 'burden' of workers who were considered unproductive. This was a result, not a cause, of the scheme, as in considering the role of sheltered employment, the Tomlinson Committee had taken evidence that trying to compete in open industry was bad for these disabled men. This view was also consistent with those expressed by existing voluntary workshops and those groups representing disabled people, who, as has been shown, were actively campaigning for further sheltered employment provision.[185] Whatever one might now think of the concept of sheltered employment, there is no evidence that in advocating a national scheme, the MOL was seeking to sacrifice the needs of the disabled people who would be employed in it in order to placate industry. Once again therefore, we must look elsewhere for the driving force behind Remploy's creation.

182 Ibid.

183 Bolderson, *Social Security, Disability and Rehabilitation*, p. 113; Bolderson, 'The Origins of the Disabled Persons Employment Quota and its Symbolic Significance'.

184 TNA LAB 20/91, 'Note of Discussion with Representatives of the British Employers' Confederation and the Trades Unions Congress on 12th October 1943, on the Draft Heads of Bill Providing for Employment of Disabled Persons' (12.10.1943); 'Minute extract of Mr Wiles', (17.09.1943).

185 'Unemployment Insurance', *The Times* (05.03.1932); 'Occupational Therapy', *The Times* (06.09.1937); 'A Thought for Armistice Day', *The Manchester Guardian* (11.11.1938); 'War-Disabled Men's Pensions', *The Manchester Guardian* (04.04.1938); 'Employment for Disabled', *The Manchester Guardian* (18.08.1945).

Remploy in the Development of the DPEA: Bevin and the MOL

After an already long and distinguished career as a Trade Union leader, Ernest Bevin played a crucial role as Minister of Labour during the Second World War, maximising the efficiency of industry for the war effort.[186] Notably successful in achieving a higher level of civilian mobilisation in industry than could be matched by any of the other nations at war, Bevin worked tirelessly in this role.[187] In doing so, he was outspoken in his belief that the efforts of workers should not go unrewarded, and pushed for economic and social reform as both a wartime and postwar priority.[188] Bevin has also been described as a minister who was keen to take personal responsibility for matters and as someone 'quick to centralise much power in his own hands'.[189] His importance in the creation of the DPEA was recognised by his contemporaries and has long been noted by academics.[190] It was also Bevin who played the key role in ensuring that the provisions of the Act were to apply to all disabled people, regardless of the cause of disability.[191] That Bevin had a keen interest in the issue of rehabilitation and the employment of the disabled has been remarked upon by scholars such as Alan Bullock, who described the DPEA as legislation which was 'very close to Bevin's heart'.[192] It was a long-standing

[186] Wrigley, 'Bevin, Ernest (1881–1951), trade unionist and politician', *Oxford Dictionary of National Biography* (01.03.2008). https://www.oxforddnb.com/. Accessed 7 September 2016.

[187] Ibid.

[188] R. Page, *Revisiting the Welfare State* (Maidenhead, Open University Press, 2007), pp. 20–2.

[189] Wrigley, 'Bevin, Ernest (1881–1951), trade unionist and politician'.

[190] For contemporaries see discussions in Hansard on the Bill. For scholars see, Thane, *Foundations of the Welfare State*, pp. 224–5; M. Stephens, *Ernest Bevin: Unskilled Labourer and World Statesman 1881–1951* (London, TGWU, 1981), pp. 102–3; A. Bullock, *The Life & Times of Ernest Bevin: Volume Two, Minister of Labour 1940–1945* (London, Heinemann, 1967), pp. 288–91; Hampton, *Disability and the Welfare State in Britain*, p. 58; Bolderson, *Social Security, Disability and Rehabilitation*, pp. 107–21; Bolderson, 'The Origins of the Disabled Persons Employment Quota and its Symbolic Significance', pp. 175–7.

[191] TNA LAB 20/56, Inter-departmental Committee on the Rehabilitation and Resettlement of Disabled Persons, 'Terms of Reference' (1942); Bolderson, *Social Security, Disability and Rehabilitation*, p. 106; 'The Disabled', *The Times* (06.12.1943).

[192] Bullock, *The Life & Times of Ernest Bevin*, p. 288.

interest which, by Bevin's own admission, was generated by his years working as a trade union official, fighting to get compensation for injured workers and witnessing the plight of those too disabled to continue to work.[193] What has not been noted until now is that the importance of Bevin in the creation of Remploy specifically, is even more apparent. A significant role was played by Bevin and his MOL, both in guiding his vision of a sheltered employment scheme through the various committees and discussions with industry into the DPEA, and in the subsequent forming of the company.

Following the outbreak of the Second World War, the first mention of the idea of a scheme of sheltered employment came from Bevin himself in 1941. On 27 February, an MOL official, Mr. Tribe, attempted to clarify the intentions of the Minister regarding rehabilitation schemes to take to the inter-departmental committee which was to consider them.[194] While this discussion focused primarily on aspects of treatment and training, the final point raised saw the emergence of the idea which was to become Remploy. Bevin informed Tribe that 'consideration should be given to a revision of our policy for securing employment for disabled persons. All employers should be compelled to employ a quota of such persons and if necessary the State should set up its own factories for the employment of those who are more seriously disabled'.[195] Bevin noted however, that this was not as urgent as immediate provision for the treatment and rehabilitation of the war-disabled, and was linked closely to postwar reconstruction.[196]

It was then Bevin who drove the issue through the Tomlinson Committee. The Committee itself came about as a result of Bevin's continued pressure, and was provided with direction as to what to consider for the sheltered employment scheme.[197] Prior to its first meeting, the Committee's Joint Secretaries, Mr. Hartwell from the Ministry of Health and Mr. Gomme from the MOL, highlighted the

[193] Mr. Ernest Bevin, *Hansard* (10.12.1943), vol. 395, col. 1345.

[194] TNA LAB 20/2, 'Note by F.N. Tribe' (27.02.1941).

[195] TNA LAB 20/2, 'Rehabilitation of Disabled Persons' (27.02.1941).

[196] Ibid.

[197] TNA CAB 67/9/160, 'Rehabilitation, Training and Employment of Disabled Persons: Note by the Minister of Labour and National Service' (31.12.1941); TNA LAB 20/56, Inter-departmental Committee on the Rehabilitation and Resettlement of Disabled Persons, 'Terms of Reference' (1942); 'Minutes of the Third Meeting' (26.02.1942).

need for sheltered employment in two memoranda.[198] One of these listed those groups who were not currently provided for through the Interim Scheme, including those requiring 'employment under sheltered conditions'.[199] Another, drew attention to the question of the provision for those 'who cannot earn an economic wage or become self-supporting', and suggested possible solutions 'which the Committee will wish to consider'.[200] Three suggestions were given: firstly, 'direct employment in State factories'; alternatively, 'employment subsidised from national funds, in specialised institutions of a semi-charitable character'; and finally, 'employment in private industry subsidised from national funds'.[201] As has been noted, the Tomlinson Committee had only limited input on sheltered employment, with changes of emphasis as to the place of a national government scheme, but finally recommended its establishment. It is likely that in doing so it was simply following the overall wishes of Bevin. The Ince Committee subsequently placed the scheme firmly in the hands of the MOL.[202] The sheltered employment scheme was therefore left to the Ministry to shape into the DPEA.

Bevin's role is similarly evident in ensuring the swift passage of the DPEA at Bill stage during the liaison process with the BEC and TUC throughout 1943.[203] Bevin urged both organisations to swift action, noting 'that he was anxious to have the proposals in the [Tomlinson] Report which require legislation put in the form of heads of a Bill as soon as possible and he would be glad to have the help of the two sides in this matter'.[204] Concerned about the BEC's delay in considering

[198] TNA LAB 20/56, Inter-departmental Committee on the Rehabilitation and Resettlement of Disabled Persons, 'Note by the Joint Secretaries: R.D.1' (07.01.1942).

[199] Ibid.

[200] Ibid.

[201] Ibid.

[202] TNA LAB 20/87, Standing Rehabilitation and Resettlement Committee, 'Minutes of the Second Meeting' (04.03.1943); 'Minutes of the Seventh Meeting' (17.09.1943); TNA LAB 20/84, Standing Rehabilitation and Resettlement Committee, 'Note by the Ministry of Labour and National Service, Production work for Undertakings providing sheltered employment for severely disabled persons: S.R.R.C.28'.

[203] TNA LAB 20/91, 'Note to T.W. Phillips from TUC' (29.04.1943); 'Note to T.W. Phillips from BEC' (27.04.1943).

[204] TNA LAB 20/91, 'Extract from minutes of 36th Meeting of the Join Consultative Committee; Standing Rehabilitation and Resettlement Committee Note 5.A'.

the proposals, Bevin asked the Ince Committee to exert pressure on the Director of the BEC, Sir John Forbes Watson, in order to speed things up.[205] This was followed by letters to the BEC expressing the Minister's impatience and demand for prompt consideration.[206] In July, Bevin decided to force the issue by pushing ahead with a draft of the Bill, with Sir John informed that the Minister could not wait any longer for the two sides of industry to make their observations.[207] Bevin had spoken to Sir John and explained that his anxiety to move quickly was in order 'to see that justice is done to the men who have already been disabled in this war'.[208]

The terms of the DPEA itself placed the enacting of the sheltered employment scheme firmly in the hands of the Minister of Labour. 'Sect. 15' of the Act which contained the measure, stated that the 'nature of the facilities to be provided under this section shall be such as the Minister may determine', which could include 'one or more companies which may be formed for that purpose and incorporated under the Companies Act, 1929'.[209] At the time of the Act coming into being, the war was still ongoing and there was no intention for all aspects to be enacted right away.[210] Bevin, however, wanted the creation of the company for sheltered employment to be one of the first.[211] This was not so it could start operating factories, as this would require first the creation of the register of disabled persons which would establish eligibility, but

[205] Bolderson, *Social Security, Disability and Rehabilitation*, p. 112, suggests that this was a genuine delay due to workload. TNA LAB 20/91, 'Note to Mr. Hetherington' (19.06.1943).

[206] TNA LAB 20/91, 'Note to Mr. Bowman' (21.06.1943); 'Notes from Sir. T.W. Phillips' (21.06.1943).

[207] TNA LAB 20/91, 'Note to Mr. Hetherington' (26.07.1943); 'Note from Sir. T.W. Phillips to Sir John Forbes Watson' (30.07.1943); 'Note from Sir. T.W. Phillips to Sir Walter Citrine' (30.07.1943).

[208] TNA LAB 20/91, 'Note from Sir John Forbes Watson to Sir T.W. Phillips' (29.07.1943).

[209] DPEA, pp. 13–4.

[210] TNA LAB 20/108, 'Note for Discussion with British Employers' Confederation and Trades Union Congress'.

[211] TNA LAB 20/87, Standing Rehabilitation and Resettlement Committee, 'Minutes of the Tenth Meeting' (04.05.1944); 'Minutes of the Eleventh Meeting' (06.07.1944); TNA LAB 20/108, 'Note for Discussion with British Employers' Confederation and Trades Union Congress'.

rather it was so that work could begin on understanding the scale and type of provision needed 'in readiness to receive severely disabled persons as soon as the registration scheme is started'.[212]

Bevin was again closely involved in the initial establishment of Remploy, including in the appointment of the Board of Directors.[213] Writing to Lord Portal, a highly distinguished Air Force officer who served as Chief of the Air Staff during the Second World War, who he asked to be Chairman on 11 December 1944, Bevin explained, 'I am most anxious to have someone who will be in a position to give enough time to this work to ensure that the provision for the disabled which is to be made through the Company shall be made as efficiently and speedily as possible as soon as war circumstances permit'.[214] Again at this stage we see that Bevin would suffer few delays, with hesitancy from the Treasury and the Board of Trade in carrying out various aspects of the formation of the company resulting in swift responses which emphasised the Minister's desire 'that the Corporation should get to work as rapidly as possible'.[215]

Though it has since been forgotten, this key role played by Bevin was remembered by those directly involved. Remploy themselves honoured him for his role as the first subject of the 'Profile' section in the maiden issue of *Remploy News* in 1952.[216] The importance of Bevin was later noted by George Isaacs, an initial member of the Remploy Board and Bevin's successor as Minister of Labour in Attlee's Labour Government. He recalled in Parliament in 1959 the creation of Remploy, noting that it was Bevin who 'conceived the idea of Remploy', and 'having conceived it,

212 TNA LAB 20/108, 'Note for Discussion with British Employers' Confederation and Trades Union Congress'; TNA LAB 20/113, 'Note from Mr. Gomme to Mr. Glen' (01.05.1944); TNA LAB 20/108, 'Note from Miss Hill to All Regional Training Officers' (06.06.1944); ' Note from Mr. Gomme to Miss Hill' (10.05.1944).

213 Numerous notes in TNA LAB 20/113 indicate discussions with the Minister on all aspects of the establishment of the Corporation, including appointments to the Board.

214 TNA LAB 20/113, 'Note from Ernest Bevin to Lord Portal' (11.12.1944). D. Richards, 'Portal, Charles Frederick Algernon, Viscount Portal of Hungerford (1893–1971), air force officer', *Oxford Dictionary of National Biography* (06.01.2011). https://www.oxforddnb.com/. Accessed 3 February 2016.

215 TNA LAB 20/113, 'Note to Mr Wiles' (08.03.1945); 'Note from Mr Wiles' (09.03.1945); 'Note to Mr Wiles' (28.02.1945); 'Note from Mr Dalton to Mr Hale' (24.01.1945); 'Note to Mr Hale' (28.04.1945); 'Note to Mr Barton' (22.03.1945). For 'Articles of Association' see TNA BM 4/1.

216 'Profile', *Remploy News*, 1 (December, 1952).

he discovered that he had some brilliant brains in the Ministry to help him to bring it into operation'.[217] He then noted that following the passing of the DPEA, 'Ernie Bevin set about establishing the corporation'.[218]

Given the central importance of Bevin and his MOL in creating Remploy, it is important to note that the motives behind this provide further cause to dismiss the notion that it was simply about placating industry through the segregation of unproductive workers. Bevin justified his insistence on a comprehensive rehabilitation and employment scheme on both the loss of manpower for the country if disabled people did not work, and through the idea that gaining employment would, for the disabled persons also mean 'their restoration to a fuller life'.[219] Similarly in outlining the proposed scheme in the Commons, Bevin's Parliamentary Secretary, George Tomlinson echoed these remarks, noting the ultimate aim of assisting disabled people wherever possible 'to live a full, free and happy life'.[220] Bevin also noted that he was motivated by his years of experience seeing the lack of welfare and employment for disabled workers, stating 'I have seen these men crippled in our streets, and I have had it on my conscience'.[221] There is no reason to doubt his motives in this case.

It is clear, therefore, that Bevin played the key role in the creation of Remploy. It was he who placed his vision of a national state scheme of sheltered employment on the agenda and drove the issue through the deliberations of the committees and discussions with industry. The DPEA itself left the establishment of the scheme to the Minister of Labour, and Bevin did not shirk from this task. The question of how to implement Remploy and the form it should take, however, remained undecided.

[217] Mr Isaacs, *Hansard* (21.07.1959), vol. 609, cc. 1135–94.

[218] Ibid.

[219] TNA CAB 71/5, 'Minister of Labour and National Service, Memorandum to Lord President's Committee, LP(41)182' (4.11.1941).

[220] Mr. Tomlinson, *Hansard*, (10.12.1943), vol. 395, cc. 1260.

[221] Mr. Bevin, *Hansard* (10.12.1943), vol. 395, cc. 1345–1346.

A Predetermined Purpose?

While the vision of a national state scheme of sheltered employment was being championed by Bevin and the MOL through to the passing of the DPEA, the specifics of what kind of scheme it would be and how it would function remained unresolved.[222] Miss Hill, a MOL official, was tasked with preparing a potential outline for the scheme in June 1944.[223] This focused mainly on the 'activities of the Company once it is formed' and touched on a wide range of areas including suggestions regarding eligibility, wages and existing voluntary provision.[224] In terms of the 'Provision to be made under the Company', the outline suggested that this would involve the creation of 'a network of centres each serving a restricted area'.[225] These centres would be residential, though they would also accommodate daily workers, and would consist of workshops, hostel, offices and storerooms.[226] Acknowledging that disabled people would not want to be moved too far from their communities, the outline recommended that the centres be situated 'in or near towns'.[227] In terms of the work itself, the outline recommended that the focus should be given to light industries using 'non-bulky materials' in 'clean operation', and if possible, which lend themselves to 'sitting work'.[228] Such general recommendations were not intended to be binding and indeed would later be extensively modified.

A key point at this stage was attempting to establish something of the scale of need. In considering this, while acknowledging the difficulty in obtaining reliable figures, the outline estimated that 'about 1500

[222] 'Rehabilitation Plans', *The Times* (03.05.1943).

[223] TNA LAB 20/108, 'Note from Miss Hill to Mr Gomme' (23.05.1944); 'Note from Miss Hill' (21.06.1944); 'Employment Under Special Conditions, Outline of a Scheme under Section 15 of the Disabled Persons (Employment) Act, 1944, E.M.D. 5565' (June, 1944).

[224] TNA LAB 20/108, 'Employment Under Special Conditions, Outline of a Scheme under Section 15 of the Disabled Persons (Employment) Act, 1944, E.M.D. 5565' (June, 1944).

[225] Ibid.

[226] Ibid.

[227] Ibid.

[228] Ibid.

severely disabled persons' required sheltered employment.[229] It was noted however, that 'it must be recognised that the Company will probably only learn the true extent of the problem after it has commenced its activities, or at any rate after a trial run in one or two areas'.[230] Hill wrote to MOL regional officers in June 1944 for 'general observations and advice' and a 'considered estimate' of the numbers requiring sheltered employment to aid in the preparation of the company.[231] To begin with, Hill requested from each region 'some figures as to the number in the area not at present provided for and likely to need, and qualify for, the special facilities under Sect. 15', and to have these divided into '(a) those willing to work in a residential sheltered workshops, (b) those willing to attend a workshop within daily travelling distance, (c) those capable only of employment in their own homes'.[232] Responses offered a wide range of estimates.[233] The Scotland Regional Office, for example, gave detailed figures which estimated that for category '(a)' there would be '742 men', '154 women', '23 juveniles'; for category '(b)' '2927 men', '599 women' and '116 juveniles'; and for category '(c)' '506 men', '265 women' and '151 juveniles'.[234] Whereas, the Wales Regional Office estimated for category '(a)' '85 persons'; for '(b)' '440 persons'; and for '(c)' '70 persons'.[235]

Overall, the responses indicated two things: firstly, that the potential extent of the problem was far larger than previously envisaged; and secondly, that the preference was overwhelmingly for non-residential workshops.[236] In terms of the former, the scale of the problem clearly took the MOL by surprise, especially with regards to Scotland.[237] In a

229 Ibid.

230 Ibid.

231 TNA LAB 20/108, 'Note from Miss Hill to All Regional Training Officers' (06.06.1944); 'Note from Miss Hill to Mr Gomme' (23.05.1944).

232 TNA LAB 20/108, 'Note from Miss Hill to All Regional Training Officers' (06.06.1944).

233 See TNA LAB 20/108, 'Summary of Replies from T.R.O's' (13.07.1944).

234 TNA LAB 20/108, 'Note to Miss Hill' (12.06.1944); (03.08.1944).

235 TNA LAB 20/108, 'Note to Miss Hill' (16.06.1944).

236 Ibid.; TNA LAB 20/108, See responses to Miss Hill.

237 This was discussed further in correspondence between Miss Hill and Mr Card of the Scotland Regional Office; TNA LAB 20/108, 'Note to Mr Card' (08.08.1944); 'Note to Miss Hill' (29.08.1944).

note to another MOL official, Hill exclaimed that 'we must do something to provide work for these people, even if in advance of the general scheme'.[238] She suggested appointing a Managing Director of the Company 'at once and turn him loose on Scotland to experiment'.[239] In terms of the type of centre to be established, Hill noted that 'it seems fairly clear from the replies in general that there will have to be a large number of small workshops within daily travelling distance'.[240] This was discussed further with the head of the MOL's training schemes, in July 1944, who 'considered that the vast majority of men would prefer to remain in their own homes and attend a non-residential centre'.[241] The MOL therefore established that the scheme should not involve residential settlement, but rather local centres, representing the only example of any real predetermined operational policy.

As time went on without any firm resolutions on many of the other specifics of the company, a concerned Hill wrote to fellow MOL official, Mr Gomme, on the 1 September 1944:

> with the approaching end of the war in the western theatre, ought we not to speed up preparations for completing our Scheme under Section 15…I don't know when the Register is likely to be set up, but there is so much to be done, that we ought to go ahead.[242]

Further limited consideration did eventually take place in January the following year, including discussions on general issues such as eligibility, working hours and wages.[243] This time Gomme expressed some alarm, explaining to a colleague that 'we have not yet worked out the policy we intend to follow under Section 15'.[244] In order to discuss this with the NACED, which had by then been established to consider and monitor

[238] TNA LAB 20/108, 'Note from Miss Hill' (30.08.1944).

[239] Ibid.

[240] TNA LAB 20/108, 'Note from Miss Hill to Mr Greenhough' (1944).

[241] TNA LAB 20/108, 'Note from Miss Hill' (07.07.1944).

[242] TNA LAB 20/108, 'Note from Miss Hill, Further Points Arising on Sect. 15' (01.09.1944).

[243] TNA LAB 20/108, 'Questions of a General Nature relating to Legal Points, Policy and Procedure which require consideration in connection with the implementation of Sect. 15 of the Disabled Persons (Employment) Act 1944'.

[244] TNA LAB 20/584, 'Note from Mr Gomme to Mr Taylor' (10.01.1945).

the implementation of the various measures contained in the DPEA, Gomme produced a draft memorandum to facilitate discussions.[245] A further meeting of MOL officials took place in April 1945, which considered the topics of eligibility and wages.[246] Although the MOL clearly put significant effort into considering how the scheme should run, lacking the expertise and necessary information, it was not able to produce a substantial plan and even what it propose continued to be in the form of suggestions rather than iron-clad rules. Bevin had informed the NACED that, in terms of the company, 'the Ministry did not claim a monopoly of ideas', and he hoped that they would offer suggestions.[247] It is therefore apparent that prior to the first meeting of its Board of Directors on 30 May 1945, many of the specifics of how Remploy should function remained undecided.[248]

Conclusions

This chapter has clarified numerous aspects relating to the creation of Remploy, which further serves to enhance our understanding of the birth of the welfare state. Contrary to the popular view of Remploy as a direct response to the conditions of the Second World War, the importance of a number of both long- and short-term factors is evident. The idea of a national government scheme of sheltered employment was not unique to the Second World War and had, along with other key measures of the DPEA, been considered in the aftermath of the previous war. The issue remained prominent throughout the interwar period as part of the wider campaign for further provision for disabled ex-servicemen. Remploy did not simply appear as a result of the Second World War, but was rather

[245] TNA LAB 20/584, 'Draft of Memorandum for National Advisory Council' (January, 1945). At the third meeting of the NACED on 24 May 1945, it was decided to appoint a Standing Committee on Sheltered Employment, TNA LAB 20/1100, NACED, 'Minutes of the Third Meeting' (24.05.1945); NACED, 'Minutes of the Sixth Meeting' (29.11.1945).

[246] TNA LAB 20/108, 'Note of a meeting held in Mr. Taylor's room on 5 April 1945' (05.04.1945).

[247] TNA LAB 20/1100, NACED, 'Minutes of the First Meeting' (30.01.1945).

[248] TNA BM 4/1. The Disabled Persons Employment Corporation would be renamed 'Remploy' the following year.

the culmination of longer term aspirations. While attempting to visualise developments in policy had the war not occurred is fraught with difficulty, given Bevin's importance in the creation of Remploy, and his insistence that it was not the war which led him to do so, it seems likely that, given the opportunity, he would have formulated a national sheltered employment scheme along the same lines. Whether there would have been sufficient political will to then put the scheme into practice is less clear. While not generating the idea of Remploy, the Second World War provided an advantageous moment, both politically and practically, to introduce such a scheme as an element in the wider vision for postwar Britain. As such, the case of Remploy supports the school of thought espoused by historians such as Laybourn, Lowe, Gladstone and Thane, in which the importance of a number of factors, including, but not limited to, the Second World War, are credited for the creation of the welfare state.[249] This warns us against any notion of considering the war as marking a clean break with what had gone before. This has important implications, particularly in the current historiography of disability in which wars in general, and the two World Wars of the twentieth century in particular, provide much of the focus. While this attention is understandable and certainly valid, the findings of this chapter demonstrate the importance of longer term developments in forming disability policy and the need to cross these convenient period divides in twentieth-century disability historiography.

It is apparent that Remploy's development was quite distinct from the other aspects of the DPEA. This provides an important qualification to any over-simplification of Remploy as simply another component within this legislation and thus of presenting the DPEA as a single unified programme targeting 'disabled people' as a homogeneous group. Given the nature of the DPEA as a landmark piece of legislation in disability policy, it is important to fully consider the various aspects it incorporated and how they were formulated and enacted, if we are to properly understand the history of disability across the period. Importantly, the notion of the Government designing Remploy as a means to segregate the severely disabled in order to placate industry has been shown to be misplaced. Demand for sheltered employment was widespread and included groups

[249] See Laybourn, *The Evolution of British Social Policy and the Welfare State*, pp. 209, 223; Lowe, *The Welfare State in Britain Since 1945*, pp. 16–7; Gladstone, *The Twentieth-Century Welfare State*, p. 51; Thane, 'Voluntary Action in Britain Since Beveridge'.

representing the interests of disabled people. Similarly, the records examined testify to the importance of the 'welfare' of severely disabled people in the minds of those forming the scheme. Undoubtedly paternalistic, and whether misplaced or not, and whatever one now thinks of sheltered employment, it was clearly considered desirable at the time, and it certainly appears that those involved in Remploy's creation, including Bevin, believed it was desired by, and in the best interests of, those it was intended to cater for. The case of Remploy therefore supports Anderson's assertion that the DPEA itself was created with the 'best interests of disabled people' in mind, as this was understood at the time, and further highlights the importance of understanding the development of disability policy in its historical context.[250]

In the particular case of Remploy, the role played by Bevin was vitally important. It was he who first considered creating a national scheme of sheltered employment during the war, and he and his MOL officials who pushed the measure through the various committees considering the wider DPEA proposals. The sheltered employment scheme outlined in the DPEA reflected his vision and the Act specifically left it to the Minister to enact, a role to which Bevin applied himself fully. A common view of the politics of the wartime Coalition Government, has suggested that the Conservatives were not seen as the party of future peacetime planning, with Churchill's insistence on a focus on the war effort.[251] Examination of this has focused on discussion of the Beveridge proposals, however, as the case of Remploy has shown, we can also see this in the sphere of disability employment, with the DPEA, and Remploy in particular, resulting from the efforts of Labour's Bevin. More generally, this also highlights the importance of key officials such as Bevin in the creation of the welfare state, and the continued role of individual political agency in policy development in the twentieth century.

Finally, it is apparent that there was no clear direction as to how Remploy should operate at its inception. We should be wary therefore of attributing a set function as inherent in its formation, or presenting it as a coherent scheme from its birth. This also highlights the danger of seeing

[250] Anderson, 'British Women, Disability and the Second World War', p. 48; Anderson, 'Turned into Taxpayers', p. 470.

[251] A. Thorpe, 'Myth and Counter-myth in Second World War British politics', in C. Williams and A. Edwards (eds.) *The Art of the Possible: Politics and Governance in Modern British History, 1885–1997* (Manchester, Manchester University Press, 2015), p. 129.

the creation of the welfare state as a singular event in which a coherent and static set of measures were considered and enacted. Beyond a general remit to provide a non-residential form of sheltered employment on a national scale, no aspect of Remploy's function was firmly determined prior to its creation. Remploy thus began to operate with fundamental questions about its purpose unresolved.

CHAPTER 3

'Human vs Economic', Contesting the Purpose of Remploy

Introduction

References to Remploy across disciplines have tended to carry the assumption that it operated as a cohesive unified scheme with a distinct purpose.[1] However, there have been differing views on what this primary purpose was. The dominant narrative espoused by Barnes, Shah and Priestley, and implied by Millward, suggests that Remploy's primary purpose during the

[1] For example, A. Borsay, *Disability and Social Policy in Britain Since 1750: A History of Exclusion* (Basingstoke, Palgrave Macmillan, 2005), p. 135; S. Wheatcroft, *Worth Saving: Disabled Children During the Second World War* (Manchester, Manchester University Press, 2013), p. 168; S. Humphries and P. Gordon, *Out of Sight: The Experience of Disability 1900–1950* (Plymouth, Northcote House, 1992), p. 138; L. Bryder, *Below the Magic Mountain: A Social History of Tuberculosis in Twentieth-Century Britain* (Oxford, Clarendon Press, 1988), p. 237; A. Land, R. Lowe and N. Whiteside, *The Development of the Welfare State 1939–1951: A guide to documents in the Public Record Office* (London, HMSO, 1992), pp. 203–4; P. Bridgen and R. Lowe, *Welfare Policy Under the Conservatives 1951–1964* (London, PRO, 1998), p. 262; S. Shah and M. Priestley, *Disability and Social Change: Private Lives and Public Policies* (Bristol, Policy Press, 2011), p. 139; E. Topliss, *Provision for the Disabled* (Oxford, Basil Blackwell, 1979), pp. 55–6; T. Jeffries, 'The Remploy Resource', *Industrial Management & Data Systems*, vol. 86, no. 1/2 (1986), p. 7; A. Kochan, 'Remploy: Disabled and Thriving', *Assembly Automation*, vol. 16, no. 1 (1996); J. Anderson, "Turned into Taxpayers': Paraplegia, Rehabilitation and Sport

© The Author(s), under exclusive license to Springer Nature Switzerland AG 2025

A. Holroyde, *Sheltered Employment and Disability in the British Welfare State*, New Directions in Welfare History,
https://doi.org/10.1007/978-3-031-87876-3_3

period of the classic welfare state was regarded as 'humanitarian rather than economic'.[2] This 'golden age' of Remploy operating as a social service was then brought to an end by the Thatcher governments of the 1980s, with a fundamental change of focus to maximising its commercial efficiency. An alternate view has been offered by Lonsdale and Topliss, who argued that an 'uneasy compromise' always existed within Remploy between humanitarian and economic considerations.[3] As with virtually all considerations of Remploy, such statements are not based on detailed research on the company and serve to support wider conclusions about the development of disability policy in Britain. With Remploy as the prime example of sheltered employment across disciplines, it is important that this fundamental aspect is understood. This chapter will therefore consider the vital question of how Remploy's primary function was understood in this period, prior to the election of the Conservative Government in 1979. As well as examining developments in overall policy, it will also consider how this was reflected at the local factory level. This is important in order to ascertain the degree to which Remploy operated as a coherent scheme with a uniform experience across locations, and in understanding how central policy was felt within the factory itself.

Consideration of the primary purpose of Remploy will focus upon the views of governments, Parliament and the Remploy Board of Directors. From examination of the records it is clear that in a similar vein

at Stoke Mandeville, 1944–56', *Journal of Contemporary History*, vol. 38, no. 3 (2003), p. 469; E. Elsey, 'The Rehabilitation and Employment of Disabled Ex-Servicemen after the Two World Wars', unpublished PhD Thesis, University of Teesside (1994), pp. 276–7; M. Oliver, *The Politics of Disablement* (Basingstoke, Macmillan, 1990), pp. 88–9; M. Hyde, 'Sheltered and Supported Employment in the 1990s: The Experiences of Disabled Workers in the UK', *Disability & Society*, vol. 13, no. 2 (1998), pp. 199–215; M. Reiss, *Blind Workers Against Charity: The National League of the Blind of Great Britain and Ireland, 1893–1970* (London, Palgrave Macmillan, 2015), p. 140; J. Anderson, *War, Disability and Rehabilitation in Britain: 'Soul of a Nation'* (Manchester, Manchester University Press, 2011), pp. 183–5; H. Bolderson, *Social Security, Disability and Rehabilitation: Conflicts in the Development of Social Policy 1914–1946* (London, Jessica Kingsley Publishers, 1991), pp. 109–110.

[2] C. Barnes, *Disabled People in Britain and Discrimination* (London, C. Hurst & Co., 2000), p. 73; Shah and Priestley, *Disability and Social Change*, pp. 138–40; G. Millward, 'Invalid Definitions, Invalid Responses: Disability and the Welfare State, 1965–1995', unpublished PhD Thesis, London School of Hygiene and Tropical Medicine (2013), pp. 184–5.

[3] S. Lonsdale, *Work and Inequality* (Harlow, Longman, 1985), p. 138; Topliss, *Provision for the Disabled*, pp. 55–7.

to the nationalised industries, though Remploy's day-to-day running was largely left to the management of the company's Board, there was always a large measure of government control through the MOL in terms of overall policy (with a representative of the Ministry attending every Board meeting), and the Treasury which supervised finances.[4] Remploy did not produce a profit at any point during the period considered here, and therefore was reliant on government funding. As such, governments of the period always had to determine the level of financial support given to Remploy and thus had a great deal of influence on overall policy and the scope of the company's activities. An examination of Remploy therefore provides a new case study to consider in the long-running debate over the existence and extent of a consensus in welfare policy between the two main political parties in the period. Considerations of disability policy in this debate have been few and focused solely upon welfare in terms of cash benefits, with both Millward and Hampton proposing the existence of a 'consensus in action' with a continuity in terms of the response to the needs of disabled people, if not in ideological position.[5] In a recent entry into this debate, Toye has called for historians to move away from the traditional aspects of welfare policy which have been considered and examine previously unexplored areas.[6] This chapter will therefore do so by exploring the case of Remploy.

The chapter will begin with an examination of policy across three periods. The first section considers the period of Labour government from 1945 to 1951 as Remploy was being established, and this is then followed by the period of Conservative governments, from 1951 to 1964. Finally, developments from the return of Labour to power in 1964, through to 1979 will be considered. The chapter will then examine how Remploy functioned at the local factory level and whether this reflected policy, resulting in a coherent, cohesive national scheme.

[4] P. Dorey, *British Politics Since 1945* (Oxford, Blackwell, 1995), p. 9.

[5] Millward, 'Invalid Definitions, Invalid Responses', p. 284; J. Hampton, *Disability and the Welfare State in Britain: Changes in Perception and Policy 1948–79* (Bristol, Policy Press, 2016), p. 244.

[6] R. Toye, 'From "Consensus" to "Common Ground": The Rhetoric of the Postwar Settlement and its Collapse', *Journal of Contemporary History*, vol. 48, no. 1 (2012), p. 23.

Developments in Policy, 1945–1951

The Remploy Board of Directors met for the first time on 30 May 1945, just over a month before Clement Attlee would come to lead the new Labour Government which would establish what is considered the British welfare state.[7] The Board was initially comprised of 8 members, which would grow to 12 by 1951, and was described as 'representing industry, trade unions and those with knowledge of employing disabled people'.[8]

From the beginning, the Board were clear that their understanding was that the purpose of Remploy was to provide 'genuine employment' and establish a viable long-term business for its severely disabled employees. There was to be no place for either charity or rehabilitative occupational therapy.[9] For the Board, the aim of the company was 'to provide productive and worthwhile work' in a way which resembled a 'normal' industrial operation as closely as possible.[10] This goal was reflected in the name adopted for the company's sites. Initial discussions about names included suggestions such as 'King George's Workshops'.[11] These were rejected in favour of the term 'British Factories'—later 'Remploy Factories'—with the deliberate use of 'factory' to distinguish them from charitable sheltered employment which commonly used the term 'workshop', and so as to 'encourage in the disabled workers the feeling that they were working in an industrial concern of some importance'.[12] Similarly, Remploy was

[7] The National Archives (TNA) BM 10/1, Remploy Limited, 'A Review of the working of the Company during its first seven years' (March, 1953), p. 3; TNA BM 8/1, Disabled Persons Employment Corporation Limited, 'Minutes of the First meeting of the Board of Directors' (30.05.1945).

[8] See TNA BM 8/1 and BM 8/2. See also, Remploy Limited, *Golden Jubilee*, (April, 1995).

[9] TNA BM 10/1, Remploy Limited, 'A Review of the working of the Company during its first seven years' (March, 1953), p. 47.

[10] Ibid.

[11] TNA BM 8/1, Disabled Persons Employment Corporation Limited, 'Minutes of the Fifth Meeting of the Board of Directors' (25.09.1945); 'Minutes of the Sixth Meeting of the Board of Directors' (31.11.1945).

[12] TNA BM 8/1, Disabled Persons Employment Corporation Limited, 'Minutes of the Eighth Meeting of the Board of Directors' (29.01.1946); TNA BM 10/1, Remploy Limited, 'A Review of the working of the Company during its first seven years' (March, 1953), p. 4. For decision to use 'British Factories' see TNA BM 8/1, Disabled Persons Employment Corporation Limited, 'Minutes of the Eighth Meeting of the Board of Directors' (29.01.1946). For decision to only use the term 'Remploy Factory', see TNA

to avoid the handicrafts and production of novelty items which were traditionally associated with charitable organisations and instead 'produce articles which were worth while making and would be up to ordinary standards and thus marketable without any indication that they were the product of disabled persons'.[13] This desire to operate as a 'normal' commercial company as much as possible, and provide this 'genuine employment' was also reflected in the Board's concern about the financial performance of the early factories.[14]

It would be wrong, however, to suggest that the Board completely disregarded the concept of Remploy's role as one of a welfare or social service. Their understanding appears to have been that the purpose of Remploy was to provide a viable business *and* a social service and that these were, in fact, one and the same. The service Remploy offered was in providing 'genuine employment' in which the workers could feel they were part of the productivity of the nation in a meaningful way and had earned their weekly pay packet as much as anyone else.[15] This concept of 'genuine employment' was therefore of central importance for the Board, and to best achieve it they felt the company should begin to establish itself as a robust commercial operation by concentrating provision in the 'bigger industrial towns' with 10 or 12 factories.[16]

This view appears to have been at odds with the MOL's emphasis on the purely social service aspect of the scheme, revealing contesting views on the function of Remploy from its beginning. For the MOL, Remploy was to be *the* solution to the 'problem' of employment for the severely disabled and was to rapidly establish provision based entirely upon the level of need. Such sentiments were expressed frequently by the new Minister of Labour, George Isaacs, a former chairman of the

BM 8/1, Disabled Persons Employment Corporation Limited, 'Minutes of the Fifteenth Meeting of the Board of Directors' (24.09.1946).

[13] TNA BM 8/1, Disabled Persons Employment Corporation Limited, 'Minutes of the First Meeting of the Board of Directors' (30.05.1945).

[14] TNA BM 8/1, Disabled Persons Employment Corporation Limited, 'Minutes of the Twenty-Ninth Meeting of the Board of Directors' (27.01.1948); 'Minutes of the Thirty-Second Meeting of the Board of Directors' (27.04.1948).

[15] TNA BM 10/1, Remploy Limited, 'A Review of the working of the Company during its first seven years' (March, 1953), p. 63.

[16] TNA BM 8/1, Disabled Persons Employment Corporation Limited, 'Minutes of the First meeting of the Board of Directors' (30.05.1945).

TUC, who announced the commencement of Remploy to parliament in November 1945 in terms of this perception, stating that it was 'making preparations to provide sheltered employment to whatever extent may be found necessary'.[17] Isaacs had himself been one of the initial members of the Remploy Board prior to his appointment as Minister of Labour.[18] This was a very brief period of only several months during which time he attended three board meetings. There is no evidence that while a member of the Board he was opposed to the views expressed about the desired direction of the company, though it is apparent that once he became Minister, his opinion and that of the Board diverged. When later asked if the factories were designed to be profitable, Isaacs replied that while it was hoped that they would work at a profit, financial losses were expected and acceptable, noting 'the main purpose of these workshops is to provide employment'.[19]

With overall policy ultimately determined by the MOL, it was on this basis that far more factories were planned than had been initially envisaged by the Board. Following the opening of the first factory in Bridgend at the end of April 1946, Isaacs revealed plans for 60 Remploy factories.[20] The following year, in addition to the 6 already in operation, a further 98 were proposed.[21] By the end of the year the target given was 107 factories, and in early 1949 this had increased once more to 140.[22] Nor were

[17] Mr. George Isaacs, *Hansard* (08.11.1945), vol. 415, cc. 1590–2; TNA BM 8/1, Disabled Persons Employment Corporation Limited, 'Minutes of the Fourth Meeting of the Board of Directors' (28.08.1945); H. Pemberton, 'Isaacs, George Alfred (1883–1979), trade unionist and politician', *Oxford Dictionary of National Biography* (23.09.2004). https://www.oxforddnb.com/. Accessed 22 April 2016. These sentiments were echoed by Mr. Ellis Smith, Parliamentary Secretary to the Board of Trade, Mr. Ellis Smith, *Hansard* (22.11.1945), vol. 416, cc. 754. For details of Ellis Smith see J.M. Bellamy and J. Saville (eds.), *Dictionary of Labour Biography, Vol. 9* (Palgrave Macmillan: Basingstoke, 1993), pp. 265–8.

[18] TNA BM 8/1, Disabled Persons Employment Corporation Limited, 'Minutes of the Fourth Meeting of the Board of Directors' (28.08.1945).

[19] Mr. George Isaacs, *Hansard* (02.12.1947), vol. 445, cc. 186–8.

[20] Mr. George Isaacs, *Hansard* (03.05.1946), vol. 422, cc. 453-542; TNA BM 8/1, Disabled Persons Employment Corporation Limited, 'Minutes of the Eleventh Meeting of the Board of Directors' (30.04.1946).

[21] Mr. George Isaacs, *Hansard* (17.04.1947), vol. 436, cc. 34–5.

[22] Mr. George Isaacs, *Hansard* (02.12.1947), vol. 445, cc. 186–8; TNA BM 8/1, Disabled Persons Employment Corporation Limited, 'Minutes of the Forty-First Meeting of the Board of Directors' (23.02.1949).

the figures for planned factories a final limit, as the Minister suggested that if a need remained in any area, 'further factories will be established'.[23] The approach appears to have been on planning a Remploy factory wherever the need had been established or even expressed. It is evident that when dealing with the regular queries from MPs about the possibility of opening a factory in an area, Isaacs consistently answered that one would be forthcoming in the area or close to it, or that it would be considered.[24] His Parliamentary Secretary, Ness Edwards, went further in stating that the intention was 'to continue building this type of factory throughout the country until we have provided sheltered employment for all persons requiring it'.[25] The approach of the MOL was therefore rapid expansion based upon delivering a social service of sheltered employment to all those in need, with no serious consideration of commercial efficiency.

The evidence suggests MPs commonly shared this view of Remploy. In addition to the regular discussion in the Commons of the general issue of employment for disabled people, questions were frequently asked about the Remploy factory programme. Following the official opening ceremony for the Bridgend Factory in November 1946, a much publicised occasion attended by Isaacs, the calls for more factories began in earnest and continued with regularity for the next several years.[26] March 1947, for example, saw no less than 7 instances of MPs calling for further factories.[27] The demand was for rapid expansion in order to prevent severely

[23] Mr. George Isaacs, *Hansard* (26.11.1946), vol. 430, cc. 1388–9.

[24] See for example; Mr. George Isaacs, *Hansard* (05.03.1946), vol. 420, cc. 164; Mr. George Isaacs, *Hansard* (17.10.1946), vol. 427, cc. 239; Mr. George Isaacs, *Hansard* (22.10.1946), vol. 427, cc. 347–8; Mr. George Isaacs, *Hansard* (05.11.1946), vol. 428, cc. 203–4; Mr. George Isaacs, *Hansard* (05.11.1946), vol. 428, cc. 203–4; Mr. George Isaacs, *Hansard* (12.12.1946), vol. 431, cc. 1333–4.

[25] Mr. Ness Edwards, *Hansard* (21.03.1947). vol. 435, cc. 816–26.

[26] TNA BM 8/1, Disabled Persons Employment Corporation Limited, 'Minutes of the Fifteenth Meeting of the Board of Directors' (24.09.1946). From October 1946 to June 1949 there are over 50 instances recorded in Hansard of questions being asked about Remploy provision.

[27] Mr. Wilkes, *Hansard* (04.03.1947), vol. 434, cc. 29; Mr. David Thomas, *Hansard* (10.03.1947), vol. 434, cc. 963-1094; Mr. Wilkes, *Hansard* (17.03.1947), vol. 435, cc. 152-64; Sir Ian Fraser, *Hansard* (19.03.1947), vol. 435, cc. 416-526; Mr. Chetwynd, *Hansard* (21.03.1947), vol. 435, cc. 816-26; Mr. Robens and Mr. David Jones, *Hansard* (21.03.1947), vol. 435, cc. 816-26.

disabled people from being left to 'rot in their cottages'.[28] Continuous pressure was placed upon Remploy and the MOL from MPs, encouraged by the responses of the latter, to provide more factories.[29]

It is noteworthy that the overwhelming majority of the interest expressed in Remploy, in terms of official parliamentary proceedings recorded in Hansard, came from Labour MPs, with only a handful of queries from Conservatives.[30] Labour did enjoy a large majority in government at this time, with 393 MPs compared to the 213 Conservatives.[31] Remploy as a concept was also more in keeping with the ideological make-up of the Labour Party at this time, reflecting its wider commitment to full employment, nationalisation, central planning and welfare. While Hansard cannot reveal all the discussions which take place among politicians, and Isaacs himself claimed that Remploy was under pressure to expand 'from all quarters of the House', the discrepancy is striking.[32]

There were therefore differing visions of how Remploy should function from its very beginning, with the Board wishing to establish Remploy as a commercial enterprise, and the MOL, reflecting also the expressed views of many MPs, demanding instead it offer provision to match the need. With direction ultimately determined by the MOL, it was this latter policy which was adopted and which led to the rapid expansion of Remploy. While the planned figure of 140 factories was not to be reached, Remploy ended its first 7 years with 91 factories spread out over the country, which would essentially remain the company's overall footprint across the period considered here, employing over 5800 disabled people.[33]

[28] Mr. N. Edwards, *Hansard* (05.12.1950), vol. 482, c. 314.

[29] Isaacs noted the pressure, TNA LAB 20/453, 'Note from G. Isaacs to S. Cripps' (10.02.1949). Remploy also, TNA BM 8/1, Disabled Persons Employment Corporation Limited, 'Minutes of the Fortieth Meeting of the Board of Directors' (26.01.1949).

[30] Examination of the records of *Hansard* revealed that in the period up to June 1949 there were 56 instances of queries about Remploy by Labour MPs, 3 from Conservative MPs, and 1 from a Unionist MP.

[31] R. Lowe, *The Welfare State in Britain Since 1945* (Basingstoke, Palgrave Macmillan, 2005), p. 90.

[32] TNA LAB 20/453, 'Note from G. Isaacs to S. Cripps' (10.02.1949). Remploy also noted this, TNA BM 8/1, Disabled Persons Employment Corporation Limited, 'Minutes of the Fortieth Meeting of the Board of Directors' (26.01.1949).

[33] TNA BM 10/1, Remploy Limited, 'A Review of the working of the Company during its first seven years' (March, 1953), p. 34.

The Board complained at an early stage that Isaacs was being far too optimistic in the promises he was making about the speed and extent of expansion, and commented frequently upon the severe difficulties this posed in terms of costs, organisation and logistics.[34] In addition to these practical problems, was the perceived danger to the Board's vision of 'genuine employment'. The worry, expressed by the Executive Director of Remploy, Air Commodore G.O. Venn, who had been appointed following his retirement from the post of Director of Personal Services at the Air Ministry, was that workers 'would be inclined to think that as they were in government factories it would not be necessary for employees to work hard, or for them to keep good time'.[35] Such concerns were increased after comments were made by Isaacs, including at the opening ceremony for the Bridgend factory, that 'it would not matter if the factories did not pay for themselves'.[36] It was later reported that the workers at Bridgend were 'using that statement as an excuse for slow work'.[37] At other factories too it was reported that there were employees 'of the opinion that once they were in the job they had no need to worry'.[38] In response, the Board asked for Isaacs to 'issue a statement which will call for a greater effort by the severely disabled employed in Remploy Factories'.[39]

Tensions came to a head in 1949, sparked by the financial results for the previous year which showed an overall loss of approximately £387,000.[40] This led the Chancellor of the Exchequer, Sir Stafford

[34] See for example, Ibid.; Remploy Limited, We *Have a Part to Play*, (28.09.1988). For Government acknowledgement see 'Loss By Remploy Limited: Ministry's Reply to Criticism', *The Times* (30.08.1952).

[35] TNA BM 8/1, Disabled Persons Employment Corporation Limited, 'Minutes of the Sixteenth Meeting of the Board of Directors' (29.10.1946); TNA LAB 20/120, MOL, 'Note on The Disabled Persons Employment Corporation Limited' (1945).

[36] TNA BM 8/1, Disabled Persons Employment Corporation Limited, 'Minutes of the Eighteenth Meeting of the Board of Directors' (28.01.1947).

[37] Ibid.

[38] Ibid.

[39] Ibid.; TNA BM 8/1, Disabled Persons Employment Corporation Limited, 'Minutes of the Twenty-Sixth Meeting of the Board of Directors' (28.10.1947); 'Minutes of the Nineteenth Meeting of the Board of Directors' (25.02.1947).

[40] TNA BM 8/1, Disabled Persons Employment Corporation Limited, 'Minutes of the Forty-First Meeting of the Board of Directors' (23.02.1949); TNA LAB 20/453, 'Statement of Income and Expenditure for the nine months ended 31st December 1948'.

Cripps, to raise concerns at the amounts involved and in a letter to the MOL, these 'misgivings' on the 'large amount provided for deficits' were expressed.[41] Described by Morgan as 'the high Anglican prophet of austerity', Cripps had been appointed Chancellor following the fuel and convertibility crises of 1947, which had served to limit the bold 'socialist advance' pursued by his predecessor, and pursued an agenda of restraint in public expenditure.[42] Though he stopped short of demanding a reduction in funding for Remploy, Cripps asked that the Board be warned that in future 'a report will be required containing justification for charges at the present rate if they are to continue'.[43] In reply, Isaacs came to their defence, and highlighted the efforts being made to make the factories 'as nearly self-supporting as can be'.[44] The efforts he described were based on increasing sales, with no suggestion of halting the expansion.[45] Thus the concern expressed by the Treasury did not initially persuade Isaacs to change course.

The concerns of the Chancellor were, however, shared by the Board themselves, and at a meeting in February 1949, the newly appointed Chairman, Sir Robert Burrows, whose background was in industry, expressed his dismay at Remploy's 'heavy expenditure'.[46] The problem, as far as he could see, was that the pressure to open new factories meant

[41] TNA LAB 20/453, 'Note from E. Hale to T.W.F. Dalton' (31.01.1949). M. Hill, *The Welfare State in Britain: A Political History since 1945* (Aldershot, Edward Elgar Publishing, 1993), p. 42.

[42] K.O. Morgan, *Britain Since 1945: The People's Peace, 3rd Edition* (Oxford, Oxford University Press, 2001), pp. 29, 67, 70; D. Fraser, *The Evolution of the British Welfare State*, 4th Edition (Basingstoke, Palgrave Macmillan, 2009), p. 267; K. Laybourn, *The Evolution of British Social Policy and the Welfare State, c.1800–1993* (Keele, Keele University Press, 1995), p. 231; P. Clarke & R. Toye, 'Cripps, Sir (Richard) Stafford (1889–1952), politician and lawyer', *Oxford Dictionary of National Biography*, (06.01.2011). https://www.oxforddnb.com/. Accessed 26 July 2019.

[43] TNA LAB 20/453, 'Note from E. Hale to T.W.F. Dalton' (31.01.1949).

[44] TNA LAB 20/453, 'Note from G. Isaacs to S. Cripps' (10.02.1949).

[45] Ibid.

[46] TNA BM 8/1, Disabled Persons Employment Corporation Limited, 'Minutes of the Forty-First Meeting of the Board of Directors' (23.02.1949). See records of appointment of Sir Robert in TNA LAB 20/120.

that the company could not consolidate its position to improve production or reduce losses.[47] The Board agreed with this assessment and it was decided that the Chairman would write to Isaacs to ascertain 'whether he considers we should postpone the opening of further factories or whether, in his opinion, the work of the Corporation in employing severely disabled persons justified these very heavy losses'.[48] The aim was to obtain a 'definite statement of policy' as to what function the company was to serve—was its role as a business or a social service to be given priority?[49] Isaacs' first reaction was not to endorse the desired pause in the expansion but to instead strengthen the company to deal with it better.[50]

This would change however, the following month, as Sir Robert engaged in a meeting with Sir Edward Bridges at the Treasury.[51] An experienced and prominent civil servant, Sir Edward had served as Permanent Secretary to the Treasury and Head of the Civil Service since 1946.[52] During this meeting, Sir Robert made the Board's feelings on the direction of Remploy clear, and in terms of his own views, explained that 'he did not wish to be associated with an organisation which was losing a very large amount of money'.[53] Stressing the view of the Board that they should consolidate Remploy's position, Sir Robert said he 'was anxious that they should not be pressed to go too fast'.[54] Sir Edward, confirming that the Treasury was greatly concerned at the rate of expansion 'as this meant additional losses', provided assurances that the Chancellor would press Isaacs on the matter further.[55]

[47] TNA BM 8/1, Disabled Persons Employment Corporation Limited, 'Minutes of the Forty-First Meeting of the Board of Directors' (23.02.1949).

[48] Ibid.

[49] Ibid.

[50] TNA LAB 20/453, 'Note to Secretary' (25.02.1949).

[51] TNA LAB 20/453, 'Note from G. Ince' (24.03.1949); TNA BM 8/1, Disabled Persons Employment Corporation Limited, 'Minutes of the Forty-Second Meeting of the Board of Directors' (30.03.1949).

[52] R. Chapman, 'Bridges, Edward Ettingdene, first Baron Bridges (1892–1969), civil servant', *Oxford Dictionary of National Biography* (12.01.2018). https://www.oxforddnb.com/. Accessed 26 July 2019.

[53] TNA LAB 20/453, 'Note from G. Ince' (24.03.1949).

[54] Ibid.

[55] Ibid.

As promised, Cripps wrote to Isaacs later in the month, forcefully expressing concern that Remploy was expanding 'faster than would be justified on consideration of economic production'.[56] In addition, he echoed the view presented to him by Sir Robert of the importance of providing 'genuine employment', noting that the 'main benefit of employment to a disabled man is that it gives him a sense of usefulness and of pulling his own weight'.[57] Arguing against the building of factories based on an area's need alone, he stressed that 'some regard must be paid to commercial prospects, and to the inevitable limits on the capacity of the Corporation's organisation'.[58]

Supported by the Board, the Treasury had expressly challenged the policy towards Remploy directed by the MOL. It has been suggested by historians such as Laybourn, that the battles over expenditure within the Labour Government, which would famously culminate in the resignation of the Minister of Health, Aneurin Bevan, over the introduction of prescription charges in the NHS, first emerged in the autumn of 1949 following the decision to devalue the pound.[59] It is apparent, however, that an earlier skirmish occurred between the Treasury and the MOL some months before this over the direction of Remploy.

Following this direct intervention by the Chancellor, and thus facing opposition from both the Board and Treasury, Isaacs relented and it was decided that the position of Remploy would be jointly examined by the company, the MOL and the Treasury, and an agreed future programme established.[60] With the Board and Treasury allied in their desires, a 'slow down' was agreed, with a delay to the completion of factories already in progress wherever possible and a limit to the opening of new factories from 1951 to 'about 12 a year'.[61] Isaacs announced the policy change in the House of Commons on 7 July 1949. Stressing the arguments which had been made by the Board and subsequently adopted by the Treasury

[56] TNA LAB 20/453, 'Note from S. Cripps to G. Isaacs' (29.03.1949).

[57] Ibid.

[58] Ibid.

[59] Laybourn, *The Evolution of British Social Policy and the Welfare State*, p. 231; Morgan, *Britain Since* 1945, pp. 73–4, 100–103.

[60] TNA LAB 20/453, 'Note from A.F.A. Sutherland to Col. Robertson' (04.04.1949).

[61] TNA BM 8/1, Disabled Persons Employment Corporation Limited, 'Minutes of the Forty-Fifth Meeting of the Board of Directors' (29.06.1949); TNA LAB 20/453, 'Slowing Down of Remploy Factory Programme'.

that it would be a 'false kindness to the severely disabled to jeopardise the success of the Corporation by over-hasty expansion at the present stage', Isaacs informed the House that there would be 79 factories in operation by the end of the year and 'some slowing down thereafter'.[62] A final programme for factory building was later completed which anticipated 74 factories to be in operation by the end of the year, at least 20 more during 1950 and a further 46 by 1954.[63]

Having achieved their aim, the Board focused fully upon consolidating Remploy as a business as its expansion was slowed. While keeping in mind the 'great importance of the well-being of the disabled employees', the reduction of the losses was to become the Board's 'constant endeavour' in order to 'keep down the charge on the country's revenue'.[64] This resulted in new initiatives including efforts to increase the monitoring of factories, the establishment of standard product lines, the creation of a dedicated sales division and the introduction of mechanisation.[65] Such measures had a limited effect on the company's commercial efficiency. The Board did credit the slowdown with having a positive effect with a general upward trend in production and sales.[66] However, problems persisted and by the summer of 1951, with the company requiring an additional £300,000 subvention from the Treasury, the position was described as 'still far from satisfactory'.[67]

Nor had the new policy direction laid the issue of Remploy's central purpose to rest. Interest in Remploy from MPs remained, and there were continued requests for factories for individual constituencies and a general

[62] Mr. G. Isaacs, *Hansard*, 466 cc176-8 (07.07.1949); TNA LAB 20/453, 'Remploy Factories Memo; Note D.P.802/1949' (27.06.1949).

[63] TNA LAB 20/453, Remploy Limited, 'Copy of Statement circulated by Headquarters, Ministry of Labour and National Service to Regional Controllers' (03.10.1949); Remploy Limited, 'Executive Director's Report No. 44' (21.09.1949).

[64] TNA BM 8/2, Remploy Limited, 'Minutes of the Sixtieth Meeting of the Board of Directors' (20.12.1950); 'Minutes of the Fifty-Eighth Meeting of the Board of Directors' (25.10.1950).

[65] See Board Meetings throughout TNA BM 8/1.

[66] TNA BM 8/2, Remploy Limited, 'Minutes of the Sixtieth Meeting of the Board of Directors' (20.12.1950).

[67] TNA BM 8/2, Remploy Limited, 'Minutes of the Sixty-Sixth Meeting of the Board of Directors' (27.06.1951); 'Minutes of the Sixty-Eighth Meeting of the Board of Directors' (26.09.1951).

extension of the Remploy programme.[68] As before, such comments and requests came overwhelmingly from Labour MPs.[69] There was also the beginning of concern expressed that the focus on commercial efficiency in Remploy was not compatible with its perceived role as a social service.[70] Isaacs himself, following his replacement as Minister of Labour by Bevan, spoke of Remploy as 'a matter very dear to me', and continued to emphasise his view of the social value of the company's work, which 'could not altogether be measured in terms of money'.[71]

In a sign of things to come, however, the emphasis on Remploy's commercial efficiency was to quickly become greater than the Board had intended. In January 1950, soon after the agreed pause in expansion championed by the Board, its submitted expenditure estimates for the year were returned from the MOL with a demand for capital expenditure cuts which would drastically alter even the reduced building programme.[72] In negotiations with the MOL, Remploy's previous stance was reversed as it had to plead for agreement to proceed with planned factories at Springburn and Maesteg.[73] The MOL reply, which followed the re-election of the Labour Government on a manifesto of consolidation of welfare and continued restraint in public spending, made it clear that any further expansion was dependent on an increase in sales figures

[68] See for example, Mr. Mainwaring, *Hansard* (24.11.1949), vol. 470, cc. 578–644; Mr. A. Edward Davies, *Hansard* (13.07.1950), vol. 477, cc. 1709–18; Mr. H. Hynd, *Hansard* (13.03.1951), vol. 486, cc. 1336–423; Mr. MacPherson, *Hansard* (28.03.1950), vol. 473, cc. 21; Mr. L. Hale, *Hansard* (18.04.1950), vol. 474, cc. 15–6; Mr. G. Thomas and Mr. Isaacs, *Hansard* (24.10.1950), vol. 478, cc. 330; Sir Ian Fraser and Mr. A. Bevan, *Hansard* (25.01.1951), vol. 483, cc. 297; Dr. King, Mr. R. Morley and Mr. A. Bevan, *Hansard* (01.02.1951), vol. 483, cc. 1063–4; Mr. H. Hynd, *Hansard* (08.03.1951), vol. 485, cc. 84–5.

[69] Examination of Hansard reveals that from July 1949 there were then 23 queries about Remploy from Labour MPs and 3 from Conservative MPs.

[70] Mr. John McKay and Mr. Lee, *Hansard* (24.07.1951), vol. 491, cc. 180–1.

[71] Mr. Isaacs, *Hansard* (23.01.1951), vol. 483, cc. 77–108. TNA BM 8/2.Remploy Limited, 'Minutes of the Sixtieth Meeting of the Board of Directors' (20.12.1950).

[72] TNA BM 8/1, Remploy Limited, 'Minutes of the Fiftieth Meeting of the Board of Directors' (04.01.1950).

[73] TNA BM 8/1, Remploy Limited, 'Minutes of the Fifty-First Meeting of the Board of Directors' (22.02.1950).

from the company to justify it.[74] With the outbreak of the Korean War later in the year bringing costs for rearmament and ongoing battles within the Cabinet over the priorities of welfare expenditure, the final Attlee Government has been characterised as being jaded and lacking in new ideas.[75] Against this backdrop, the new approach to Remploy would not be reconsidered.

By the end of this period of Labour Government, therefore, the importance of Remploy's commercial efficiency was already established. Contrary to the notion that a business imperative only appeared in the 1980s to override a previous focus on the welfare aspect of Remploy, this was present from the very beginning and was initially endorsed, even championed, by its Board of Directors. Contesting this view, the drive of the MOL to position Remploy as a primarily social service, established based upon need alone, was defeated by the combined efforts of the company and a Treasury pursuing a policy of austerity in the face of economic difficulties. Though a number of MPs still challenged this view, the Board achieved their aim of establishing the company's purpose as one of providing 'genuine employment', through operating as much as possible as a commercially viable business and thereby reducing the cost to the Exchequer. By the end of the Attlee governments, this view was fully adopted by the MOL. This saw the beginning of the link between the scope of the company and its economic performance alongside governments' welfare expenditure priorities.

Developments in Policy, 1951–1964

Though the Conservative Party had attacked the costs of welfare during its time in opposition, following its election to government in 1951, political expediency and the influence of the 'One Nation Tories', who saw the welfare state 'as a necessary part of economic and social cohesion', ensured that there was no widespread dismantling of the postwar

[74] Ibid. In the end Remploy was allowed to proceed with the new factories but not the proposed extensions, TNA BM 8/1, Remploy Limited, 'Minutes of the Fifty-Second Meeting of the Board of Directors' (29.03.1950). Morgan, *Britain Since 1945*, p. 84.

[75] B. Coxall and L. Robins, *British Politics Since the War* (Basingstoke, Macmillan, 1998), p. 21; Laybourn, *The Evolution of British Social Policy and the Welfare State*, p. 234.

settlement established under Labour.[76] There was, however a firm grip on all public spending and the imposition of expenditure cuts on public services during times of economic difficulty.[77] For Remploy, this meant that the approach taken by the Labour Government prior to the election was to become firmly entrenched, and the economic pinch upon the company, in common with welfare expenditure generally, was to become a tight squeeze under the successive Conservative governments which followed.[78]

The agenda was set almost immediately with the company's expenditure estimates for 1952–53 reduced under directives from both the MOL and the Treasury.[79] The minutes of Remploy Board meetings throughout this period of Conservative government reveal a near continuous pressure to reduce expenditure.[80] Primarily this was the result of edicts passed down to the MOL from the Treasury, who noted that the former had been continuously 'exercised' to keep funding to Remploy 'to a minimum'.[81] While sympathetic to the financial pressures this placed upon the Board, the view of the MOL was largely aligned with the need to maximise commercial efficiency, with the opinion that it was up to the company to do more to reduce its continuous financial losses.[82] This position was then further endorsed by a report from the Select

[76] Hampton, *Disability and the Welfare State in Britain*, p. 51; Coxall and Robin, *British Politics Since the War*, p. 22; Morgan, *Britain since 1945*, pp. 112–3; Fraser, *The Evolution of the British Welfare State*, p. 289; R. Page, *Revisiting the Welfare State* (Maidenhead, Open University Press, 2007), pp. 52–7.

[77] Page, *Revisiting the Welfare State*, pp. 52–7; Hampton, *Disability and the Welfare State in Britain*, p. 51; Coxall and Robin, *British Politics Since the War*, p. 22; Morgan, *Britain since 1945*, pp. 112–3; Fraser, *The Evolution of the British Welfare State*, p. 289.

[78] Hampton, *Disability and the Welfare State in Britain*, p. 51.

[79] TNA BM 8/2, Remploy Limited, 'Minutes of the Sixty-Ninth Meeting of the Board of Directors' (31.10.1951); 'Minutes of the Seventy-Second Meeting of the Board of Directors' (30.01.1952).

[80] See TNA BM 8/1, BM 8/2, BM 8/3 for these minutes.

[81] TNA LAB 20/929, 'Remploy Memorandum by Treasury' (1955); 'Note to Sir Brunel Cohen' (03.11.1955); 'Note from Mr. P.H. St. John Wilson to Dame Mary Smieton' (15.03.1956); 'Note from Mr. P.H. St. John Wilson to Mr J. R. Wade, D.P.2747/1955' (13.04.1956); 'Note from Mr. St. John Wilson to Mr. J Wade, D.P. 2747/1955' (17.03.1956); TNA BM 8/2, Remploy Limited, 'Minutes of the One Hundred and Fourteenth Meeting of the Board of Directors' (16.11.1955).

[82] TNA LAB 20/929, 'Note from Mr. St. John Wilson' (31.11.1956); 'Note from Mr. Slater to Mr. St. John Wilson' (19.08.1955); 'Notes for Minister (to be read in

Committee on Estimates in 1952, which judged Remploy purely in terms of its commercial efficiency and was highly critical of its management and organisation.[83] Remploy was presented as a failing business which was costing the Exchequer a large, and increasing, amount of money.[84] The publication of the report caught the attention of the press with numerous headlines focused upon the amount of money 'lost' by the company.[85] A more measured assessment came in the 1956 report of the Committee of Inquiry on The Rehabilitation, Training and Resettlement of Disabled Persons (Piercy Committee), established to provide a full review of the progress of the provisions of the DPEA. This report stressed the valuable welfare role Remploy played beyond its financial results, yet it also emphasised the importance of productivity and evoked the concept of 'genuine employment' in distinguishing this kind of sheltered employment provision from purely occupational welfare.[86]

As a result of the establishment of the new policy, the temporary 'slow down' in expansion agreed upon under the previous Labour Government became an indefinite halt under the Conservatives. The new Minister of Labour, Sir Walter Monckton, a former solicitor-general and only recently elected MP appointed with the task of preventing industrial unrest, announced in the Commons in 1953 that despite the widely held view that more factories were needed, any further expansion would have to be justified by Remploy's commercial performance, and would be subject to the favourable economic conditions of the country in general to

conjunction with the letter of 3rd November to Sir Brunel Cohen)' (03.11.1955); 'Note from Mr. St. John Wilson to Dame Smieton' (08.12.1955).

83 *Fourth Report from the Select Committee on Estimates,* 162 (1952), paras. 22–30, pp. xii-xv; TNA BM 8/2, Remploy Limited, 'Minutes of the Seventy-Third Meeting of the Board of Directors' (27.02.1952).

84 Ibid., para. 30, p. xv; paras. 292–3, p. 22.

85 TNA LAB 20/ 653, 'State Company for Disabled Loses Heavily', *The Nottingham Journal* (30.04.1952); '£2 M. Loss On Factories For Disabled', *Daily Telegraph* (30.04.1952); 'Yearly Loss Of £380 On Each Disabled Workers', *Manchester Guardian* (30.04.1952); 'State Firm For Disabled Censured, *Daily Mail* (30.04.1952); 'Firm Training Disabled "Overspends", *News Chronicle* (30.04.1952).

86 *Report of the Committee of Inquiry on The Rehabilitation Training and Resettlement of Disabled Persons*, 9883 (1956); Topliss, *Provision for the Disabled*, pp. 55–7; Reiss, *Blind Workers Against Charity,* pp. 138–40.

fund the increase in cost.[87] By 1960 the MOL would decide that there was still no justification for the opening of any new factories on these grounds.[88] As well as ending the expansion in the number of factory sites, the tight control on expenditure was reflected in terms of employee numbers. With each employee in Remploy effectively working at a loss, this became a key area to reduce expenditure. By October 1954, Remploy was employing 6676 workers.[89] In order to secure a desired reduction in expenditure for the following year, the MOL demanded that Remploy reduce its employee numbers to 6000 'as soon as possible'.[90] This was not to be achieved through dismissals, but by allowing the natural 'run down' through not replacing workers who left for reasons such as securing work in open employment, sickness, or death.[91] This reduction was considered by the Board to have been extremely damaging to the company, both in terms of production and morale and was a policy imposed upon them by the Conservative Government, entirely for economic reasons and without their support.[92]

[87] TNA LAB 20/929, 'Letter from Sir Walter Monckton to Sir Robert Burrows' (16.01.1954); TNA BM 10/2, Remploy Limited, 'A Brief Outline of the Birth and Early Development of Remploy Limited' (May, 1979), p. 21; M. Pugh, 'Monckton, Walter Turner, first Viscount Monckton of Brenchley (1891–1965), lawyer and politician', *Oxford Dictionary of National Biography* (06.01.2011). https://www.oxforddnb.com/. Accessed 20 January 2017.

[88] TNA BM 8/2, Remploy Limited, 'Minutes of the One Hundred and Sixty-Third Meeting of the Board of Directors' (16.03.1930).

[89] TNA BM 8/2, Remploy Limited, 'Minutes of the One Hundred and Second Meeting of the Board of Directors' (27.10.1954); TNA BM 10/2, Remploy Limited, 'A Brief Outline of the Birth and Early Development of Remploy Limited' (May, 1979), p. 21.

[90] TNA LAB 20/929, 'Letter from J.R. Wade to John Wilson' (25.05.1955); 'Remploy Memorandum by Treasury' (1955); TNA BM 8/2, Remploy Limited, 'Minutes of the One Hundred and Eighth Meeting of the Board of Directors' (04.05.1955); 'Minutes of the One Hundred and Sixth Meeting of the Board of Directors' (23.02.1955); TNA BM 10/2, Remploy Limited, 'A Brief Outline of the Birth and Early Development of Remploy Limited' (May, 1979), p. 21.

[91] TNA BM 8/2, Remploy Limited, 'Minutes of the One Hundred and Eighth Meeting of the Board of Directors' (04.05.1955); 'Minutes of the One Hundred and Sixth Meeting of the Board of Directors' (23.02.1955).

[92] TNA BM 8/2, Remploy Limited, 'Minutes of the One Hundred and Eighth Meeting of the Board of Directors' (04.05.1955); 'Minutes of the One Hundred and Sixth Meeting of the Board of Directors' (23.02.1955); TNA BM 10/2, Remploy Limited, 'A Brief Outline of the Birth and Early Development of Remploy Limited' (May, 1979), p. 21.

In November 1955, against a backdrop of a severe balance of payments crisis and a mandate to cut public expenditure, the Treasury set out its own views on establishing the scope of Remploy's activities with a focus on reducing its cost to the Exchequer, the establishment of a fixed total amount available to Remploy over a given period, and the target for the company to reduce the loss per head to the average wage of its disabled employees.[93] Under the first of these '5 year plans', Remploy would receive an annual revenue grant of £2,500,000 and an average annual capital spending limit of £200,000.[94] Expansion was now possible, though the financial formula would remain the same, thus explicitly linking the scope of Remploy to its commercial performance.[95] Remploy did not manage to keep in line with this funding plan, requiring several additional grants in the following years, though these were always fiercely opposed by the Treasury and subject to reductions.[96] The target or measure of keeping the company losses in line with wages paid to its disabled workers also continued. Both Barnes and Millward noted the existence of this particular target in the 1980s, but this was not a new development under the Thatcher Government geared towards economic rationalisation.[97] Rather, this target and policy were in place from this point in 1955, and remained the key measure of Remploy's efficiency throughout the period.

The improvement of Remploy's commercial efficiency also became more explicitly expressed as a goal in Parliament.[98] The Conservatives adopted the view initially expressed by the Board and endorsed by

[93] TNA LAB 20/929, 'Remploy Memorandum by Treasury' (1955). Coxall and Robins, *British Politics Since the War*, p. 22; H. Glennerster, *British Social Policy: 1945 to the Present*, 3rd Edition (Oxford, Blackwell Publishing, 2007), pp. 78–9.

[94] TNA LAB 20/929, 'Note from Sir W. Monckton to Sir Brunel Cohen, D.P.2747/1955' (16.12.1955).

[95] Ibid.

[96] TNA BM 8/2, Remploy Limited, 'Minutes of the One Hundred and Thirty-Fourth Meeting of the Board of Directors' (18.09.1957); 'Minutes of the One Hundred and Thirty-Fifth Meeting of the Board of Directors' (02.10.1957); 'Minutes of the One Hundred and Forty-First Meeting of the Board of Directors' (19.03.1958); 'Minutes of the One Hundred and Forty-Ninth Meeting of the Board of Directors' (17.12.1958).

[97] Barnes, *Disabled People and Discrimination,* p. 73; Millward, 'Invalid Definitions, Invalid Responses', pp. 184–5.

[98] See for example the debate on 'Remploy Factories', *Hansard* (19.07.1955), vol. 544, cc. 270–331.

Labour, that Remploy should provide 'genuine employment' in order to be worthwhile.[99] The Conservative governments at this time have been characterised as remaining committed to the welfare state, largely out of political necessity rather than sincere belief in its aims, but only in terms of maintenance and management.[100] This appears to be reflected in the case of Remploy, as though they remained committed to supporting the company, there was always very strict expenditure management, and a constant pressure to reduce the cost to the Exchequer.

The Remploy Board itself, while unable to reverse the overall policy, did show attempts to negotiate within this framework. They had wanted the initial temporary halt on expansion in 1949 to allow them to consolidate the business, but were not in agreement with the indefinite 'standstill order', expressing a desire instead to open as many as 20 further factories in 1952.[101] The Chairman at this time, Sir Robert Burrows, noted that under the Government economy drive, Remploy had been 'clamped down' against its wishes.[102] There was a clear demarcation here between the view of the Board, which had wanted a 'slow down', and the Conservative Government which had demanded a total halt.

Remploy became increasingly focused on improving its commercial efficiency, with the appointment of a new Managing Director, Mr Sam Green, in 1952.[103] His appointment to Remploy generated some publicity, and indeed some apprehension, with one national newspaper describing him as 'a company doctor wielding a surgeon's knife'.[104] Following his appointment, Remploy underwent a significant reorganisation on commercial lines, which included transitioning from a geographical to trade based organisation, the imposition of new sales targets and

[99] Ibid; Sir Peter Bennett, *Hansard* (06.05.1952), vol. 500, cc. 342–52.

[100] Hill, *The Welfare State in Britain*, pp. 46–7; Fraser, *The Evolution of the British Welfare State*, p. 289.

[101] Sir Peter Bennett, *Hansard* (06.05.1952), vol. 500, cc. 342–52; *Fourth Report from the Select Committee on Estimates,* 162 (1952), paras. 282–7, p. 2.

[102] *Fourth Report from the Select Committee on Estimates,* 162 (1952), paras. 282–7, p. 21; TNA LAB 20/929, 'Remploy Memorandum by Treasury' (1955).

[103] TNA BM 8/2, Remploy Limited, 'Minutes of the Seventy-eighth Meeting of the Board of Directors' (30.07.1952).

[104] TNA BM 10/2, Remploy Limited, 'A Brief Outline of the Birth and Early Development of Remploy Limited' (May, 1979), p. 19.

a public relations push.[105] The loss of some non-disabled staff was also involved, as was the closure of the factory at Maesteg which had been deemed uneconomical.[106] Despite all attempts, such efforts were to prove a question of limiting financial losses rather than generating any profit.

The growing emphasis placed on commercial efficiency was not absolute, nor did it preclude consideration of the welfare needs of disabled workers. The Board supported and encouraged a range of social and welfare activities within factories, established a welfare fund to aid sick or injured workers, rejected the suggestion that some factories be placed on 'short-time' to save money, or that large numbers of workers be 'laid off' due to shortages of work.[107] There were also occasional calls from members of the Board to reduce the focus on the commercial aspects of the company. At the annual general meeting in November 1958, the Chairman commented that it was disappointing that 'people were apt to view Remploy from a purely financial standpoint and failed to appreciate that the function of the Company was to employ productively as many severely disabled persons as possible'.[108] Overall, the perception among the Board members appears to have been that Remploy should provide sheltered employment for as many disabled people as possible, but should maximise productivity in order to reduce losses and make this goal viable.[109] Attempting to balance these objectives, and determine precisely where the emphasis should lie, often resulted in tensions

[105] Ibid., p. 20; TNA BM 8/2, Remploy Limited, 'Minutes of the Seventy-ninth Meeting of the Board of Directors' (24.09.1952).

[106] 'Remploy Factories', *Hansard* (03.02.1953), vol. 510, cc. 1633–5.

[107] TNA LAB 20/929, 'Note from Mr Wade to Mr. St. John Wilson' (29.05.1956); 'Notes P.O.3258/1953' (7–11.06.1956); 'Note from Mr. St. John Wilson to Mr Wade' (14.06.1956); TNA BM 8/2, Remploy Limited, 'Minutes of the One Hundred and Twenty-Third Meeting of the Board of Directors' (19.09.1956); 'Minutes of the One Hundred and Thirty-Fourth Meeting of the Board of Directors' (18.09.1957); TNA BM 10/2, Remploy Limited, 'A Brief Outline of the Birth and Early Development of Remploy Limited' (May, 1979), p. 29.

[108] TNA BM 8/2, Remploy Limited, 'Minutes of the Thirteenth Annual General Meeting' (19.11.1958).

[109] TNA LAB 20/929, 'Letter from Sir Walter Monckton to Sir Robert Burrows' (16.01.1954); 'Sir Brunel Cohen's Notes, D.P.2747/55' (09.11.1955); 'Note from Mr Wade to Mr St. John Wilson, D.P.2747/1955' (03.04.1956). See minutes of Board meetings throughout the period covered here in TNA BM 8/2, BM 8/3, BM 8/49, BM 8/79 and BM 8/80.

between the Conservative governments and Remploy, especially when it came to unexpected demands for reductions in expenditure.[110]

In terms of activity among MPs in the Commons, the announcement of the halt to the Remploy programme did little to quell continued demands for further expansion. Hampton has suggested that during the 1950s, governments felt little pressure to increase 'statutory provision' for disabled people.[111] Remploy marks a clear exception to this. The period of Conservative government from 1951–1964 saw repeated calls from MPs for further factories and regular criticism of policy towards Remploy. A typical example was the statement from the Labour MP for Rhondda West, Iorwerth Thomas, who called for further factories for the severely disabled, claiming 'there can be no justification at all, whatever government is in power, for holding back on this serious problem'.[112] There were also concerns raised about the focus on improving production efficiency, with the prominent back-bench Labour MP, John Paton, condemning in 1952 the growing trend of considering Remploy from a purely commercial perspective, contrary to what he considered the 'proper standpoint' of its role as a social service.[113]

As under the Attlee Government, examination of the records of Hansard reveal that interest in Remploy came almost entirely from the Labour Party, with well over 100 instances of Labour MPs commenting on Remploy, asking for further provision or a reversal of policy, during the period of Conservative Government up to 1964, compared to only a handful of Conservatives.[114] Hansard can of course only provide a limited view of political discourse among MPs and it is possible that Conservative MPs were asking for further provision through other channels. Once again however, the disparity remains striking and it is certainly clear that

[110] See numerous examples in TNA BM 8/2 and TNA BM 8/3. See also NA BM 10/2, Remploy Limited, 'A Brief Outline of the Birth and Early Development of Remploy Limited' (May, 1979).

[111] Hampton, *Disability and the Welfare State in Britain*, p. 65.

[112] Mr. Iorwerth Thomas, *Hansard* (04.02.1952), vol. 495, cc. 650–759; Mr. G. Thomas, *Hansard* (17.06.1952), vol. 502, cc. 991–2.

[113] Mr. John Paton, *Hansard* (06.05.1952), vol. 500, cc. 342–52; D. Howell, 'Paton, John (1886–1976), politician', *Oxford Dictionary of National Biography* (24.05.2008). https://www.oxforddnb.com/. Accessed 14 May 2018.

[114] See *Hansard* references to Remploy.

in terms of official discussion in the Commons it was Labour MPs who were raising the issue.

The Labour Party during this period of opposition has been characterised as being paralysed by its own internal divisions.[115] Nevertheless, the topic of Remploy became a ripe means to challenge the Government. Although there were a series of debates upon Remploy in the 1950s, the most significant wave of such attacks occurred in 1955. This began with two major debates in February during which Labour MPs admonished the Government for reducing support for Remploy and ignoring its social service role.[116] This continued in June, following a general election which had seen the Conservatives increase their majority, with Labour's future leader and later Prime Minister, Harold Wilson, condemning the Government for the lack of any new intake of workers in Remploy, describing it as 'mean' and indicative of its 'policy in social affairs'.[117] The following month saw a further major debate with a proposed motion by Labour to call 'upon the Government to remove the present restrictions and to provide facilities for extending the activities of Remploy in such a way as to absorb large numbers of disabled persons'.[118] This was highlighted in the press as an important attack by the opposition.[119] The debate opened with a lengthy statement by the prominent Labour MP, Ian Mikardo. Associated with the 'Bevanite Left' of the Labour Party, Mikardo was a signatory of the 1947 *Keep Left* pamphlet, which criticised the Attlee Government's timidity in office, and wrote *The Second Five Years* in 1948, which proposed a radical programme for a subsequent Labour administration.[120] During his address, Mikardo strongly criticised the Conservative Government's attitude to Remploy, closing with the remark that 'they should be ashamed of themselves...the Government's behaviour in this

[115] N. Deakin, *The Politics of Welfare: Continuities and Change* (London, Harvester Wheatsheaf, 1994), p. 42; Morgan, *Britain Since 1945*, p. 145.

[116] See 'Remploy Scheme', *Hansard* (17.02.1955), vol. 537, cc. 546–50; 'Remploy Scheme', *Hansard* (24.02.1955), vol. 537, cc. 1419–24.

[117] Mr. Harold Wilson, *Hansard* (10.06.1955), vol. 542, cc. 144–240.

[118] Mr. Ian Mikardo, *Hansard* (19.07.1955), vol. 544 cc. 270–331.

[119] 'Lively Debates Promised on Coal and Remploy: Labour M.P.s look for Tory split', *The Manchester Guardian* (18.07.1955).

[120] T. Dalyell, 'Mikardo, Ian [known as Mik] (1908–1993), politician', *Oxford Dictionary of National Biography* (25.05.2006). https://www.oxforddnb.com/. Accessed 27 July 2019.

matter is unworthy of the leaders of a decent and civilised community'.[121] Despite a defeated motion in this instance, comments from Labour MPs continued in a similar vein, and illustrate that there was significant support in the Labour Party for a reversal of policy towards Remploy.[122]

Developments in Policy, 1964–1979

The election of Labour, finally united under Wilson, in 1964 did see an initial relaxation in the severe financial pressure which had been on the company. This Labour Government has been characterised as having had great aspirations which were ultimately undermined by economic difficulties once in power, though it remained a 'more generous spender on social policy' than the preceding Conservative governments.[123] Hampton has suggested that the political climate at this time was favourable towards increasing welfare provision for disabled people, with Labour open to reviewing social services following the rediscovery of poverty, and the growth of the 'poverty lobby' of campaigning groups which included prominent disability groups such as the DIG and the DA.[124]

For Remploy, new '3 year plans' were introduced which allowed for a steady increase in employees, and which seem to have been agreed without much dispute.[125] Throughout the Board meeting minutes from this period, there is a visible contrast with the constant discussions of pressure from the MOL to reduce expenditure under the preceding Conservative governments.[126] However, it is difficult to credit the reduction in pressure on Remploy entirely to the change of government or any such wider factors, as, unlike the situation under the Conservatives,

[121] Mr. Ian Mikardo, *Hansard* (19.07.1955), vol. 544 cc. 270–331.

[122] See *Hansard* references to Remploy.

[123] Hill, *The Welfare State in Britain*, pp. 63–86.

[124] Hampton, *Disability and the Welfare State in Britain*, p. 88.

[125] TNA BM 8/3, Remploy Limited, 'Minutes of the Two Hundred and Sixteenth Meeting of the Board of Directors' (20.01.1965); 'Minutes of the Two Hundred and Seventeenth Meeting of the Board of Directors' (17.02.1965); 'Minutes of the Two Hundred and Nineteenth Meeting of the Board of Directors' (21.04.1965); 'Minutes of the Two Hundred and Twenty-Fourth Meeting of the Board of Directors' (20.10.1965); 'Minutes of the Two Hundred and Twenty-Seventh Meeting of the Board of Directors' (19.01.1966).

[126] See TNA BM 8/2, BM 8/3.

the commercial position of Remploy at this time was relatively robust.[127] Indeed such was the strength of the company in September 1965 that the possibility was expressed that it could increase its employee numbers to 6850 by the end of the year without needing any assistance from the Treasury.[128]

Any hope that the election of a Labour government would result in the kind of policy change called for while the Party was in opposition, with the emphasis shifting to operating Remploy more as a social service and with an expansion to meet the growing level of need, was to ultimately prove to be misplaced. Responding to the economic situation retained its primacy in determining the extent of Remploy's activities, with the MOL restricting expenditure and abandoning plans for further expansion late in 1965 due to the worsening economic conditions, which were to similarly affect other forms of social expenditure.[129] When asked directly in the Commons if the Government would attempt to move away from Remploy being run as a business and return to a social service, the response was an emphatic 'no', and echoed the original view of the Remploy Board, subsequently adopted by Conservative governments, in saying that the 'greatest service to the severely disabled men and women employed by Remploy is the provision of employment which approximates as nearly as possible to work in ordinary industry'.[130] Similarly, when asked to give a statement on policy towards Remploy, the Labour Government's response, while noting the wish to see further expansion, made clear this was based on the goal of increasing 'production

[127] TNA BM 8/3, Remploy Limited, 'Minutes of the Two Hundred and Twenty-Third Meeting of the Board of Directors' (15.09.1965); 'Minutes of the Two Hundred and Twenty-Fourth Meeting of the Board of Directors' (20.10.1965); 'Minutes of the Two Hundred and Twenty-Seventh Meeting of the Board of Directors' (19.01.1966); 'Minutes of the Two Hundred and Twenty-Ninth Meeting of the Board of Directors' (17.03.1966).

[128] TNA BM 8/3, Remploy Limited, 'Minutes of the Two Hundred and Twenty-Third Meeting of the Board of Directors' (15.09.1965); 'Minutes of the Two Hundred and Twenty-Ninth Meeting of the Board of Directors' (17.03.1966).

[129] TNA BM 8/3, Remploy Limited, 'Minutes of the Two Hundred and Twenty-Fourth Meeting of the Board of Directors' (20.10.1965); 'Minutes of the Two Hundred and Twenty-Ninth Meeting of the Board of Directors' (17.03.1966). Laybourn, *The Evolution of British Social Policy and the Welfare State*, p. 242; Hampton, *Disability and the Welfare State in Britain*, p. 242.

[130] Mr. Heffer and Mr. Marsh, *Hansard* (23.11.1964), vol. 702, cc. 130w.

and sales' to justify it.[131] This was again reiterated in 1968, with the desire expressed to increase provision under Remploy, 'if the opportunity affords and there is a necessity for it'.[132] The 'opportunity' to do so was the economic circumstances by which the scope of Remploy was then determined, regardless of which of the two major parties was in power.

Following the return of a Labour Government in 1964, and with no change in policy, we see an end to any meaningful political debate over Remploy. Contrary to the general trend identified by Hampton of a greater incidence of discussions of welfare for disabled people in the Commons at this time, there was a clear reduction in the case of Remploy.[133] Hansard reveals a number of occasions of MPs asking for further provision, or to relax the emphasis on productivity, but these were few and far between.[134] From this point onwards the majority of questions relating to Remploy, which still overwhelmingly came from Labour MPs, tended to focus on requests for information or on isolated issues such as wages or government contracts.[135] By this point the fundamental policy questions about Remploy had been answered, with the return of Labour to power the agenda was fixed, and neither party could claim, as one MP noted, a 'monopoly of virtue' while in government regarding the company.[136] There was acceptance on all sides that the commercial strength of the company was of key importance and that economic factors relating to both the country and Remploy itself were to dictate its reach.

This underlying policy was to remain throughout the period considered here. A common pattern is apparent with regards to Remploy under subsequent governments, with the strength of the company and the circumstances of the wider economy dictating the scope and what expansion, if any, took place. Each government expressed the wish to expand when times were good, yet would ultimately curtail this when times were bad, resulting in something of a 'stop–go' policy—a term used to describe

[131] Mr. Iorwerth Thomas and Mr. Gunter, *Hansard* (15.11.1965), vol. 720, cc. 18-19w.

[132] Mr. Walker, *Hansard* (21.10.1968), vol. 770, cc. 863–4.

[133] Hampton, *Disability and the Welfare State in Britain*, p. 102.

[134] Mr. Alec Jones and Mr. Roderick, *Hansard* (01.05.1972), vol. 836, cc. 11–2; Mr. Roderick, *Hansard* (30.01.1974), vol. 868, cc. 126-7w; Mr Donald Stewart, *Hansard* (17.06.1976), vol. 913, cc. 741–55.

[135] See *Hansard* references to Remploy.

[136] Mr. Harold Walker, *Hansard* (21.10.1968), vol. 770 cc.863–4.

the economic management of the period generally.[137] Thus with the financial position of the company proving strong, the Labour Government re-elected in 1966 could endorse expansion with an increase in employee numbers and with the possibility raised of further factories.[138] By 1969 however, with poor trading results, a lack of available work, and rising wages leading to an estimated shortfall of £1 million, this expansion was curtailed and the building of further factories abandoned.[139] With Remploy recovering in 1971, the Conservative Government elected the previous year under Edward Heath, similarly announced a policy of bold expansion.[140] This was against a backdrop of greater attention for the needs of disabled people generally as a result of the publicity given to the passing of the Chronically Sick and Disabled Persons Act in 1970, which comprised a number of measures for the welfare of disabled people, and the Thalidomide Scandal of 1972, in which *The Sunday Times* exposed the efforts of the distributer of the drug 'Distival', which had caused limb and organ malformations in more than 400 children, to avoid paying compensation, provoking public outrage.[141] Once again, however, this expansion was to be curtailed in the face of the economic and industrial relations crisis in 1973.[142]

Labour had moved to the Left following its defeat in 1970, promising further nationalisation in its 1973 programme, and had developed an ambitious plan to deliver further sheltered employment as part of a 'new

[137] D. Kavanagh and P. Morris, *Consensus Politics from Attlee to Major,* 2nd Edition (Oxford, Blackwell, 1994), p. 38.

[138] For numerous discussions at Board level see records of meetings 1966–1968 in TNA BM 8/3 and BM 8/49. TNA BM 10/2, Remploy Limited, 'A Brief Outline of the Birth and Early Development of Remploy Limited' (May, 1979), p. 29. Mr Coleman and Mr Gunter, *Hansard* (17.05.1966), vol. 728, cc. 237w; Mr Probert and Mr Fernyhough, *Hansard* (28.05.1968), vol. 765, cc. 202-3w; Mr Probert and Mr Fernyhough, *Hansard* (23.07.1968), vol. 769, cc. 104w.

[139] See records of meetings 1969–1970 in TNA BM 8/49.

[140] See records of meetings 1970–1973 in TNA BM 8/49. Mr. Ashley and Mr. Heath, *Hansard* (25.02.1971), vol. 812, cc. 842–3; Mr. Ashley and Mr. Dudley-Smith, *Hansard* (01.07.1971), vol. 820, cc. 557–8.

[141] Hampton, *Disability and the Welfare State in Britain*, pp. 154–68; Lowe, *The Welfare State in Britain Since 1945*, p. 283.

[142] See Board meeting minutes for 1973–1974 in TNA BM 8/49.

comprehensive disabled employment service'.[143] At the same time, the DE was undertaking a full review of sheltered employment provision, considered in greater detail in Chapter 6, which raised the possibility of greatly expanding Remploy's role. Once in government in 1974, Labour did indeed announce plans for the expansion of Remploy with a progressive increase in employees and building programme to create new factories.[144] As before, and as with Labour's other plans, this was to be curtailed in the face of increasing inflation and the severe financial crises of the mid-1970s, culminating in the imposition of 'cash limits' on Remploy in 1976 and tight control on expenditure remaining for the rest of the period, again in common with all aspects of public expenditure.[145]

As before, the Remploy Board attempted to work within the overall policy to maximise the number of disabled people it could employ and demonstrated some attempts to mitigate the emphasis on commercial performance.[146] The Managing Director appointed in 1974, Mr. Oliver Philpot, was particularly notable in this regard, continuously pushing for further expansion of the company as a priority and resisting calls for cuts from the Government.[147] Thus when faced with the limits on public expenditure in 1976 owing to the financial crisis, and with Remploy failing to keep its loss below the amount paid in wages, he continued to decry any demands for cuts as deplorable and stressed repeatedly his belief that too much emphasis was being placed upon the 'commercial objective'. Though he was unsuccessful in preventing cuts to the company and the imposition of cash limits on its expenditure, he continued to state that in his view Remploy was 'primarily a social service'.[148] The period saw

[143] Hampton, *Disability and the Welfare State in Britain*, p. 145; Kavanagh & Morris, *Consensus Politics from Attlee to Major*, pp. 28–9.

[144] See Board meeting minutes for 1974–1975 in TNA BM 8/49 and BM 8/79.

[145] See records of meetings 1975–1979 in TNA BM 8/79 and BM 8/80; Hill, *The Welfare State in Britain*, pp. 106–11.

[146] TNA BM 8/3, Remploy Limited, 'Minutes of the Two Hundred and Thirty-Fourth Meeting of the Board of Directors' (22.09.1966); 'Minutes of the Two Hundred and Thirty-Seventh Meeting of the Board of Directors' (22.12.1966); TNA BM 8/79, 'Minutes of the Three Hundred and Thirty-Third Meeting of the Board of Directors' (13.09.1975); TNA BM 10/2, Remploy Limited, 'A Brief Outline of the Birth and Early Development of Remploy Limited' (May, 1979), p. 29.

[147] See Board meeting records for 1974–1976 in TNA BM 8/49 and BM 8/79.

[148] TNA BM 8/79, Remploy Limited, 'Minutes of the Three Hundred and Thirty-Fourth Meeting of the Board of Directors' (16.10.1975); 'Minutes of the Three Hundred

continued discussion among the Board as to how the company should balance what they perceived as its dual role as social service and business, with one member highlighting in 1976 the constant embroilment of the company in this question of 'human vs. economic'.[149] A firm vision within the Board on how to balance this function was never satisfactorily established, as the Hailey Report, published by Remploy in 1980 to attempt to clarify the issue, made it clear that confusion over where the precise emphasis should lie, continued.[150]

While amounts of funding and levels of financial pressure may have varied, for successive governments, Remploy's commercial performance was always important, as were the economic circumstances of the country generally which dictated the amount each was willing to spend to fund the company's activities as part of their wider public expenditure priorities. Though it had remained a point of political debate into the 1960s, there was to be no return at any point to the initial view of the MOL in the 1940s of operating Remploy purely as a social service, with its level of provision based upon need alone. Both Conservative and Labour governments expressed the wish to see the company expand, yet this was always linked to commercial and economic factors which ultimately curtailed such plans. The same justification for this approach was adopted by both parties through use of the Remploy Board's original conception of providing 'genuine employment'. In terms of this fundamental link between economic performance and Remploy's scope, justified by this concept of 'genuine employment', a consensus in the approach to the company across governments is evident. Working within this overall policy, the Board continued to consider how best to navigate Remploy between what it considered its dual objectives. Having established for the first time how the function of Remploy developed and was understood

and Thirty-Seventh Meeting of the Board of Directors' (22.01.1976); 'Minutes of the Three Hundred and Thirty-Eighth Meeting of the Board of Directors' (19.02.1976); 'Minutes of the Three Hundred and Thirty-Ninth Meeting of the Board of Directors' (18.03.1976); 'Minutes of the Three Hundred and Fortieth Meeting of the Board of Directors' (22.04.1976); TNA BM 8/83, Remploy Limited, 'Managing Director's Report No. 262' (April, 1976).

149 TNA BM 8/79, Remploy Limited, 'Minutes of the Three Hundred and Forty-Seventh Meeting of the Board of Directors' (16.12.1976).

150 TNA BM 10/48, Remploy Limited, 'Objectives and Criteria of Success' (July, 1980), p 62.

at a policy level, this chapter will now consider the 'reality' of how the company functioned at the local factory level.

The Local Factory Level

The initial desire of the Board to establish 'genuine employment' does not seem to have been reflected in the early factory environments themselves. To meet the MOL's wish for rapid expansion, and exacerbated by the shortage of materials and capital expenditure cuts in factory building in postwar Britain, many Remploy 'factories' were established in a wide range of less-than-ideal premises.[151] Proposed sites included empty cinemas, skating rinks, chapels and buildings suffering subsidence from underground mine workings.[152] Some were former voluntary sheltered workshop buildings or government training centres.[153] Many were old and dilapidated, were designed for temporary use only, were split over separate areas or floors, or shared amenities with other companies.[154] The Bridgend factory, itself a former Royal Ordnance factory, was actually split over two buildings half-a-mile apart, and was referred to by Remploy's Executive Director as a perpetual 'embarrassment to the Company'.[155] Poorer still was the Cleator Moor 'factory', which in reality consisted of four wooden huts, one of which, the main workshop, was originally built to temporarily house prisoners of war.[156] Board members

[151] TNA BM 8/1, Disabled Persons Employment Corporation Limited, 'Minutes of the Twenty-Fifth Meeting of the Board of Directors' (30.10.1947).

[152] Remploy Limited, *We Have a Part to Play* (28.09.1988); TNA BM 10/1, Remploy Limited, 'Review of the working of the Company during its first seven years' (March, 1953), p. 13; TNA LAB 20/453, MOL, 'Disabled Persons (Employment) Act, 1944: Memorandum for Disablement Advisory Committees, Disabled Persons Employment Corporation ltd, D.A.C. Memo. No.18' (November, 1948), p. 1.

[153] 'What type of factory do you work in?', *Remploy News*, 13 (December, 1953).

[154] Ibid.

[155] 'Remploy Factory, Bridgend', *Remploy News*, 1 (December, 1952); TNA BM 10/1, Remploy Limited, 'A Review of the working of the Company during its first seven years' (March, 1953), p. 14.

[156] 'The Factory on the Moor', *Remploy News*, 2 (January, 1953).

who performed factory visits frequently commented on the poor condition or suitability of the premises they found.[157] The Glasgow site, for example, was described as 'unsuitable for use as a factory', while the Stockton factory was condemned as 'dismal'.[158]

The factories Remploy wanted to use, were those built to its own specification by the Ministry of Works.[159] These were all on one floor with 'airy well-heated workshops, good canteens and kitchens which provided a hot mid-day meal, out-buildings for wheelchairs in many cases and often with pleasant frontages'.[160] However, as can be seen in Table 3.1, by 1952 when there were 91 Remploy factories, less than half were these custom-designed premises.

As time went on and policy focused more fully on commercial efficiency and 'genuine employment', the adopted premises continued to be replaced by the custom-built factories.[161] Due to the costs involved,

Table 3.1 Types of Remploy factory premises, 1952

Built by the Ministry of Works for Remploy	38
Ex-government training centre premises	23
Premises acquired and adapted	20
Sheltered workshops taken over	5
Ex-Royal Ordnance factories	3
Board of Trade factories	2

Source TNA BM 10/1, Remploy Limited, 'A Review of the working of the Company during its first seven years' (March, 1953), p. 34

[157] See for example, TNA BM 8/1, Disabled Persons Employment Corporation Limited, 'Minutes of the Thirty-Second Meeting of the Board of Directors' (27.04.1948); 'Minutes of the Thirty-Sixth Meeting of the Board of Directors' (29.09.1948); 'Minutes of the Thirty-Eighth Meeting of the Board of Directors' (24.11.1948); 'Minutes of the Forty-Fourth Meeting of the Board of Directors' (25.05.1949).

[158] TNA BM 8/1, Disabled Persons Employment Corporation Limited, 'Minutes of the Thirty-Eighth Meeting of the Board of Directors' (24.11.1948); 'Minutes of the Forty-Fourth Meeting of the Board of Directors' (25.05.1949).

[159] TNA BM 10/7, Ministry of Works, 'British Factories for Disabled Persons Employment Ltd: Model Plans' (June, 1946).

[160] 'What type of factory do you work in?', *Remploy News*, 13 (December, 1953).

[161] For information on premises see TNA BM 3/32.

this was done piecemeal and as such, problems continued.[162] The Neath factory, for example, was reported to be in such a poor state by the early 1970s that workers were raising concerns about their own safety.[163] A 1976 internal report highlighted the continued use of adopted sites with unsuitable facilities for disabled people, which it claimed was leading to low morale among workers.[164] Echoing the original complaints from nearly 30 years earlier, the report also suggested that some premises were 'basically unsuitable' for productive work, with dispersed work areas, sometimes across multiple floor levels.[165] This was the case with the Blackburn factory, which also had 'holes in the roof' which meant it was 'regularly flooded'.[166] The intention was to press the Government for permission to move out of 'all the remaining unsuitable premises' as soon as possible.[167] By the end of 1979, however, of 88 Remploy factories then in operation, 26 remained non-purpose built premises.[168] It is clear therefore, that despite the rhetoric around the function of Remploy being to provide 'genuine employment' and the attempts to promote commercial efficiency, this was not always reflected in terms of the factory itself, with wide variation in quality and suitability throughout the period.

There were also challenges in securing and providing the 'genuine' work desired. This was particularly problematic in the early years of

[162] TNA BM 8/3, Remploy Limited, 'Minutes of the One Hundred and Seventy-Fifth Meeting of the Board of Directors' (20.04.1961); 'Minutes of the Two Hundred and Twenty-Third Meeting of the Board of Directors' (15.09.1965); 'Minutes of the Two Hundred and Forty-Third Meeting of the Board of Directors' (22.06.1967); 'Minutes of the Two Hundred and Forty-Ninth Meeting of the Board of Directors' (18.01.1968); TNA BM 8/49, 'Minutes of the Two Hundred and Fifty-Fifth Meeting of the Board of Directors' (18.07.1968); 'Minutes of the Three Hundred and Thirteenth Meeting of the Board of Directors' (21.11.1973); TNA BM 8/79, 'Minutes of the Three Hundred and Twenty-Eighth Meeting of the Board of Directors' (20.03.1975); 'Minutes of the Three Hundred and Sixty-Second Meeting of the Board of Directors' (21.04.1978).

[163] TNA BM 3/32, 'Note from Personnel Director, Neath Factory' (31.08.1972).

[164] TNA BM 8/83, Remploy Limited, 'Appendix to Board Report no. 266 "The Location of Uneconomic Factories"' (September, 1976).

[165] Ibid.

[166] Ibid.

[167] Ibid.

[168] TNA BM 3/67, Remploy Limited, 'Report on Employment of Disabled People in Remploy—1979: Appendix 1' (September, 1979).

Remploy's operation, with a chronic lack of orders and materials.[169] The latter was to prove particularly frustrating, with the Hull factory receiving an order for 2800 doors which, because of the difficulty in obtaining suitable materials, was withdrawn and given to another firm.[170] Worker 'idle time' was a significant and persistent issue. With the reduction of employee numbers to reflect available work not an option, in many factories, workers were turning up regardless of whether or not there was anything to do and being paid to do so.[171] This was not only contrary to the Board's goal of 'genuine employment' but was considered one of the chief reasons for the company's financial losses.[172] Remploy had no reserved lines of production and had to tender commercially. It had always been assumed however, from the Tomlinson Report onwards, that government departments would form a significant proportion of the company's market.[173] This assumption proved to be false however, with Remploy often bemoaning the scarcity of such orders.[174] Many factory managers were forced to take orders for whatever work could be found. One result of this was that much of the initial work undertaken ended up being the kind of low-skilled busy work the Board had expressly wished to avoid. One of the very first Remploy employees, later recalled that the Bridgend factory 'was a bit of a shambles to start with – there wasn't any proper work sorted out for us. We had to go round the factory picking

[169] TNA BM 8/1, Disabled Persons Employment Corporation Limited, 'Minutes of the Twenty-Second Meeting of the Board of Directors' (27.05.1947); TNA LAB 20/453, 'Four Year Progress of the Disabled Persons Employment Corporation, D.P.802/1949'.

[170] TNA LAB 20/453, 'Ministry of Labour Note, D.O.802/1949' (27.06.1949).

[171] TNA BM 8/1, Disabled Persons Employment Corporation Limited, 'Minutes of the Twenty-Second Meeting of the Board of Directors' (27.05.1947).

[172] Ibid.; TNA BM 8/1, 'Minutes of the Twenty-Ninth Meeting of the Board of Directors' (27.01.1948).

[173] Mr. Chetwynd, *Hansard*, 449, col. 781–2 (13.04.1948); *Report of Inter-departmental Committee on the Rehabilitation and Resettlement of Disabled Persons*, 6415 (1943), para. 90–91, p. 34. See also the minutes of the Board of Directors in TNA BM 8/1.

[174] TNA BM 8/1, Disabled Persons Employment Corporation Limited, 'Minutes of the Thirty-First Meeting of the Board of Directors' (06.04.1948); TNA LAB 20/444, Disabled Persons Employment Corporation Limited, 'Executive Director's Report No. 34' (21.10.1948).

up bits of metal which we made into petrol floats for cars'.[175] A further example was given by an employee in the Dundee factory, who recalled how the factory manager would travel around the local farms collecting broken items for the staff to repair.[176] Seeking such ad hoc work meant that factories would often have numerous short-term small-scale jobs going on at the same time within a factory.[177] This made production efficiency virtually impossible with employees having to be constantly re-trained, and factories re-tooled, to meet the demands of a diverse range of orders.[178]

The ending of the initial period of expansion and subsequent focus on commercial efficiency brought some improvement. Remploy was restructured from a geographical to a trade grouping with some standard products lines introduced.[179] In doing so, Remploy attempted to focus on the national market and large-scale orders.[180] The desired new production lines included the sole manufacturing and sales rights for the Swedish *Lundia* shelving range, which remained a key product for decades.[181] There were also attempts to secure an international market and by the early 1960s Remploy was exporting goods, including furniture, travel bags, protective clothing and knitwear, to 35 countries.[182] We should not overstate this standardisation and move to new trades. Despite the reorganisation into trade groups, there remained significant variation in the precise type of work undertaken in each factory, and it

[175] Quoted in 'A Living Tale', *Remploy News: Golden Jubilee Special* (April, 1995).

[176] Remploy Limited, *We Have a Part to Play* (28.09.1988).

[177] TNA BM 8/1, Disabled Persons Employment Corporation Limited, 'Minutes of the Twenty-Second Meeting of the Board of Directors' (27.05.1947).

[178] TNA BM 10/1, Remploy Limited, 'A Review of the working of the Company during its first seven years' (March, 1953), pp. 14–5; TNA LAB 20/453, 'Note to Mr Maher' (27.05.1949).

[179] TNA BM10/2, Remploy Limited, 'A Brief Outline of the Birth and Early Development of Remploy Limited' (May, 1979), p. 20.

[180] TNA BM 10/1, Remploy Limited, 'A Review of the working of the Company during its first seven years' (March, 1953), pp. 7–8.

[181] TNA BM10/2, Remploy Limited, 'A Brief Outline of the Birth and Early Development of Remploy Limited' (May, 1979), p. 21.

[182] Ibid.

was common for them to change trades in response to economic conditions.[183] Incorporating a range of trades across its organisation meant that Remploy was always vulnerable to market fluctuations.[184] Government contracts continued to be in short supply and tendered with very slight margins.[185] This was particularly galling given the focus on commercial efficiency espoused by successive governments, which were then seen to be unsupportive in the case of providing this kind of work. For most factories a steady stream of work was never permanently secured and as a result, instances of short-term ad hoc work, including that found locally by factory managers, continued to be undertaken and idle time for workers continued to be a significant problem.[186] There was always therefore significant variation in whether the work undertaken in each local factory was commercially efficient or reflective of the concept of 'genuine employment'.

Given that much of Remploy's operation varied at the local level, the position of manager was key in determining how a factory functioned. In one sense there were the practical issues already addressed, such as how effective they were in organising the factory premises and how able they were to secure work when local sourcing was needed. They would also determine to a significant extent the level of focus on productivity or welfare in the factory through their management and relationship with

[183] See TNA BM 6, and in Board Meetings, see TNA BM 8. For specific examples, see Board Meetings for May 1958, February 1959 in BM 8/2; May 1965, December 1966 in BM 8/3; April 1969, September 1971, October 1971, February 1972, March 1972, April 1972, December 1974 in BM 8/49; May 1975, September 1975, July 1977, October 1977, January 1978, February 1978 Mar 1978, April 1978 in BM 8/79.

[184] TNA BM10/2, Remploy Limited, 'A Brief Outline of the Birth and Early Development of Remploy Limited' (May, 1979), p. 23.

[185] *Fourth Report from the Select Committee on Estimates,* 162 (1952), para. 190, pp. 15–16. See also TNA BM 8/2, Remploy Limited, 'Minutes of the One Hundred and Eighth Meeting of the Board of Directors' (04.05.1955); 'Minutes of the One Hundred and Nineteenth Meeting of the Board of Directors' (18.04.1956); 'Minutes of the One Hundred and Fortieth Meeting of the Board of Directors' (19.02.1958); 'Minutes of the One Hundred and Forty-Fourth Meeting of the Board of Directors' (18.06.1958); TNA BM 8/3, 'Minutes of the Two Hundred and Thirty-Seventh Meeting of the Board of Directors' (22.12.1966).

[186] See minutes of Board meetings in TNA BM 8, for example, December 1966 in BM 8/3; April 1969, September 1971, October 1971, February 1972, March 1972, April 1972, December 1974 in BM 8/49; May 1975, September 1975, July 1977, October 1977, January 1978, March 1978, April 1978 in BM 8/79.

the disabled workers. As might be expected, cases where this balance was well struck, with productive factories and a happy workforce, do not make as notable a mark in the archival records as where issues arose. We do see some examples in *Remploy News*, a regular newsletter produced by the company, which was keen to emphasise the well-being of employees with a focus on social and welfare activities.[187] The views and experiences of the disabled workforce themselves are not easy to ascertain. A letter, written in 1952 was presented to the Board from a worker at the St Helen's factory who wished to thank the company, 'in appreciation for all that has been done for me'.[188] Describing her initial hesitance at working in a factory, she notes that she soon felt comfortable and engaged in her work:

> Soon confidence in myself returned, and now I go merrily on, feeling that again life is worthwhile. We disabled people do appreciate all that is being done for us by Remploy. We are all so happy, working in our pleasant, modern factory, with 'music while you work', at jobs specially chosen for us. So, days at Remploy pass quickly by with a smile and a song.[189]

There may well have been factories which reflected this image, and while well-being and productivity are not mutually exclusive concepts, the overall impression from the records is that managers were in most cases focused upon maximising the productivity of the factory and operating them as commercially as possible.[190] This appears to have been the case for the simple reason that it was on the basis of productivity and economic efficiency that factories and their managers were ultimately judged by Remploy's Head Office.[191] The rhetoric described earlier in this chapter from Board members of the need to balance this with the well-being of employees, particularly following the appointment of Mr

[187] See *Remploy News* in TNA BM 6. See also 'Steady Growth of Sheltered Employment', *Financial Times,* (07.04.1970).

[188] TNA BM 8/4, 'Letter to Mr McDonnell' (16.12.1952).

[189] Ibid.

[190] TNA LAB 20/444, Disabled Persons Employment Corporation Limited, 'Executive Director Circular 7A/1' (06.10.1948).

[191] TNA BM 3/47, Remploy Limited, 'Area Liaison Officer to Personnel Director: Disabled People Entry Standard for Employment in Remploy Ltd' (27.01.1975); 'Pontefract Area Liaison Officer to Personnel Director: Disabled People Entry Standard for Employment at Remploy Limited' (28.01.1975); 'Report on a Mentally Disabled Teach-in' (05.12.1974).

Philpott as Managing Director in the 1970s, who himself suggested that from his visits to factories there was too much focus on the commercial aspect, seems not to have been reflected in the reality for factory managers.[192] This point was emphasised in an internal report in 1980, with managers complaining of a continuing disconnect between the policy espoused by the Board, and the reality of their day-to-day dealings with Head Office.[193] A factory manager could therefore do all they could to promote the well-being of employees, but ultimately the systems in place to judge their performance were based on commercial factors.

We do see instances of disabled workers themselves expressing concern, either directly, or through reports to the press or local MP. This was particularly prevalent in the aftermath of the productivity drive of the early 1950s.[194] The Labour MP John McKay raised concerns in the Commons in 1951 at reports of 'dissatisfaction in the Remploy Factory at Wallsend', owing to pressures to increase factory productivity.[195] A further case was reported the following year and in April 1954, a letter was sent to 'all Members of Parliament, the Board of Directors of Remploy and to the National Press', from the employees of the Croydon Factory, complaining about the productivity pressures in the factory.[196] Further instances punctuate the period, with an employee at the Aberdeen factory writing to his MP in 1960 to complain about harsh conditions in the factory, and in 1972 a letter reached the Managing Director from workers at the Bolton Factory, calling for the dismissal of the manager 'before we are at rock bottom'.[197] Occasionally this dissatisfaction did lead to industrial action. In 1960, unrest was reported in the Barking factory, with the employees

[192] TNA BM 8/79, Remploy Limited, 'Minutes of the Three Hundred and Thirty-Seventh Meeting of the Board of Directors' (22.01.1976); TNA BM 10/48, Remploy Limited, 'Objectives and Criteria of Success' (July, 1980), p. 62.

[193] TNA BM 10/48, Remploy Limited, 'Objectives and Criteria of Success' (July, 1980), p. 62.

[194] See TNA LAB 43/204; TNA BM 8/23, 'Note from Works Manager to Controller, Woodworking Group' (28.03.1955).

[195] Mr. John McKay, *Hansard* (24.07.1951), vol. 491, cc. 180–1.

[196] Mr. G. Thomas, *Hansard* (17.06.1952), vol. 502, cc. 991–2; TNA BM 8/2, Remploy Limited, 'Minutes of the Ninety-Seventh Meeting of the Board of Directors' (28.04.1954).

[197] TNA BM 8/2, Remploy Limited, 'Minutes of the One Hundred and Sixty-Sixth Meeting of the Board of Directors' (15.06.1960); TNA BM 8/84, 'Letter to Managing Director' (1976).

intending to go on strike.[198] In 1970 there was a strike at the Swansea factory lasting 'nearly two days', and in 1976 the Motherwell factory, described as one with 'a history of militancy', went on a 'go-slow'.[199] While such incidents were alarming and indicate the existence of resistance from some workers to productivity pressures, they were understood by the Board at the time to be isolated incidents rather than representing widespread dissatisfaction.

The examples here highlight the localised nature of Remploy. Wide variation in terms of environment, work and conditions were particularly notable in the early days of the company, and despite some standardisation, clearly continued. Overall, it is apparent that there was no uniform 'Remploy factory experience', and it did not function as a fully cohesive scheme. In one case, a disabled worker may have attended a modern purpose-built factory and engaged in meaningful, regular and satisfying work on a standard product line under a considerate manager. In another case, a disabled worker may have attended a poor-quality adapted building, engaged in some simple busy work with time spent idle and placed under pressure from a factory manager desperate to improve their commercial performance for Head Office.

Conclusions

It is clear from the analysis undertaken here that any notion that Remploy commenced with a clear and uncomplicated purpose is misplaced. There were different visions of its primary objectives, in terms of where the emphasis should lie, which continued to be contested as the company began to operate. Furthermore, contrary to the idea that Remploy existed as a humanitarian concern throughout this period, only to suffer harsh economic rationalisation under Thatcher Governments in the 1980s, it is apparent that commercial efficiency was highlighted as a key component for Remploy from the beginning. This was the view of the Board

[198] TNA BM 8/2, Remploy Limited, 'Minutes of the One Hundred and Sixty-Second Meeting of the Board of Directors' (17.02.1960); 'Minutes of the One Hundred and Sixty-Third Meeting of the Board of Directors' (16.03.1960).

[199] TNA BM 8/49, Remploy Limited, 'Minutes of the Two-Hundred and Seventy-Second Meeting of the Board of Directors' (19.02.1970); TNA BM 8/79, 'Minutes of the Three Hundred and Fortieth Meeting of the Board of Directors' (22.04.1976).

of Remploy themselves, and indeed something central to their understood conception of the company providing 'genuine employment'. This was not, however, the initial view espoused by the MOL and MPs who instead demanded the rapid expansion of the company as a social service meeting the need for providing sheltered employment for all those eligible to receive it. However, with costs rising, and with the expansion of the company making the concept of 'genuine employment' unworkable, the Remploy Board and the Treasury were aligned in demanding a slowdown from the MOL and succeeded in attaining it. Thus, as early as the 1950s the commercial efficiency of Remploy, in concert with the prevailing economic conditions, had become a paramount issue in determining its development.

This did lead to protest from the Labour Party during its period in opposition in the 1950s and early 1960s. Contrary therefore, to the view that disabled people were only discovered 'politically' from the 1960s, it is clear that in the form of Remploy, disability was part of a significant policy debate much earlier.[200] Once in government however, Labour was to adopt the same policy towards Remploy and thereby end any serious reconsideration of its purpose. The pattern emerged of each government seemingly valuing Remploy and expressing the wish to see it expand, but the commercial strength of the company, and the expenditure limits of each government when faced with economic difficulties, ultimately curtailing such expansion. Thus, the 'stop–go' approach to public spending which characterised the period more generally, certainly applies to Remploy.[201] As such we can see that in terms of a consensus, though financial support and pressure to reduce costs varied, the fundamental principle established by 1950 that Remploy's commercial strength, and economic conditions generally, were always to limit its scope remained the case for each party in government. Despite some continued opposition to this in Parliament, the overall policy for sheltered employment was set. Such findings support the notion of a 'consensus in action' in

[200] J. Hampton, 'Discovering Disability: The General Classes of Disabled People and the Classic Welfare State, 1948–1964', *The Historian*, vol. 75, no. 1 (2013), pp. 70–1; Hampton, *Disability and the Welfare State in Britain*, pp. 8, 50; S. Sainsbury, 'Disabled People and the Personal Social Services', in D. Gladstone, (ed.) *British Social Welfare: Past, Present and Future* (London, UCL Press, 1995), pp. 183–8; E. Younghusband, *Social Work in Britain: 1950–1975* (London, Allen and Unwin, 1978), pp. 210–11.

[201] Kavanagh and Morris, *Consensus Politics from Attlee to Major*, p. 38.

disability policy, with both parties ultimately following the same approach when in government, if not demonstrating a unified ideology, for much of the period.[202]

Working within this overall policy, the Board did attempt to expand provision and expressed a wish to mitigate the emphasis on commercial efficiency to a degree. Peter Dorey has suggested that the Boards of nationalised industries commonly faced difficulties in attempting to operate their company as a business in the market economy while being under overall ministerial responsibility.[203] He suggested that this often resulted in a 'messy' compromise as they were thus 'sometimes put in a position whereby they were simultaneously expected to act both as a commercial enterprise and as a social or public service'.[204] This echoes something of the apparent difficulties faced by the Remploy Board. It seems therefore, the description of an 'uneasy balance' between humanitarian and economic aims described by Lonsdale and Topliss, is apt when considering the discussions which occurred at Board level within Remploy.[205]

The common justification for the overall policy towards Remploy was through reference to a conception of it needing to provide 'genuine employment' in order to be of value to its disabled employees, with commercial efficiency an apparent key requisite for this. It was this concept, initially espoused by the Board, which subsequently became entrenched as a core aspect of this kind of sheltered employment, distinguishing such provision from alternative forms relating to occupational therapy and rehabilitation. Incorporating an emphasis on commercial efficiency to deliver this 'genuine employment', aligning with 'open industry' as much as possible, was necessary to unlock the benefits of productive work for both the individual worker and the company. For the Board, this appears to have stemmed from a genuine belief that this was a crucial aspect of Remploy's service to its disabled employees. It is not possible to gauge the degree to which this sentiment was genuinely shared by the successive governments which evoked it, but it does not seem overly

202 Millward, 'Invalid definitions, invalid responses', pp. 165, 284; Hampton, *Disability and the Welfare State in Britain*, p. 244.

203 Dorey, *British Politics Since 1945*, p. 9.

204 Ibid.

205 Lonsdale, *Work and Inequality*, p. 138; Topliss, *Provision for the Disabled*, pp. 55–7.

cynical to suggest that this could also be a useful justification to limit expenditure and press for financial savings from the company.

It is clear however, that this policy of commercial efficiency to provide 'genuine employment' was not always reflected in terms of the reality at factory level. There was always wide local variation in Remploy factory environments, work and conditions which belie any assumption that Remploy represented a cohesive scheme with central policy reflecting a uniform factory reality. Workers in Remploy could clearly experience a very different type of sheltered employment depending on their locality. The overall emphasis in terms of individual factory performance, however, remained one of commercial efficiency, which was keenly felt by many factory managers.

CHAPTER 4

'If We Do Not Want a Man, We Do Not Take Him', Eligibility, Recruitment and Retention

Introduction

Remploy provided the vast majority of sheltered employment in Britain during the period examined here. While there is no complete breakdown of how many disabled people were employed by the company overall during this time, as those that left for various reasons were replaced, the figures available suggest that by 1979, Remploy had provided sheltered employment for more than 40,000 disabled people.[1] The composition of Remploy's workforce has largely been taken for granted by academics across disciplines as being 'disabled people', 'severely disabled' people', or in the case of Borsay, Bolderson and Thane, disabled people who were deemed unproductive workers.[2] The assumption is that Remploy

[1] The National Archives (TNA) BM 3/67, Remploy Limited, 'Report on Employment of Disabled People in Remploy—1979: Appendix 9'; TNA BM 10/2, Remploy Limited, 'A Brief Outline of the Birth and Early Development of Remploy Limited' (May, 1979), p. 30; TNA BM 10/53, Remploy Ltd, 'Remploy Facts' (1986), p. 3.

[2] J. Hampton, 'Discovering Disability: The General Classes of Disabled People and the Classic Welfare State, 1948–1964', *The Historian*, vol. 75, no. 1 (2013), p. 80; L. Bryder, *Below the Magic Mountain: A Social History of Tuberculosis in Twentieth-Century Britain* (Oxford, Clarendon Press, 1988), p. 237; S. Wheatcroft, *Worth Saving: Disabled Children During the Second World War* (Manchester, Manchester University Press, 2013), p. 168; M. Hyde, 'Sheltered and Supported Employment in the 1990s: The Experiences

© The Author(s), under exclusive license to Springer Nature Switzerland AG 2025

A. Holroyde, *Sheltered Employment and Disability in the British Welfare State*, New Directions in Welfare History,
https://doi.org/10.1007/978-3-031-87876-3_4

simply, and successfully, followed the remit established for it by the DPEA in employing those designated severely disabled, referred to as 'Section II'. The degree to which Remploy functioned as a catch-all scheme for severely disabled people, has important implications for our understanding of disability in postwar Britain as there is a widely held image of the welfare state excluding disabled people, and the other measures of the DPEA failing to live up to their initial promise.[3] This is also important when we consider that securing 'full employment' among the general population was a key element in the classic welfare state settlement, and has been seen as a major achievement by scholars such as Lowe, Glennerster and Page.[4] This chapter will therefore consider whether this

of Disabled Workers in the UK', *Disability & Society*, vol. 13, no. 2 (1998), p. 200; P. Bridgen and R. Lowe, *Welfare Policy Under the Conservatives 1951–1964* (London, PRO, 1998), pp. 262–3; H. Bolderson, *Social Security, Disability and Rehabilitation: Conflicts in the Development of Social Policy 1914–1946* (London, Jessica Kingsley Publishers, 1991), p 109; E. Topliss, *Provision for the Disabled* (Oxford, Basil Blackwell, 1979), p. 56; M. Reiss, *Blind Workers Against Charity: The National League of the Blind of Great Britain and Ireland, 1893–1970* (London, Palgrave Macmillan, 2015), p. 139; E. Elsey, 'The Rehabilitation and Employment of Disabled Ex-Servicemen after the Two World Wars', unpublished PhD Thesis, University of Teesside (1994), pp. 276–7; J. Anderson, "Turned into Taxpayers': Paraplegia, Rehabilitation and Sport at Stoke Mandeville, 1944–56', *Journal of Contemporary History*, vol. 38, no. 3 (2003), p. 469; C. Barnes, *Disabled People in Britainand Discrimination* (London, C. Hurst & Co., 2000), p. 71; A. Land, R. Lowe and N. Whiteside, *The Development of the Welfare State 1939–1951: A Guide to Documents in the Public Record Office* (London, HMSO, 1992), p. 204; M. Mantin, 'Coalmining and the National Scheme for Disabled Ex-Servicemen after the First World War', *Social History*, vol. 41, no. 2 (2016), p. 170; A. Borsay, *Disability and Social Policy in Britain Since 1750: A History of Exclusion* (Basingstoke, Palgrave Macmillan, 2005), p. 135; H. Bolderson, 'The Origins of the Disabled Persons Employment Quota and its Symbolic Significance', *Journal of Social Policy*, vol. 9, no. 2 (1980), p. 178; P. Thane, *Foundations of the Welfare State, 2nd Edition* (London, Longman, 1996), p. 225.

[3] Hampton, 'Discovering Disability', pp. 75–7; J. Hampton, *Disability and the Welfare State in Britain: Changes in Perception and Policy 1948–79* (Bristol, Policy Press, 2016); p. 1; Bolderson, 'The Origins of the Disabled Persons Employment Quota and its Symbolic Significance', pp. 170–2; A. Roulstone and S. Prideaux, *Understanding Disability Policy* (Bristol, Policy Press, 2012), pp. 26–32; Hyde, 'Sheltered and Supported Employment in the 1990s', p. 200.

[4] R. Lowe, *The Welfare State in Britain Since 1945* (Basingstoke, Palgrave Macmillan, 2005), pp. 80–1, 115–9; R. Page, *Revisiting the Welfare State* (Maidenhead, Open University Press, 2007), p. 38; D. Fraser, *The Evolution of the British Welfare State*, 4th Edition (Basingstoke, Palgrave Macmillan, 2009), pp. 267–8; H. Glennerster, *British Social Policy: 1945 to the Present*, 3rd Edition (Oxford, Blackwell Publishing, 2007), p. 5; K. Laybourn, *The Evolution of British Social Policy and the Welfare State, c.1800–1993* (Keele, Keele

was indeed achieved for the Section II population through sheltered employment.

In some cases, descriptions of Remploy's workforce have highlighted particular groups. One enduring view holds that Remploy provided employment primarily for ex-service personnel, a cohort considered to have received preferential treatment in terms of welfare and employment.[5] Anderson highlighted Remploy as part of the continued 'special treatment' afforded to this group.[6] Anderson further suggested that Remploy concentrated on providing employment for those with particular disabilities, specifically 'pulmonary tuberculosis, congenital deformities, heart and lung disease, and epilepsy'.[7] In all these descriptions of Remploy, it is assumed that the production workforce consisted entirely of disabled people. This is also implicit in descriptions of sheltered employment as 'segregated employment', and was the long-standing belief within Remploy itself as an aspect of its past which distinguished the company from its international equivalents for whom the inclusion of non-disabled people in the workforce was the norm.[8] By contrast, Topliss claimed in 1979 that the inclusion of a proportion of non-disabled workers in the

University Press, 1995), p. 241; S. Sainsbury, 'Disabled People and the Personal Social Services', in D. Gladstone, (ed.) *British Social Welfare: Past, Present and Future* (London, UCL Press, 1995), p. 184.

[5] See for example, BBC News 'What are Remploy workers doing now?', (31.11.2014). http://www.bbc.co.uk/news/uk-29843567. Accessed 16 August 2024; R. Slorach, *A Very Capitalist Condition: A History and Politics of Disability* (London, Bookmarks, 2016), p. 141; W. Gagen, 'Remastering the Body, Renegotiating Gender: Physical Disability and Masculinity during the First World War, the Case of J.B. Middlebrook', *European Review of History*, vol. 14, no. 4, pp. 536–7; J. Bourke, *Dismembering the Male: Men's Bodies, Britain and the Great War* (London, Reaktion Books, 1996), pp. 37–9; Hampton, *Disability and the Welfare State in Britain*, pp. 53–4.

[6] J. Anderson, *War, Disability and Rehabilitation in Britain: 'Soul of a Nation'* (Manchester, Manchester University Press, 2011), p. 183.

[7] Ibid.

[8] G. Millward, 'Invalid Definitions, Invalid Responses: Disability and the Welfare State, 1965–1995', unpublished PhD Thesis, London School of Hygiene and Tropical Medicine (2013), pp. 184–5; S. Humphries and P. Gordon, *Out of Sight: The Experience of Disability 1900–1950* (Plymouth, Northcote House, 1992), p. 138; Wheatcroft, *Worth Saving*, p. 168; Slorach, *A Very Capitalist Condition*, p. 141; Hyde, 'Sheltered and Supported Employment in the 1990s', p. 200; Barnes, *Disabled People in Britain and Discrimination*, p. 74.

production workforce was 'always envisaged' for Remploy.[9] This chapter will explore this aspect of Remploy by addressing the fundamental question of who was employed by the company and the basis upon which this occurred.

This will begin with an exploration of statutory eligibility for sheltered employment under the terms of the DPEA, and an analysis to determine whether 'full employment' for severely disabled people was achieved. The chapter will then consider how recruitment for Remploy was undertaken and address the question of retention once employment was gained. The case presented by Anderson that Remploy focused on employing people with specific disabilities will then be analysed, through exploration of what was referred to by the company as its 'disability mix'. Finally, the chapter will explore the assumption that Remploy only employed disabled people in its production workforce.

Eligibility Under the Terms of the DPEA

Gaining entry to Remploy involved a specific process which all potential workers had to follow. The initial step was registering as 'disabled' upon the Disabled Persons' Employment Register, which has itself received only limited attention from historians.[10] The register was the voluntary mechanism established by the DPEA for accessing any of its provisions—including sheltered employment. Even at this stage there were regulations limiting who could join the register. First, a person had to be considered disabled as defined by the Act, which stated that:

> 'Disabled person' – means a person who, on account of injury, disease or congenital deformity, is substantially handicapped in obtaining or keeping employment, or in undertaking work on his own account, of a kind which apart from that injury, disease or deformity would be suited to his age, experience and qualifications.[11]

[9] Topliss, *Provision for the Disabled,* pp. 55–6.

[10] Borsay, *Disability and Social Policy in Britain Since 1750*, p. 135; Topliss, *Provision for the Disabled*, p. 49.

[11] DPEA, para. 1.

The Act further stipulated that a person's disability must be likely to last for 6 months or more, that the person must be at least 14 years old, be resident in Great Britain, and be willing to undertake training or employment.[12] Those disqualified from registering included disabled people undergoing treatment under the Lunacy and Mental Treatments Acts, prisoners, full-time hospital patients and those deemed to be of 'bad character'.[13] It was also possible to be removed from the register for refusal to attend training, rehabilitation or employment once offered.[14]

This legislative framework remained largely the same throughout the period covered here, and indeed into the 1990s.[15] The only significant changes were that from 1958, a person's disability had to be likely to continue for 12 months instead of 6, and in 1959, mentally-ill patients were no longer disqualified from registering.[16] Such changes provide an important example of how 'disability' can be defined and how this can change over time.[17] Here we see an example of what Millward has referred to as a 'bureaucratic' conception of disability, as one defined for purposes of policy and legislation.[18] This conception in particular is not

[12] DPEA, para. 7; Statutory Rule and Order (1945), No. 938 in Bolderson, *Social Security, Disability and Rehabilitation*, p. 117.

[13] Ibid.; See also TNA LAB 20/109.

[14] Statutory Rule and Order (1945), No. 938 in Bolderson, *Social Security, Disability and Rehabilitation*, p. 117.

[15] TNA BM 10/34, Remploy Limited, 'Report of the Working Party on the Mix of Disabilities Employed by Remploy', p. 9; TNA ET 2/32, ESA, 'The Disabled Persons Register' (1977). DE, *The Net Exchequer Costs of Sheltered Employment*, Research Paper No. 69 (1989), p. 3; Borsay, *Disability and Social Policy in BritainSince 1750*, p. 135; Topliss, *Provision for the Disabled*, p. 49; Bolderson, *Social Security, Disability and Rehabilitation*, p. 170; A. Holroyde, 'Sheltered Employment and Mental Health in Britain: Remploy c.1945–81', in S.J. Taylor and A. Brumby (eds.), *Healthy Minds in the Twentieth Century: In and Beyond the Asylum* (Palgrave Macmillan, 2020), pp. 113–35.

[16] *Disabled Persons Employment Act 1958* amendments. Bolderson, *Social Security, Disability and Rehabilitation*, p. 117.

[17] See Millward, 'Invalid Definitions, Invalid Responses', pp. 14–20; G. Millward, 'Social Security Policy and the Early Disability Movement—Expertise, Disability, and the Government, 1965–77', *Twentieth Century British History*, vol. 26, no. 2 (2015), p. 281; Sainsbury, 'Disabled People and the Personal Social Services', pp. 183–4; J.E. Bickenbach, *Physical Disability and Social Policy* (Toronto, University of Toronto Press, 1993), pp. 20–3; T. Moreton, 'Sheltered Employment: Gateway or 'road block"?, *Personnel Review*, vol. 21, no. 6 (1992), p. 40.

[18] Millward, 'Invalid Definitions, Invalid Responses', p. 43.

static, as can been seen here with a shifting boundary in what was accepted as 'disabled' in terms of the aims of the legislation, with the introduction of a previously excluded group in those mentally-ill patients. While such stipulations meant that some disabled people would be excluded from registering and thereby excluded from Remploy, it is worth noting the relatively broad definition of 'disability' enshrined in the Act.

In addition to those automatically excluded, there were a large number of disabled people who, despite being eligible, chose not to register. In a study published in 1979, Topliss noted a 'steady decline in total numbers on the register since the peak year of 1950'.[19] Figures indeed show that from this peak of 936,196 people on the register, both employed and unemployed, in 1950, by 1961 this had dropped to 666,454, and by 1977 had reduced again to 532,402.[20] Remploy themselves estimated that by 1979 the overall number of people who were likely eligible for registration was over 1 million.[21] Several reasons have been suggested, both by Remploy at the time, and others such as Topliss since, as to why eligible disabled people chose not to register. Chief among these were that they may not have been aware of the need to do so; that they felt it was unnecessary based on their own circumstances; that they saw little benefit from what was offered; that they could receive more money in the form of cash benefits by not working; or that they disliked the idea and associated stigma of being identified as 'disabled'.[22] As Topliss suggested, such reasons might be less applicable to severely disabled people, as they were less likely to be able to find employment without joining the register.[23]

[19] Topliss, *Provision for the Disabled*, p. 50.

[20] TNA BM 10/34, Remploy Limited, 'Report of the Working Party on the Mix of Disabilities Employed by Remploy, Table 4.1: Analysis of Disabled Register' (June, 1981), p. 11.

[21] TNA BM 10/48, Remploy Limited, 'Objectives and Criteria of Success' (July, 1980), p. 18.

[22] TNA BM 10/34 Remploy Limited, 'Report of the Working Party on the Mix of Disabilities Employed by Remploy' (June, 1981), pp. 9–10; TNA BM 8/3, Remploy Limited, 'Minutes of the One Hundred and Eightieth Meeting of the Board of Directors' (18.10.1961); TNA BM 3/47, 'Note from Cardiff Area Liaison Officer to Personnel Director' (28.01.1975); TNA LAB 20/1429, DE, 'Sheltered Employment: A Draft Consultative Document' (October, 1973), p. 33; TNA BM 3/71, Remploy Limited, 'Report on Factory Managers Meeting "B"' (May, 1979). Topliss, *Provision for the Disabled*, p. 51; B. Gleeson, *Geographies of Disability* (London, Routledge, 1999), p. 132.

[23] Topliss, *Provision for the Disabled*, p. 51.

However, while there might be fewer disabled people who would be designated as Section II who chose not to register, there was still likely to have been a significant number.

In order to be eligible for employment in Remploy, a person, having been able and willing to join the register, had then to be assessed as being Section II and therefore as someone requiring sheltered employment. The decision to classify disabled persons as being either Section I (considered able to gain some form of work in 'open employment') or Section II was taken by MOL officials in the position of Disablement Resettlement Officers (DROs). Based in local employment exchanges, DROs categorised disabled persons as either Section I or II using medical reports and guidelines produced and distributed by the Ministry.[24] Unfortunately, there are no records pertaining to the actual assessment. However, a MOL circular from 1946 outlined the steps for determining if someone was Section II, stating the DRO should take into account submitted medical evidence, the person's employment history and the results of ongoing efforts to place them in employment.[25] A doctor involved in the process claimed that the medical evidence provided to DROs was based on a comprehensive examination of the person, with a resulting report evaluating stamina, capacity for work, physical and functional ability and any potentially harmful environmental conditions.[26] A specimen medical report form for use by DROs from 1945 corresponds to this outline.[27] A disabled person was thereby defined as being Section II based entirely upon a combination of the opinions of medical professionals and bureaucrats. The former assessed their physical capacity, with the latter complementing this with their employment history and prospects, and ultimately deciding their categorisation. There is no mention in any record of the opinion of disabled people themselves having had any impact upon this assessment.

[24] TNA BM 10/12, Remploy Limited, 'Report of a Survey of Remploy Undertaken by Organisation and Methods Division of H.M. Treasury' (June, 1955), para. 6. For medical reports see TNA LAB 20/173, SEC, 'Minutes of the Ninth Meeting' (12.11.1946). Also see Anderson, *War, Disability and Rehabilitation in Britain*, pp. 196–7; Topliss, *Provision for the Disabled*, pp. 52–4.

[25] TNA LAB 20/215, MOL, 'Training and Employment Under Special Conditions of Registered Disabled Persons Who Are Severely Disabled' (1946).

[26] 'Work for the Disabled', *The Times* (20.10.1952).

[27] TNA LAB 20/127, MOL, 'Specimen, D.P.1 form' (1945).

The inadequacies of this system of administration have been briefly highlighted by Anderson, who noted that DROs were not medical professionals and only initially underwent a three-day training course, which was clearly insufficient to provide the knowledge required to interpret the medical report and determine the employment prospects for disabled candidates.[28] From further examination, it is apparent that the initial introduction of the register was met with a wide variation across localities in the numbers assessed as being Section II.[29] The MOL initially attempted to combat this by circulating more detailed instructions on assessment, creating a new position of District Disablement Resettlement Officer to oversee the training of DROs, and promoting closer involvement with medical professionals to assist in cases of uncertainty.[30] This does not appear to have been successful, with continued variation in assessments prompting further concerns.[31] The issue was eventually raised in Parliament in 1957 by the Labour MP Edward Evans. With a background in 'blind and deaf teaching' and having served as the Chairman of the Minister of Health's Advisory Committee on Handicapped Persons in 1949 as well as then being Chairman of the National Institute for the Deaf, Evans spoke with some authority when bemoaning the quality of training DRO's received.[32]

The MOL made further attempts to improve training during the 1960s, with a surviving outline of the basic training programme revealing an extended timetable over 20 days which included a mixture of talks on legislation and processes, as well as visits to hospitals, Remploy and other sheltered workshops.[33] There were also additional courses made

[28] Anderson, *War, Disability and Rehabilitation in Britain*, p. 197. See also TNA LAB 20/189 and LAB 20/241 for MOL concerns.

[29] TNA LAB 20/253, Disabled Persons Employment Corporation Limited, 'Regional Representatives Conference Minutes' (18.12.1945); TNA LAB 20/173, SEC, 'Minutes of the Ninth Meeting' (12.11.1946).

[30] TNA LAB 20/253, Disabled Persons Employment Corporation Limited, 'Regional Executive Officers' Conference No. 4' (19.02.1946); Anderson, *War, Disability and Rehabilitation in Britain*, p. 197. See also TNA LAB 20/127, MOL, 'Survey of DRO Placing Work' (May, 1950).

[31] TNA LAB 20/381, NACED, 'Special Survey of the Disabled Live File' (15.04.1948).

[32] Mr Edward Evans, *Hansard* (07.06.1957), vol. 571 cc. 1595; 'Obituary: Mr. Edward Evans', *The Times* (31.03.1960).

[33] TNA LAB 20/1140, MOL, 'Basic Training of D.R.Os' (1965).

available to DROs, including a medical course which provided sessions on a wide range of relevant topics such as 'Diseases of the Chest', with the aim to better understand the effects of specific conditions on employment prospects.[34] Aside from this increase in training, the overall system remained essentially unchanged into the 1990s.[35] Local variations in designation also continued throughout the period, with Remploy noting in 1980 that the decision remained 'personally with the DRO' and therefore varied 'significantly, between one DRO and another'.[36]

Eligibility for employment with Remploy was therefore limited in terms of legislation and policy, and was subject to local variation in the implementation of this by gatekeepers in the form of DROs. Remploy was not open to all 'severely disabled' people, but only to a select group who complied with the definitions and stipulations of the DPEA, chose to register, and were then deemed to be Section II. This reveals a significant barrier to accessing Remploy, but having been assessed as Section II, such persons were then supposedly eligible for a place in sheltered employment.

'Full Employment' for Section II People?

The concept of 'full employment' for the general working population was a key aspect of the classic welfare state, providing the foundation for the contributory social security system and was an understood and accepted priority for each government of the period.[37] It has also been highlighted by academics as a genuine achievement, with employment maintained at

[34] TNA LAB 20/1140, MOL, 'Programme for D.R.O. Training Course at St. James's Hospital, Leeds' (June, 1965).

[35] Topliss, *Provision for the Disabled*, p. 53; Barnes, *Disabled People in Britain and Discrimination*, p. 71.

[36] TNA BM 10/48, Remploy Limited, 'Objectives and Criteria of Success' (July, 1980), pp. 19, 26; TNA LAB 20/173, SEC, 'Minutes of the Ninth Meeting' (12.11.1946); TNA LAB 20/707, Remploy Limited, 'Note to Mr Taylor' (30.03.1949); TNA BM 3/47, Remploy Limited, 'Disabled People Entry Standards into Remploy Limited' (03.02.1975); Topliss, *Provision for the Disabled*, p. 53.

[37] Lowe, *The Welfare State in Britain Since 1945*, pp. 115–9; D. Gladstone, *The Twentieth-Century Welfare State* (Basingstoke, Palgrave Macmillan, 1999), p. 70; B. Coxall and L. Robins, *British Politics Since the War* (Basingstoke, Macmillan, 1998), pp. 50–1.

a 'historically high level'.[38] The DPEA effectively created a distinct population group in terms of employment—those designated as Section II. Any notion that Remploy achieved similar results for this population can be refuted very simply. Chapter 3 has already indicated how employee numbers in Remploy fluctuated in response to economic and political demands, and, as Table 4.1 indicates, Remploy did not provide employment for all those registered as Section II at any point during the period considered here.

Although Remploy was the chief provider of sheltered employment, it was not the only option available. The 'mixed economy' of sheltered employment will be considered more fully in Chapter 6, but it is referenced here to consider the overall level of unemployment for the discrete population of Section II people. Table 4.2 indicates the numbers employed by both Remploy and the combination of the various other providers of sheltered employment. With the data available it is then possible to crudely calculate the percentage of Section II people who were unemployed from 1957 to 1978. This can then be compared with the unemployment levels of the general population, which during the period when 'full employment' was pursued as policy prior to the severe financial crises of the mid-1970s which saw the abandonment of this principle, rarely reached 3%.[39] The contrast with the level of unemployment for Section II people is striking, with unemployment for this group showing a low-point of 34.9% and an increasing trend for much of the period, reaching a high-point of 53.3% in 1972. These people, unable to secure a place in sheltered employment, might find themselves signposted to occupational therapy centres, industrial rehabilitation units, or other welfare

[38] Lowe, *The Welfare State in Britain Since 1945*, pp. 80–1, 115–9.; Page, *Revisiting the Welfare State*, p. 38; Fraser, *The Evolution of the British Welfare State*, pp. 267–8; Glennerster, *British Social Policy*, p. 5; Laybourn, *The Evolution of British Social Policy and the Welfare State*, p. 241.

[39] H. Pemberton, 'The Transformation of the Economy', in P. Addison and H. Jones (eds.) *A Companion to Contemporary Britain 1939–2000* (Oxford, Blackwell, 2005), p. 192; Lowe, *The Welfare State in Britain Since 1945*, pp. 317–8.

Table 4.1 Registered section II personnel employed by Remploy compared to unemployed, 1946–1979

Year	*Section II employed by Remploy*[40]	*Section II registered unemployed*[41]
1946	164	12,390
1947	322	10,655
1948	866	10,850
1949	2477	11,583
1950	4467	8183
1951	5407	–
1952	5812	7117
1953	6021	6889
1954	6332	5124
1955	6581	4575
1956	6132	3950
1957	6083	3702
1958	6185	–
1959	6156	4199
1960	6303	4313
1961	6203	4543
1962	6359	4864
1963	6291	5511

(continued)

[40] For 1946 Executive Director Reports in TNA LAB 20/187, LAB 20/399. For 1947–79, TNA BM 10/2, Remploy Limited, 'A Brief Outline of the Birth and Early Development of Remploy Limited: Appendix B' (May, 1979).

[41] For 1946, TNA LAB 20/187, 'Executive Director's Report No. 15, Appendix H (19.11.1946). For 1947, Mr. Isaacs, *Hansard* (09.12.1947), vol. 445 cc.843–4. For 1948–49, TNA LAB 20/707, MOL, 'Great Britain totals of registered disabled persons' (April, 1949). For 1950, Mr Frederick Lee, *Hansard* (20.02.1951), vol. 484 cc. 1031–3. For 1952, TNA LAB 20/591, MOL, 'Number of Unemployed Registered Disabled Persons' (October, 1952). For 1953, TNA LAB 43/268, 'Note on Letter dated 17th May' (May, 1956). For 1954, TNA BM 8/5, MOL, 'National Advisory Council: Table B'. For 1955, Mr. Watkinson, *Hansard* (24.02.1955), vol. 537 cc. 1425–6. For 1956, Mr. Iain Macleod, *Hansard* (28.02.1956), vol. 549 cc.98–9W. For 1957, Mr. Robert Carr, *Hansard* (13.12.1957), vol. 579 cc. 1708. For 1959–61, TNA LAB 20/1071, MOL, 'Unemployed Registered Disabled Persons by Age Groups'. For 1962, Mr. Green, *Hansard* (16.04.1962), vol. 658 cc. 12–3w. For 1963–73, TNA LAB 20/1429, DE, 'Sheltered Employment: A Draft Consultative Document: Table VIII' (October, 1973). For 1974, Mr. Harold Walker, *Hansard* (20.03.1975), vol. 888 cc. 536–42w. For 1975–76, TNA BM 10/48, Remploy Limited, 'Objectives and Criteria of Success: Appendix 6' (July, 1980). For 1977–79, TNA BM 10/34, Remploy Limited, 'Report of the Working Party on the Mix of Disabilities Employed by Remploy, Table II' (June, 1981), p. 13.

Table 4.1 (continued)

Year	*Section II employed by Remploy*	*Section II registered unemployed*
1964	6519	5978
1965	6823	6141
1966	6817	6382
1967	6817	7533
1968	7179	8630
1969	7447	9602
1970	7505	10,013
1971	7518	11,120
1972	7746	12,105
1973	7959	11,164
1974	8077	10,989
1975	8308	11,101
1976	8514	11,457
1977	7972	10,901
1978	7894	9719
1979	8030	8314

Sources See footnotes

programmes.[42] Some may have been able to secure work in open employment, but for many it would mean reliance upon whatever cash benefits their individual circumstances entailed, if at all.[43]

These figures are also far higher than those for disabled people generally. Unemployment levels for disabled people tended to be higher than the general population over the period, with Hampton suggesting that they were at times 'three to four times greater', and figures showing that by 1975 the unemployment rate for disabled people generally was 13–14%.[44] The disparity between these figures and those for Section II people specifically highlights the need to examine groupings such as 'disabled

[42] TNA LAB 20/1429, DE, 'Sheltered Employment: A Draft Consultative Document' (October, 1973), p. 32. See also TNA ET 2/32. S. Shah and M. Priestley, *Disability and Social Change: Private Lives and Public Policies* (Bristol, Policy Press, 2011), pp. 138–9.

[43] Hampton, *Disability and the Welfare State in Britain;* Lowe, *The Welfare State in Britain Since 1945,* p. 146; J. Gulland, *Gender, Work and Social Control: A Century of Disability Benefits* (Palgrave Macmillan, 2019).

[44] Hampton, *Disability and the Welfare State in Britain,* p. 196.

Table 4.2 Breakdown of unemployment for section II and UK population average, 1957–1978

Year	*Employed in sheltered workshops*			*Section II registered unemployed*	*Percentage unemployed*	
	Remploy	*Other sheltered workshops*	*Total in sheltered workshops*		*Section II*	*UK average*
1957	6083	814	6897	3702	34.9%	1.6%
1958	6185	909	7094	–	–	2.2%
1959	6156	1132	7288	4199	36.6%	2.3%
1960	6303	1167	7470	4313	36.6%	1.7%
1961	6203	1181	7384	4543	38.1%	1.6%
1962	6359	1319	7678	4864	38.8%	2.1%
1963	6291	1460	7751	5511	41.6%	2.6%
1964	6519	1792	8311	5978	41.8%	1.7%
1965	6823	2022	8845	6141	41%	1.5%
1966	6817	2023	8840	6382	41.9%	1.6%
1967	6817	2208	9057	7533	45.4%	2.5%
1968	7179	2408	9605	8630	47.3%	2.5%
1969	7447	2444	9891	9602	49.3%	2.5%
1970	7505	2625	10,130	10,013	49.7%	2.7%
1971	7518	2748	10,266	11,120	52%	3.5%
1972	7746	2880	10,626	12,105	53.3%	3.8%
1973	7959	3165	11,124	11,164	50.1%	2.7%
1974	8077	3277	11,354	10,989	49.2%	2.6%
1975	8308	3170	11,478	11,101	49.2%	4.2%
1976	8514	3228	11,742	11,457	49.4%	5.7%
1977	7972	3410	11,382	10,901	48.9%	6.2%
1978	7894	3577	11,471	9719	45.9%	6.1%

Sources TNA BM 10/48, Remploy Limited, 'Objectives and Criteria of Success: Appendix 5' (1980), p. 73; The Government Statistical Service, *Unemployment statistics from 1881 to the present day* (1996). https://www.ons.gov.uk/. Accessed 5 July 2019

people' more closely, as in this case it is clear that the unemployment rate for those disabled people designated Section II was higher still.

The 'achievement' of full employment, considered so central to the classic welfare state, was therefore not extended to the severely disabled, either in terms of Remploy specifically, nor in terms of sheltered employment generally. Fulfilling the requirements to be eligible under the DPEA for sheltered employment was no guarantee of a place either in a Remploy factory or any of the alternatives. This chapter will now address this question of who was selected for Remploy and how this selection was carried out.

Ex-Service Personnel

As was indicated in Chapter 2, part of Bevin's role in the formation of the DPEA was in ensuring the measures contained in the Act were not to be limited based upon of the origin of disability. What was included in the Act, however, despite Bevin's objections, was Clause 16 stating that if the measures could not 'for the time being be provided for all persons in need of them', then preference would be given to ex-service men and women.[45] This meant that where demand for places in a Remploy factory outpaced those available, ex-service personnel should have been given priority. This does seem to have been the initial intention of Remploy's senior management as in his first report as Executive Director in July 1945, Air Commodore Venn explained that he had expressed the keenness of the company to engage disabled ex-servicemen during a meeting with MOL officials.[46] This emphasis continued in reports of Venn's initial fact-finding visits to various sheltered workshops and training schemes, as well as in discussions with representatives of the War Office and Air Ministry.[47] The preference was also noted in the guidelines for the setting up of a Remploy factory and in the official MOL guidance for local employment officers.[48] As well as reflecting the terms of the DPEA, such a focus is unsurprising at the close of the war and during the process of demobilisation.

As Remploy factories began to operate however, this sentiment appears to have quickly dissipated, with the notion of a preference vanishing from

[45] DPEA.

[46] TNA LAB 20/187, Disabled Persons Employment Corporation Limited, 'Executive Director Report No. 1' (23.07.1945).

[47] See Executive Director reports in TNA LAB 20/187, for example, 'Executive Director Report No. 4'; 'Executive Director Report No. 5'.

[48] TNA LAB 20/187, Disabled Persons Employment Corporation Limited, 'Executive Director Report No. 8, Appendix "G", Notes by Executive Director on the Setting Up of a British Factory' (18.03.1946); TNA LAB 20/253, Disabled Persons Employment Corporation Limited, 'Minutes of the Regional Executive Officers' Conference' (19.11.1946); TNA LAB 20/201, MOL, 'Employment with the Disabled Persons Employment Corporation Limited, M.L.Circ. 139/166' (24.07.1946).

records pertaining to recruitment. There is also evidence that even from the earliest stages, the reality of recruitment diverged from any such intention. In an interview panel for the first Remploy factory at Bridgend in May 1946, which Venn himself attended and reported upon, it was clear that this 'priority' did not dictate the selection.[49] A complete breakdown of the numbers of ex-service personnel in Remploy for the period considered here is no longer extant, but what evidence there is demonstrates that the Remploy workforce was not solely composed of this group. There are only occasional instances in the reports of Remploy's Executive and Managing Directors in the 1950s in which the percentage of ex-servicemen is revealed and sparse mentions elsewhere, but it is possible to gain a sense of the numbers employed. By 1951, when Remploy was nearing the end of its period of expansion, a report revealed that of the then 5224 'severely disabled' employees in Remploy, 2242 were ex-servicemen, some 43%.[50] The following year this had dipped slightly to 42%, at a time when MOL records show there were 2774 Section II ex-service personnel unemployed..[51] In 1958 the percentage of ex-service personnel in Remploy had shrunk again to around 40%, and by 1979 this was down to 29%.[52]

It is clear therefore that ex-service personnel represented only a significant minority of the workers in Remploy. The preference enshrined in the DPEA, while initially accepted in theory, appears to have been swiftly abandoned in practice. The category of 'ex-service' also ceases to figure in records on recruitment and in the many internal reports of the company's personnel. This has important implications for the historiography of disability and the welfare state. Historians such as Anderson, Hampton

[49] TNA LAB 20/187, Disabled Persons Employment Corporation Limited, 'Executive Director Report No. 10' (20.05.1946); 'Executive Director Report No. 10: Appendix D' (20.05.1946); 'Executive Director Report No. 11: Appendix F' (18.06.1946).

[50] TNA LAB 20/43, Remploy Limited, 'Executive Director Report No. 60' (21.03.1951).

[51] TNA BM 8/13, Remploy Limited, 'Executive Director Report No. 72' (24.04.1952); TNA LAB 20/591, MOL, 'Disabled Persons (Employment) Act, 1944, Number of Unemployed Registered Disabled Persons' (October, 1952). For Remploy numbers see TNA BM 3/67, 'Appendix 2'.

[52] TNA LAB 13/1029, J. L. Edwards, 'Remploy: An Experiment in Sheltered Employment for the Severely Disabled in Great Britain', *International Labour Review*, Vol. LXXVII, No. 2 (February, 1958), p. 8; TNA BM 3/67, Remploy Limited, 'Report on Employment of Disabled People in Remploy—1979, Appendix 6'.

and Borsay have suggested that disabled ex-servicemen continued to maintain a privileged position in the postwar period, with greater success in returning to their previous jobs, of finding employment generally, of claiming more generous benefit payments in the form of war pensions, and in benefiting from a political profile and as the focus of many charitable efforts.[53] However, we can see that in the case of Remploy, this privileged position had ceased to be universal.

Selection for Entry: Factory Access

Before considering the process by which selection for Remploy took place it is necessary to consider a more practical limitation in terms of having physical access to a factory. Not everyone who registered and was deemed Section II lived within an acceptable commuting distance. The exclusion of disabled people from employment due to location and the limitations of available transport has been noted as a persistent problem by scholars such as Brendan Gleeson.[54] In the case of Remploy, each factory had a 'catchment area', but there were not enough to create full national coverage. In 1952 the Remploy Chairman, Sir Robert Burrows, noted the impracticality of providing a factory for everyone eligible, remarking that 'you cannot put factories in a lot of inaccessible places where there are disabled people'.[55]

What factories there were, were specifically situated in order for employees in the local area to 'make a daily journey to and from work to their homes using public transport'.[56] As geographers considering disability have noted however, urban infrastructure including public transport can prove extremely problematic for disabled people owing to an

[53] Anderson, *War, Disability and Rehabilitation in Britain*, pp. 187–9, 211; Elsey, 'The Rehabilitation and Employment of Disabled Ex-Servicemen after the Two World Wars', pp. 292–7; Hampton, *Disability and the Welfare State in Britain*, pp. 99, 199–209; Borsay, *Disability and Social Policy in Britain Since 1750*, pp. 160–2; Millward, 'Social Security Policy and the Early Disability Movement', p. 281; Fraser, *The Evolution of the British Welfare State*, p. 258.

[54] Gleeson, *Geographies of Disability*, p.132.

[55] *Fourth Report from the Select Committee on Estimates,* 162 (1952), para. 287, p. 21.

[56] TNA BM 10/1, Remploy Limited, 'A Review of the working of the Company during its first seven years' (March, 1953), p. 37. See also TNA LAB 13/1029, Edwards, 'Remploy: An Experiment in Sheltered Employment for the Severely Disabled in Great Britain' (February, 1958), p. 10.

underlying assumption that 'passengers are non-impaired'.[57] Remploy was aware of potential difficulties and made attempts to mitigate them including providing additional transport 'to supplement an inadequate [public transport] service'.[58] In one case this involved a factory modifying a commercial lorry to serve as a company bus.[59] As well as local initiatives, Remploy's policy was to provide commuting expenses to all employees where the cost 'exceeded 6d.' a day.[60]

In 1956, calculations were done which estimated there were 2660 unemployed Section II people nationwide who were within a suitable distance of a Remploy factory, and by 1959 this had increased to nearly 3000.[61] By the end of the period it was suggested by Remploy that approximately two-thirds of registered unemployed Section II people—some 6000—were living within a factory catchment area.[62] There were understandably large regional differences in these numbers. In 1960, for example, the North Western Region was reported to have 546 unemployed Section II people within factory catchment areas, compared to 33 people outside them; while the Eastern and Southern Region had 164 unemployed Section II people within catchment areas and 204 outside.[63] While there were therefore a number of people for whom no local factory

[57] Gleeson, *Geographies of Disability*, pp. 137–40.

[58] TNA BM 10/1, Remploy Limited, 'A Review of the working of the Company during its first seven years' (March, 1953), p. 37.

[59] TNA LAB 20/444, Disabled Persons Employment Corporation Limited, 'Remploy Factory, Barking: Transport facilities for disabled employees' (21.12.1948).

[60] TNA LAB 13/1029, Edwards, 'Remploy: An Experiment in Sheltered Employment for the Severely Disabled in Great Britain' (February, 1958), p. 10; TNA BM 10/1, Remploy Limited, 'A Review of the working of the Company during its first seven years' (March, 1953), p. 37.

[61] TNA LAB 43/268, 'Note on Letter dated 17th May, 1956 from Mr Willey'; TNA LAB 20/1052, NACED, 'Analysis of the Severely Disabled Unemployed' (February, 1960); NACED, 'Analysis of the Severely Disabled Unemployed: Appendix IV' (February, 1960).

[62] TNA BM 10/48, Remploy Limited, 'Objectives and Criteria of Success' (July, 1980), p. 20.

[63] TNA LAB 20/1052, NACED, 'Analysis of the Severely Disabled Unemployed: Appendix IV' (February, 1960).

could provide employment, and who were therefore beyond the reach of the scheme, there remained a significant number of registered Section II employees within the catchment area of a Remploy factory who were not selected to work in one.

Selection for Entry: Central Recruitment Policy

Recruitment into a Remploy factory was administered at the local level, but there are some important developments in Remploy's central policy to be considered. Chapter 3 has already demonstrated the importance of maximising commercial efficiency in Remploy, and this was reflected in terms of selecting employees. There was concern among Remploy's senior management over the productivity of the workforce from the beginning. In his initial assessment of those designated as Section II, the Remploy Executive Director, Venn, lamented that the majority were old, and having not worked before had 'deteriorated to such an extent as to be virtually unemployable'.[64] However, in the first few years of its existence, prior to the slowdown policy described in Chapter 3 which would come in the late 1940s, there remained the possibility that Remploy would have to eventually cater for all those on the Section II register.[65] The question of productivity was therefore raised at this point in terms of giving preference to the most capable candidates. Therefore, while there was no notion yet of permanently excluding those considered less productive, Remploy's central policy was that recruitment should focus on getting those who were most capable into 'useful employment' first, in order to establish a 'productive atmosphere' within a factory.[66]

This approach did not last long. By 1951, alongside the focus on improving Remploy's commercial performance, and following investigations of the Section II register involving the NACED, the MOL and

[64] TNA LAB 20/187, Disabled Persons Employment Corporation Limited, 'Executive Director Report No. 1' (23.07.1945).

[65] TNA LAB 20/253, Disabled Persons Employment Corporation Limited, 'Regional Representatives Conference No. 2' (18.12.1945).

[66] TNA LAB 20/187, Disabled Persons Employment Corporation Limited, 'Executive Director Report No. 1' (23.07.1945); TNA LAB 20/444, Disabled Persons Employment Corporation Limited, 'Executive Director Circular 7A/1' (06.10.1948); TNA BM 10/1, Remploy Limited, 'A Review of the working of the Company during its first seven years' (March, 1953), pp. 39–40.

Remploy, the attitude began to develop that not all those on the Section II register were in practice 'suitable' for Remploy.[67] This 'suitability' was based on an assessment of a person's potential productivity. The Remploy Board agreed that it was reasonable that entry to a factory should be subject to a candidate's ability 'to attain a minimum percentage of a fit person's output in a similar job'.[68] This was justified both in terms of maintaining production and because it had been observed that the presence of those unable to keep pace in a factory 'tends to dishearten the more productive people'.[69] When giving evidence to the Select Committee on Estimates in 1952, the then Remploy Chairman, Sir Robert, expressed this now orthodox position, admitting that there effectively existed a third category of disability, beyond those deemed Section I and Section II in which 'there is a degree of incapacity which makes it really impossible to take a man into a factory'.[70] He explained that Remploy was currently being selective in its recruitment, noting that 'if we do not want a man, we do not take him'.[71] This position was endorsed by a MOL representative also providing evidence to the Committee, who concurred that 'Remploy are not bound to take everybody'.[72] It is not clear what precise standard was set on applicants at this time but the Executive Director did note that the company did not normally accept someone who 'cannot in the first place work a minimum of 30 hours [per week]'.[73] Remploy did not therefore simply recruit those designated as eligible under the DPEA without some selection, with productivity quickly established as the determining factor. While the DPEA recognised

[67] TNA LAB 20/1052, NACED, 'Analysis of the Severely Disabled Unemployed'; SEC, 'Unemployed Severely Disabled Persons, S.E.C.39'; TNA LAB 20/591, MOL, 'Quarterly Bulletin No. 12: Part 1—National Advisory Council on the Employment of the Disabled Meeting' (June, 1951).

[68] TNA BM 8/2, Remploy Limited, 'Minutes of the Fifty-Seventh Meeting of the Board of Directors' (27.09.1950).

[69] TNA BM 8/2, Remploy Limited, 'Minutes of the Sixty-Second Meeting of the Board of Directors' (26.02.1951).

[70] *Fourth Report from the Select Committee on Estimates*, 162 (1952), para. 203, pp. 16–7.

[71] Ibid.

[72] Ibid., paras. 204–5.

[73] TNA BM 10/1, Remploy Limited, 'A Review of the working of the Company during its first seven years' (March, 1953), p. 38.

only two categories of disability, both the Remploy Board and the MOL were united in modifying this legislation in practice to informally create a further one for those deemed too unproductive.

Once established, this acceptable level of productivity continued to be endorsed by the MOL during the Conservative governments of the 1950s, in which the subject of avoiding the recruitment of those designated 'Low Production Potentials' was regularly discussed.[74] The Conservative Minister of Labour, Iain MacLeod, who had personal experience of disability, with both himself and his wife suffering from a range of health conditions, summed up the prevailing attitude in 1956, stating that 'it would be a false kindness, and certainly very costly, to take on or retain those who are unable, and sometimes perhaps unwilling, to make any significant contribution to production'.[75] This view was also endorsed in the conclusion of two reports. In 1955, the report on Remploy by the Organisation and Methods Division of the Treasury highlighted the need for the company to employ more productive employees if it was to improve its commercial efficiency.[76] The following year saw the publication of the influential Piercy Report, which clarified the idea of sheltered workshops as being 'places of employment with as high as possible a rate of individual productivity'.[77] Sheltered employment generally was thus to be for 'those who are willing to undertake the work provided and able

[74] TNA BM 8/2, Remploy Limited, 'Minutes of a Special Meeting of the Board of Directors' (13.07.1955); 'Minutes of the One Hundred and Eleventh Meeting of the Board of Directors' (27.07.1955); TNA LAB 20/929, 'Record of Meeting' (20.07.1955); 'Note from St. John Wilson' (18.10.1955); 'Notes for Minister' (03.11.1955); 'Note from Sir Brunel Cohen to Iain MacLeod, D.P.2747/1955' (19.01.1956); 'Note from Mr. Iain MacLeod to Sir Brunel Cohen, D.P.2747/1955' (22.02.1956).

[75] TNA LAB 20/929, 'Note from Mr. Iain MacLeod to Sir Brunel Cohen, D.P.2747/1955' (22.02.1956); 'Sir Brunel Cohen's Notes, D.P.2747/55' (09.11.1955). Hampton, *Disability and the Welfare State in Britain*, p. 52; D. Goldsworthy, 'Macleod, Iain Norman (1913–1970), politician', *Oxford Dictionary of National Biography* (06.01.2011). https://www.oxforddnb.com/. Accessed 15 October 2017.

[76] TNA BM 8/6, Remploy Limited, 'Summary of Principal Comments & Recommendations made by O. & M. Division' (June, 1955); TNA LAB 20/929, 'Note from Sir Monckton to Sir Brunel Cohen, D.P.2747/1955' (16.12.1955).

[77] *Report of the Committee of Inquiry on The Rehabilitation Training and Resettlement of Disabled Persons*, 9883 (1956), p. 94.

to make a significant contribution to production'.[78] It was this concept which was to remain the guiding principle in recruitment for Remploy.[79]

The question of how to actually determine what benchmark qualified as a 'significant contribution', remained ambiguous until it was finally quantified in the 1970s. A Consultative Document produced by the DE under the Heath Government in 1973 on 'Sheltered Employment for Disabled People', which sought to spur improvements to the field of provision, suggested that a reasonable minimum productivity standard would be 'not less than one third of the output of a fit but otherwise comparable person performing similar work in ordinary industry'.[80] Though it is not clear when this was officially adopted by Remploy, and there is no record of it being discussed at Board level, in early 1975 the Personnel Director noted that the official central recruitment policy of the company was indeed a 'minimum standard on entry of one-third of that of an able-bodied person (usually interpreted as a "20 minute hour")'.[81] This was to remain the official policy well into the 1980s.[82]

The adoption of this measure was not carried without opposition, however, both from within the company and without.[83] The DE noted that the biggest single criticism it received was that the entry standard to Remploy was too high.[84] Conversely, there were regular complaints from Remploy that it was increasingly difficult to find candidates who could reach this benchmark, with Remploy's Board frequently commenting on

[78] Ibid.

[79] TNA LAB 20/1052, SEC, 'Analysis of the Severely Disabled Unemployed, S.E.C. 87' (February, 1960); TNA LAB 20/1429, DE, 'Sheltered Employment: A Draft Consultative Document' (October, 1973), para. 2.25, p 12. Topliss, *Provision for the Disabled*, pp. 55–8.

[80] TNA LAB 20/1429, DE, 'Sheltered Employment: A Draft Consultative Document' (October, 1973), para. 4.58, pp. 57–9.

[81] TNA BM 3/47, Remploy Limited, 'Personnel Director to Managing Director: Section II Employees—Entry Standards' (10.02.1975).

[82] TNA BM 3/54, Remploy Limited, 'Remploy in the Long Term' (22.04.1977), para. 2.2, p. 1; TNA BM 10/48, Remploy Limited, 'Objectives and Criteria of Success' (July, 1980), p. 8; TNA BM 10/53, Remploy Limited, 'Remploy Facts' (September, 1986), p. 9.

[83] TNA BM 10/48, Remploy Limited, 'Objectives and Criteria of Success' (July, 1980), p. 27.

[84] TNA BM 8/79, Remploy Limited, 'Minutes of the Three Hundred and Twenty-Sixth Meeting of the Board of Directors' (15.01.1975).

the lack of suitable candidates, and suggesting that only 'one in every 2 or 3 persons' on the Section II register were employable.[85] Once again the Board was aligned in its view with the DE, which agreed that within the Section II category, up to two-thirds were unsuitable for Remploy.[86]

A minimum level of productivity was therefore established as necessary for entry to a Remploy factory. This was supported by the MOL and then DE under successive governments and became entrenched in the wider understanding of what sheltered employment should provide. This policy endorsed the selection of candidates based on their ability to meet a productivity benchmark and thereby excluded those registered Section II people who could not.

Selection for Entry: Local Recruitment Practice

While there was a central policy guiding recruitment, the process itself was carried out entirely at a local level with each Remploy factory recruiting its own workforce from the local candidate pool. In each case the perceived quality of applicants could vary widely, as could the number available.[87] The general process of recruitment remained largely unchanged throughout the period considered here.[88] When vacancies arose in a Remploy factory, the designated local employment office was alerted.

[85] TNA BM 8/79, Remploy Limited, 'Minutes of the Three Hundred and Twenty-Eighth Meeting of the Board of Directors' (20.03.1975). See further references to this in Board Meeting Minutes for October 1971, November 1971, September 1973, May 1974, September 1974, October 1974, in TNA BM 8/49; January 1976, March 1978, in TNA BM 8/79. See also TNA BM 10/48, Remploy Limited, 'Objectives and Criteria of Success' (July, 1980), p. 20.

[86] TNA LAB 20/1429, DE, 'Sheltered Employment: A Draft Consultative Document' (October, 1973), para. 4.61, p 60.

[87] TNA LAB 20/173, SEC, 'Sheltered Employment Committee S.E.C.14, Appendix II' (September, 1946); TNA LAB 20/929, Remploy Limited, 'Note from Sir Brunel Cohen to Minister of Labour' (27.03.1956); TNA LAB 20/1052, SEC, 'Unemployed Severely Disabled Persons, S.E.C.39'; SEC, 'Analysis of the Severely Disabled Unemployed'.

[88] TNA LAB 20/187, Disabled Persons Employment Corporation, 'Executive Director Report No. 8, Appendix G' (18.03.1946); Disabled Persons Employment Corporation Limited, 'Executive Director Report No. 10' (20.05.1946); TNA LAB 20/201, MOL, 'Circular 139/166: Employment with the Disabled Persons Employment Corporation Limited' (24.07.1946). Mr. Isaacs, *Hansard* (23.03.1949), vol. 463 cc.39–40w; TNA BM 10/1, Remploy Limited, 'A Review of the working of the Company during its first seven years' (March, 1953), p. 39; TNA LAB 13/1029, Edwards, 'Remploy: An Experiment in Sheltered Employment for the Severely Disabled in Great Britain' (February, 1958), p. 9.

The DRO attached to that office then submitted potential applicants for an interview which was held at the factory by a panel consisting of the factory manager, factory doctor and the DRO. The DRO was present in an advisory capacity only. The final decision whether to accept or refuse an applicant rested with the manager, with the doctor providing a further medical assessment of an applicant's suitability. It was this localised panel which ultimately provided access to a Remploy Factory.

Chapter 3 has already demonstrated that individual factories could work very differently and that there was often a gulf between official Remploy policy and the realities at the local level. One Remploy Area Liaison Officer (ALO)—the level of management above factory manager—noted the disconnect between central recruitment policy and local practice, explaining that the policy was 'applied at local level at so many variances that the original decision bears no resemblance to the factual situation eventually arrived at'.[89] This was also something noted by the DE in its 1973 Consultative Document.[90] There were thus further local factors which served to define who was 'suitable' for Remploy and thereby further restrict access. The key areas examined here are variations in entry standards, methods of assessments, and an even greater emphasis on potential productivity.

The local nature of recruitment meant that the standard against which managers assessed applicants was not uniform and instead reflected the needs of the individual factory.[91] Initially, Remploy's policy was that local factory conditions were not to be given paramount importance when recruiting workers. Given the kinds of disparate work which factories undertook in the early period, this is perhaps unsurprising. Noting that managers were attempting to limit recruitment based upon finding the right candidates for specific jobs, the Executive Director issued a circular

The process was largely unchanged at least into the 1980s, TNA BM 10/53, Remploy Limited, 'Remploy Facts' (September, 1986), p. 9.

[89] TNA BM 3/47, Remploy Limited, 'Newcastle upon Tyne Area Liaison Officer to Personnel Director' (03.02.1975); 'Note from Managing Director, Disabled People' (22.01.1975).

[90] TNA 20/1429, DE, 'Sheltered Employment: A Draft Consultative Document' (October, 1973), p.71.

[91] TNA BM 10/48, Remploy Limited, 'Objectives and Criteria of Success, Appendix 9: M.I.R. Department Circular No: 1758, Sect. 4.2 Entry Standards' (20.02.1979); TNA BM 10/53, Remploy Limited, 'Remploy Facts' (September, 1986), p. 9.

in 1948 instructing them not to do this, explaining instead that 'if suitable work does not exist in the factory, it is to be found'.[92] As such, managers were encouraged to introduce additional work to suit the employees available 'even though that work may consist of chopping firewood, making clothes pegs or some other similar job'.[93]

With the emphasis shifting to commercial strength and with factory lines becoming standardised with specific production processes, this approach changed.[94] By 1952, the Remploy chairman reported that candidates for Remploy were being assessed based on their ability to perform in the particular trade of a given factory.[95] This was brought into focus with the investigation of Remploy factory entry standards instigated by the Managing Director in 1975 in response to the DE questioning the process. The Managing Director admitted that setting down a comprehensive entry standard was 'extremely hard to do' as though the standard was the '20 minute hour', he assumed that in reality it varied widely across the network of factories.[96] The responses provided to the Managing Director from the various Directors and ALOs tasked to discover the reality of the situation, indicate the continued emphasis of recruiting based on the needs of the particular factory, and the wide range of standards which this entailed.[97] The Personnel Director emphasised this and the 'large element of luck' involved in a candidate gaining entry to Remploy as their perceived ability matched the requirements of the particular factory.[98] He concluded that recruitment standards 'vary quite a lot from factory to factory and more particularly from trade to trade'.[99] This was elaborated upon by the ALO for Cardiff, who suggested that in general woodworking factories 'demand the highest standard of fitness',

[92] TNA LAB 20/444, Disabled Persons Employment Corporation Limited, 'Executive Director Circular 7A/1' (06.10.1948).

[93] TNA BM 10/1, Remploy Limited, 'A Review of the working of the Company during its first seven years' (March, 1953), p. 40.

[94] Ibid., p. 31.

[95] *Fourth Report from the Select Committee on Estimates,* 162 (1952), para. 189, p. 15.

[96] TNA BM 3/47, Remploy Limited, 'Note from Managing Director, Disabled People' (22.01.1975).

[97] See TNA BM 3/47 for responses.

[98] TNA BM 3/47, Remploy Limited, 'Personnel Director to Managing Director: Section II Employees—Entry Standards' (10.02.1975).

[99] Ibid.

and orthopaedic factories 'demand more intelligence', with packaging factories accepting a 'much lower standard' of both.[100] The Cardiff ALO also hinted at how the variation could work the other way, with applicants not wanting the particular work available at their local factory.[101]

Further variations occurred in how candidates were assessed for vacancies by the factory panel. Unfortunately, there are no complete records of interviews and assessment of candidates retained in the archives. There are, however, occasional glimpses of the criteria applied. Assessment began with the DRO selecting the candidate for the interview. In a study of the Section II register in the South London region in 1950, it was noted that DROs examined the medical and industrial records of each person and then classified them as either 'suitable', 'unsuitable', or 'possibly suitable' for their local Remploy factory.[102] The factors which were considered were the attitude to work, the employment record, the nature of the disability, travelling difficulties and age.[103] A report on the Section II register for Huddersfield in 1973 assessed candidates on similar lines.[104]

The DRO's impression of the candidate's attitude towards work appears to have been the key focus for their own assessment. Some specific examples of this appeared in a report for the MOL on the Section II register undertaken in 1956, which included extracts from DRO reports.[105] In one example, a candidate was described as follows: 'he has not worked since March 1948 and he has adapted himself to a life of idleness. The will to work is obviously missing'.[106] In some cases, this appears to have reflected a belief that the candidate did not really want employment but wished instead to rely on benefit payments. In

[100] TNA BM 3/47, Remploy Limited, 'Cardiff Area Liaison Officer to Personnel Director' (28.01.1975).

[101] Ibid.

[102] TNA LAB 20/1052, SEC, 'Unemployed Severely Disabled Persons, S.E.C.39'.

[103] Ibid.; TNA LAB 20/1429, DE, 'Sheltered Employment: A Draft Consultative Document' (October, 1973), p. 33.

[104] TNA BM 8/50, Remploy Limited, 'Note from Personnel Director: Huddersfield Factory' (03.04.1973).

[105] TNA LAB 20/1052, SEC, 'Examination of a Sample of 242 Register Disabled Persons classified as unlikely to obtain employment except under sheltered conditions, S.E.C.61' (November, 1956).

[106] Ibid.

one example the DRO remarked of a candidate that 'with his present allowances of £5 3s. 6d. per week from the National Assistance Board he appears to be quite content'.[107] Similarly of another candidate, a man aged 61, the DRO stated that 'there is in my opinion no incentive for this man, who is very badly disabled, to take employment, and I have little doubt that he has in effect retired, and will continue to draw N.A. [National Assistance] Grant until he is 65 years of age'.[108] Given that it was this subjective opinion on something as intangible as an impression of a candidates 'will to work' which was the key factor in determining entry, it is unsurprising that, as with the initial categorisation as Section II, the further categorisation of 'suitable for Remploy' was widely variable.

The role of the doctor on the interview panel was to provide a medical assessment of the candidate's ability to undertake the kind of work done in the factory to the required standard.[109] Again there are no surviving records of these assessments. There are, however, instances from the 1975 investigation of entry standards in which ALOs commented on the reliance on the doctor's judgement as to the candidate's physical and mental abilities to carry out the role.[110] With both the DRO and doctor providing advice only, the final decision as to whether to employ a candidate fell to the factory manager. The chief interest of the manager appears to have been, as with the DRO, determining the candidate's 'will to work'.[111] An example of how this was ascertained, was provided in a response to the 1975 investigation by the Cardiff ALO, who noted how he himself did so on occasions where he joined the interview panel:

[107] Ibid.

[108] Ibid.

[109] TNA LAB 20/444, Disabled Persons Employment Corporation Limited, 'Executive Director Circular 7A/1' (06.10.1948); TNA BM 10/1, Remploy Limited, 'A Review of the Company during its first seven years' (March, 1953), p. 38.

[110] TNA BM 3/47, Remploy Limited, 'Cardiff Area Liaison Officer to Personnel Director' (28.01.1975); Remploy Limited, 'L.&T.P. Director to Managing Director' (11.02.1975); TNA BM 10/53, Remploy Ltd, 'Remploy Facts' (September, 1986), p. 9.

[111] TNA BM 3/47, Remploy Limited, 'Personnel Director to Managing Director: Section II Employees—Entry Standards' (10.02.1975); Remploy Limited, 'Cardiff Area Liaison Officer to Personnel Director' (28.01.1975); Remploy Limited, 'Brixton Area Liaison Officer to Personnel Director' (29.01.1975); TNA BM 10/53, Remploy Ltd, 'Remploy Facts' (September, 1986), p. 9.

> When I attend interview panels I invariable ask the applicant, 'Do you want to work in this factory?'. A sideways glance at the DRO used to indicate 'no', because the applicant would be afraid of saying 'no' in case his dole money was reduced. Today, applicants are more honest and usually give a positive 'yes' or 'no'. This question can eliminate 5–10% of applicants. If I am still doubtful about the 'will to work', I ask, 'can you arrive at this factory by 7:30 a.m. every morning and work for 8 hours?' (4 factories in my area start at 7:30am). If the applicant has ascertained bus times you can be sure he is keen.[112]

As with the determination of the 'will to work' by the DRO, this was a purely subjective measure with no set process or standard, with the clear potential for wide variation across the factory network from manager to manager.

It was recognised that this local recruitment process was inherently flawed. The Piercy Report in 1956 noted that the interview process could not accurately reveal the true productivity potential of candidates.[113] This was highlighted later during the 1975 investigation by Remploy's Managing Director who suggested that factory managers did not always make a correct assessment of potential employees.[114] This point was raised again at the end of the period in Remploy's internal report on the company's Objectives and Criteria of Success, which called for a better pre-employment assessment procedure as an urgent area of improvement.[115]

As was shown in Chapter 3, factory managers were, in general, primarily concerned with maximising the commercial efficiency of their factory. It is not surprising therefore that concerns were raised about a tendency for managers to be 'over-selective' in recruitment from as early as 1948.[116] Even with the establishment of a minimum standard

[112] TNA BM 3/47, Remploy Limited, 'Cardiff Area Liaison Officer to Personnel Director' (28.01.1975).

[113] *Report of the Committee of Inquiry on The Rehabilitation Training and Resettlement of Disabled Persons*, 9883 (1956).

[114] TNA BM 3/47, Remploy Limited, 'Note from Secretary and Director, Disabled People: Entry Standard for Employment in Remploy Ltd' (28.01.1975).

[115] TNA BM 10/48, Remploy Limited, 'Objectives and Criteria of Success' (July, 1980), p. 30.

[116] TNA LAB 20/444, Disabled Persons Employment Corporation Limited, 'Executive Director Circular 7A/1' (06.10.1948); TNA BM 10/1, Remploy Limited, 'A Review of

of productivity as policy, the issue remained, with factory managers continually being seen as going beyond this to employ only the most productive individuals.[117] Such criticism was levelled at Remploy in the Commons in 1972 by the Labour MP Mr Caerwyn Roderick, who accused the company of being too selective and placing production efficiency over employment.[118] He repeated this in January 1974, when he was assured by the Conservative Under-Secretary of State for Employment, Mr Nicholas Scott, that 'there is no pressure on Remploy to recruit less severely disabled personnel in order to reduce losses and increase efficiency'.[119] This statement does not seem to reflect the reality for factory managers.

The responses to the investigation of entry standards in 1975 endorsed the view that many factory managers were continuing to be selective beyond the established benchmark.[120] One ALO noted that managers were 'much more concerned with their factory costs than having satisfactorily employed a particularly severely disabled person', and that 'there are too many instances of managers wanting "fit" disabled people to help them achieve their production targets'.[121] Blame was not entirely placed on factory managers themselves, as the responses made clear that they felt they were simply responding to the demands placed upon them by Head Office and the measures of performance which were based on productivity.[122] Similar conclusions in an internal report from 1980 illustrate that the problem persisted across the period.[123]

Recruitment for Remploy, undertaken at the local level, was therefore subject to wide variation and further levels of selectivity. Candidates

the Company during its first seven years' (March, 1953), p. 39; *Fourth Report from the Select Committee on Estimates*, 162 (1952), para. 177, p. 14.

117 TNA BM 8/2, Remploy Limited, 'Minutes of the One Hundred and Sixty-Fifth Meeting of the Board of Directors' (18.05.1960).

118 Mr. Roderick, *Hansard* (01.05.1972), vol. 836, cc. 11–2.

119 Mr. Roderick and Mr. Scott, *Hansard* (30.01.1974), vol. 868, cc. 126–7w.

120 See responses in TNA BM 3/47.

121 TNA BM 3/47, Remploy Limited, 'Area Liaison Officer to Personnel Director' (27.01.1975).

122 Ibid.; TNA BM 3/47, Remploy Limited, 'Pontefract Area Liaison Officer to Personnel Director' (28.01.1975).

123 TNA BM 10/48, Remploy Limited, 'Objectives and Criteria of Success' (July, 1980), p. 62.

were subject to the productivity needs of their local factory, the paternalistic and medical assessments of a panel of gatekeepers, and, finally, the whims and personality of a single factory manager. Entry to Remploy was therefore reserved for those candidates perceived to be able to make the maximum contribution to the factory's productivity. This meant that a great many severely disabled people, despite eligibility in terms of the DPEA, were excluded from gaining entry to Remploy.

Employee Retention

Demonstrating adequate productivity potential and finally securing a place in a Remploy factory was no guarantee of remaining with the company. From the opening of the first factories through to 1979, some 3838 employees were dismissed due to being 'unsuitable for further employment'.[124] As with the establishment of a benchmark of productivity for recruitment into the factory, the introduction of a similar benchmark for the existing workforce, and the termination of the employment of those unable or unwilling to reach this level, was accepted by both the Remploy Board and by the MOL/DE across successive governments.[125] As a corollary of the focus on improving the commercial efficiency of the company described in Chapter 3, there was a focus on improving the production capacity of the workforce, and the termination of employment for those who could not maintain the given standard.[126]

Remploy had always had the ability to terminate the employment of those deemed 'unemployable'—i.e. those who could no longer make an

[124] TNA BM 3/67, Remploy Limited, 'Report on Employment of Disabled People in Remploy—1979, Appendix 9'.

[125] TNA LAB 20/929, 'Record of Meeting' (20.07.1955); 'Note from Mr St. John Wilson to S. Green, D.P.2587/1955' (18.10.1955); 'Sir Brunel Cohen's Notes, D.P.2747/55' (09.11.1955); 'Note from Sir Monckton to Sir Brunel Cohen, D.P.2747/1955' (16.12.1955); TNA LAB 20/929, 'Note from Mr St. John Wilson to Mr Wade, D.P. 2747/1955' (17.03.1956); 'Note from Sir Brunel Cohen to Mr MacLeod, D.P.2747/1955' (27.03.1956).

[126] See for example, TNA BM 8/49, Remploy Limited, 'Minutes of the Two Hundred and Seventy-Sixth Meeting of the Board of Directors' (18.06.1970); 'Minutes of the Two-Hundred and Eighty-Sixth Meeting of the Board of Directors' (27.05.1971); TNA BM 8/79, 'Minutes of the Three Hundred and Thirty-Seventh Meeting of the Board of Directors' (22.01.1976); TNA BM 10/48, Remploy Limited, 'Objectives and Criteria of Success, Appendix 9: M.I.R. Department Circular No: 1758, Sect. 4.2 Entry Standards' (20.02.1979).

adequate contribution to the productivity of the factory.[127] This was greatly aided by the introduction of an employment 'trial period' in 1956 which allowed for the removal of workers who proved to be unproductive following their recruitment.[128] Even following the completion of this trial period, every worker underwent a routine medical examination every 6 months to ensure they were still capable of working in the factory.[129] By 1975 this had changed to an annual review.[130] Alongside these were continuous informal assessments made by the factory manager, and the factory doctor during their regular visits.[131]

As with initial recruitment, the worker was subject to assessment by a doctor and factory manager to determine their ability to maintain productivity. This saw the creation of a system of 'functional assessment' referred to as 'M.U.S.I.C', under which each employee was graded in terms of Mobility, Usefulness or dexterity, physical Strength, Intelligence and Consistency.[132] Similarly, each role in the factory could be graded in terms of the requirements in these areas.[133] In this way, the factory manager and doctor could attempt to create a productivity profile of each employee and each role in the factory.[134] This system remained in place until it was revised in 1972 and replaced with a new framework with the following criteria: 'ability to work: skill; application; tempo; co-operation with supervision; relationship with other employees; attitude to disability; attitude to work/motivation; attendance; punctuality; general assessment'.[135] The aspects listed indicate both the scope of assessment,

[127] TNA BM 8/1, Remploy Limited, 'Minutes of the Fifty-First Meeting of the Board of Directors' (22.02.1950).

[128] TNA LAB 43/268, 'Notes on letter from Mr Willey' (17.05.1956).

[129] TNA LAB 13/1029, Edwards, 'Remploy: An Experiment in Sheltered Employment for the Severely Disabled in Great Britain' (February, 1958), p. 9; 'Work for the Disabled', *The Times* (20.10.1952).

[130] TNA BM 3/47, Remploy Limited, 'Personnel Department Circular No: 1173' (17.01.1972).

[131] TNA BM 10/1, Remploy Limited, 'A Review of the Company during its first seven years' (March, 1953), pp. 62–3.

[132] Ibid., 'Appendix C'.

[133] Ibid.

[134] Ibid.

[135] TNA BM 3/47, Remploy Limited, 'Personnel Department Circular No: 1173' (17.01.1972).

with a combination of physical ability and general attitude towards work, and the subjective nature of many of these areas which draw comparisons with the kind of medical surveillance and moral regulation which Gulland highlighted in the context of incapacity benefits.[136]

Initially, when a factory manager wished to terminate the employment of an employee deemed unproductive, they would have to submit a rationale together with a report from the factory doctor.[137] The case was then considered by the Industrial Relation Officer and the Principal Medical Officer, with the final decision coming from the Executive Director.[138] This process was designed explicitly to 'protect the severely disabled from impatient and intolerant Managers'.[139] By 1956 the process had changed slightly, with the factory manager notifying the Trade Union Representative of the intention to dismiss the worker. Reports by the factory manager and doctor were then submitted to Head Office, alongside any Trade Union representation, to be considered by one of the company directors in consultation with the company's Chief Medical Officer.[140] Unfortunately, there are no full surviving records of such cases, however, it is possible to get a sense of how employees were assessed as being unsuitable to remain. Towards the end of 1951 a report was compiled on the 'Least Productive Employees' across the company, with the goal of determining who should not be retained.[141] Included in the file are some of the comments made by the Principal Medical Officer, for example: 'his disability has increased until he is now practically unable to perform any useful work'.[142]

The increasing focus on the need for disabled workers to maximise their productivity as a pre-requisite for continued employment led to some criticism from MPs and occasions of disputes between management and workers. This is perhaps best highlighted in the case of the

136 Gulland, *Gender, Work and Social Control.*

137 TNA BM 10/1, Remploy Limited, 'A Review of the Company during its first seven years' (March, 1953), pp. 40–1.

138 Ibid.

139 Ibid.

140 TNA LAB 43/268, 'Note to Mr Anderson M.P.' (19.07.1956).

141 TNA BM 8/13, Remploy Limited, 'Executive Director Report no. 69' (23.01.1952).

142 Ibid.

Remploy factory in Liverpool in 1954. The Labour MP, Mrs Braddock, contacted the Minister of Labour on behalf of one of her constituents working at the factory. Braddock explained that 'a Medical Officer has recently visited and informed certain of the employees that their output must considerably increase or the possibility of their being removed from the factory will be considered'.[143] She continued by making reference to the particular individual who had seen her, explaining that he 'is very badly disabled and the effect on his mental condition of these interviews is rather distressing…he informs me that he has always attempted to do the best he can in the department in which he is employed'.[144] Having been asked to look into the matter by the MOL, Remploy explained that the Company's Principle Medical Officer had visited the factory to investigate 'cases of employees of low productive potential which had been referred to Head Office', which included the individual who had seen Mrs Braddock.[145] The reply noted that 'the employees concerned admitted that they could do much better and as this was borne out by their medical assessments, they were told that they would be expected to show an improvement in their work and that the position would be reviewed in the near future'.[146] Determining whether a disabled worker was meeting their own productivity limits was not, therefore, a matter for the worker themselves. Instead, it was a combination of factory management and factory doctors who assessed the productivity level of each employee and then decided whether they were working to their capacity in a role.[147]

The 'Disability Mix'

It was briefly suggested by Anderson that Remploy concentrated on providing employment for people with particular disabilities.[148] As has been shown here, the focus for recruitment and retention was based upon individual productivity, and as such there was no specific focus on

143 TNA LAB 43/268, 'Letter from Mrs Braddock' (20.03.1954).

144 Ibid.

145 TNA LAB 43/268, 'Note from Mr Mallett to Mr Coburn' (30.03.1954).

146 Ibid.

147 TNA BM 8/2, Remploy Limited, 'Minutes of the One Hundred and Sixty-Second Meeting of the Board of Directors' (17.02.1960).

148 Anderson, *War, Disability and Rehabilitation in Britain*, p. 183.

employing people based on disability. Each factory could only recruit from the local disabled population, and this was determined based on their suitability to be productive in the job available. There were however, two important exceptions to this. The first was blind people, who were not generally employed by Remploy, nor intended to be, as they were long seen as a distinct group who had been provided for by their own legislation and specialist sheltered employment.[149] The other exception was those suffering from TB for which special Remploy factories were established. This was necessitated by the fear of contagion and the large numbers of TB cases noted as needing sheltered employment by the MOL as Remploy began to operate.[150] By 1952, 7 'Special' Remploy factories were dedicated to those with TB.[151] As the number of applicants suffering with tuberculosis declined, these factories were eventually converted in the 1960s to standard factories.[152] Beyond these specific cases, recruitment into Remploy was not based upon the inclusion or exclusion of particular disabilities within the Section II register.

Remploy's focus on productivity meant that the 'disability mix' of its employees did differ, though only marginally, from that of the Section II register itself.[153] There was, for example, a greater proportion of those in Remploy with lower limb disabilities, than those with impaired vision. The disabilities Anderson highlighted were those featured in an article published by a MOL official in 1958, which grouped the most common disabilities in Remploy at the time.[154] An internal report tracked the changing 'disability mix' from 1964 through to 1979, highlighting that the key developments were the reduction in employees suffering from TB

[149] Ibid; Reiss, *Bind Workers Against Charity*, pp. 141–3.

[150] TNA LAB 20/173, NACED, 'The employment of the infectious case of tuberculosis in industry' (1945).

[151] TNA BM 10/1, Remploy Limited, 'A Review of the Company during its first seven years' (March, 1953), pp. 19-20; TNA LAB 13/1029, Edwards, 'Remploy: An Experiment in Sheltered Employment for the Severely Disabled in Great Britain' (February, 1958), p. 8. Bryder, *Below the Magic Mountain*, p. 238.

[152] TNA BM 10/2, Remploy Limited, 'A Brief Outline of the Birth and Early Development of Remploy Limited' (May, 1979), p. 26.

[153] TNA BM 10/48, Remploy Limited, 'Objectives and Criteria of Success, Appendix No. 7' (July, 1980).

[154] Ibid; TNA BM 8/23, Remploy Limited, 'Managing Director's Report no. 30, Appendix L' (16.03.1955); TNA LAB 13/1029, Edwards, 'Remploy: An Experiment in Sheltered Employment for the Severely Disabled in Great Britain' (February, 1958), p. 8.

and the increase in employees with 'mental disabilities'.[155] As was previously noted, following the passing of the Mental Health Act in 1959, former mental hospital patients became eligible for registration and thus potentially eligible for a place in Remploy.[156] As government policy began to reflect the priority of de-institutionalisation of mental health patients, with a move to community-orientated care, Remploy was indeed considered part of this provision.[157] Remploy had, however, always included people considered severely disabled owing to mental illness.[158] The only immediate result of the passing of the 1959 Act was some limited experimentation with the more 'serious' cases of mental illness the company might be expected to cater for such as schizophrenia.[159] The real impact of the Act, in terms of Remploy, was in supporting a longer term trend of an increasing number of people on the Section II register classed as 'mentally disabled'.[160] While this did reflect a steady shift in terms of who could apply for Remploy, and prompted some discussion among the Board and senior management, it does not seem to have led to any change

[155] TNA BM 3/67, Remploy Limited, 'Report on Employment of Disabled People in Remploy, Appendix 4' (1979). TNA BM 10/48, Remploy Limited, 'Objectives and Criteria of Success' (July, 1980), p. 21.

[156] TNA BM 10/2, Remploy Limited, 'A Brief Outline of the Birth and Early Development of Remploy Limited' (May, 1979), p. 26.

[157] Ibid; TNA LAB 20/1429, DE, 'Sheltered Employment: A Draft Consultative Document' (October, 1973), pp. 33–4; Roulstone and Prideaux, *Understanding Disability Policy*, pp. 36–9; J. Welshman, 'Inside the Walls of the Hostel, 1940–74' in P. Dale and J. Melling, *Mental Illness and Learning Disability Since 1850* (Abingdon, Routledge, 2006), p. 200.

[158] TNA LAB 20/444, Disabled Persons Employment Corporation Limited, 'Executive Director Report 36: Appendix B' (18.11.1948); TNA BM 5/9, Remploy Limited, 'Factory Manager's Guide' (1949); *Fourth Report from the Select Committee on Estimates*, 162 (1952), Annex 9, p. 100.

[159] TNA BM 10/2, Remploy Limited, 'A Brief Outline of the Birth and Early Development of Remploy Limited' (May, 1979), p. 26.

[160] TNA BM 10/48, Remploy Limited, 'Objectives and Criteria of Success, Appendix No 7' (July, 1980); TNA LAB 20/1429, DE, 'Sheltered Employment: A Draft Consultative Document' (October, 1973), pp. 33–4; Mr Dudley Smith, (21.06.1972), *Hansard*, vol. 839 c.680.

in the recruitment process itself, the emphasis on productivity, or how Remploy fundamentally operated during the period considered here.[161]

Remploy's 'disability mix' was therefore a by-product of the recruitment process, not the driver behind it, and changed over time. Beyond the exceptions noted for blind people and those with TB, the fundamental question for recruitment was not a person's disability, but their ability to contribute productively to their local factory regardless of it.

The Non-Disabled Workforce

There has been a general assumption that Remploy's production workforce consisted entirely of disabled people, with the exception of Topliss, who suggested that it was 'always envisaged' that Remploy should include a proportion of non-disabled workers.[162] In terms of non-disabled workers, there were always a number of non-disabled staff members employed by Remploy in management, clerical and administrative roles, but it is apparent that there were also a significant number of non-disabled employees performing productive work on the factory floor.[163] The inclusion of this workforce, referred to as the 'fit' by Remploy, was explicitly an attempt to boost productivity.[164] This was first discussed in 1947 with the impetus coming from a visit by the Executive Director, Venn, to a sheltered workshop in London which included 'fit men' as 20% of its workforce to boost production.[165] The Board agreed that Venn should approach the Minister of Labour 'for authority to make similar arrangements'.[166]

161 TNA BM 3/70, Remploy Limited, 'Report of the Working Party on the Mix of Disabilities Employed by Remploy' (March, 1981). For more on this see Holroyde, 'Sheltered Employment and Mental Health in Britain', pp. 113–35.

162 Topliss, *Provision for the Disabled*, pp. 55–6.

163 A distinction was made between the proportion of 'fit' employees overall and those who were 'production workers', TNA BM 8/2, Disabled Persons Employment Corporation Limited, 'Minutes of the One Hundred and Fortieth Meeting of the Board of Directors' (19.02.1958); TNA BM 10/48, Remploy Limited, 'Objectives and Criteria of Success' (July, 1980), p. 72.

164 TNA BM 10/1, Remploy Limited, 'A Review of the Company during its first seven years' (March, 1953), p. 47.

165 TNA BM 8/1, Disabled Persons Employment Corporation Limited, 'Minutes of the Twenty-Fourth Meeting of the Board of Directors' (29.07.1947).

166 Ibid.

The question of the proportion of 'fit' to disabled workers was discussed, both in terms of the merits on production of a higher number, and the need to prevent it getting too high, on a number of occasions.[167] There was always, according to Remploy, the temptation to keep increasing the number of 'fit' workers to boost productivity, which was understandable given the financial pressures placed upon the company.[168] This was balanced against the understanding of the overall aim of the company being to employ severely disabled people.[169] This aim had of course already been modified somewhat to limit this to a certain section of 'productive' severely disabled people, but this was still keeping recruitment in the boundary of 'Section II' people, which the inclusion of 'fit' people was not. The agreed limit on the employment on non-Section II workers was set at 15% of the productive workforce, which was to remain the maximum allowed for the remainder of the period examined here.[170] It has not been possible to determine the actual figures for the whole period, but what evidence there is indicates that Remploy likely kept to the limit on a company level.[171] As noted however, company policy did not always reflect the factory reality, and there were instances

[167] TNA BM 8/2, Remploy Limited, 'Minutes of the One Hundred and Thirty-First Meeting of the Board of Directors' (15.05.1957); 'Minutes of the One Hundred and Fortieth Meeting of the Board of Directors' (19.02.1958); 'Minutes of the One Hundred and Forty-Sixth Meeting of the Board of Directors' (17.09.1958); 'Minutes of the One Hundred and Fifty-Seventh Meeting of the Board of Directors' (16.09.1959); 'Minutes of the One Hundred and Sixty-Sixth Meeting of the Board of Directors' (15.06.1960); 'Minutes of the One Hundred and Sixty-Ninth Meeting of the Board of Directors' (19.10.1960).

[168] TNA BM 3/55, Remploy Limited, 'Notes on MSC/Remploy Meeting' (28.07.1978).

[169] Ibid.

[170] TNA BM 10/1, Remploy Limited, 'A Review of the Company during its first seven years' (March, 1953), p. 47; TNA BM 10/48, Remploy Limited, 'Objectives and Criteria of Success, Appendix 4' (July, 1980), p. 72.

[171] TNA LAB 43/268, 'Notes on letter from Mr Willey' (17.05.1956); TNA BM 8/2, Remploy Limited, 'Minutes of the One Hundred and Fortieth Meeting of the Board of Directors' (19.02.1958); 'Minutes of the One Hundred and Forty-Sixth Meeting of the Board of Directors' (17.09.1958); TNA BM 8/32, Remploy Limited, 'Managing Director Report No. 86, Personnel Management: Appendix A' (11.04.1960); TNA BM 8/84, Remploy Limited, '"Remploy in the Long-Term", Managing Director's Basic Study Group, Appendix 4' (13.04.1977).

of individual factories exceeding the limit.[172] In 1960 there were 11 factories doing so, including two where 'fit' workers comprised 34% of the workforce.[173] Such breaches were excused where they were temporary measures required to ensure a production order was fulfilled.[174] The records also demonstrate the local variation in the employment of 'fit' personnel, with some factories employing as little as 2% and others skirting close to the limit or exceeding it.[175] In addition to non-disabled workers, Remploy also employed some 'Section I' workers, who though still disabled, were not technically eligible under the terms of the DPEA, and again appear to have been incorporated due to their increased productivity. This was only a very small number, however, peaking at 160 people in 1953 and gradually reducing over the period to reach only 20 by 1979.[176]

It is apparent therefore, that the focus of Remploy on maximising the productivity of its workforce also resulted in the employment of a number of workers who were not Section II. This is important, as the inclusion of non-disabled workers was a different concept than that of selecting the most productive disabled workers, as this openly contravened the mandate of Remploy as existing to employ the severely disabled in an explicit way. While the company-wide limit of 15% may have been maintained, this was still a significant number of 'fit' employees taking the place of Section II employees. This is also important in the understanding of Remploy as a place of 'segregated' employment. This notion of Remploy, and indeed of

[172] TNA BM 8/2, Remploy Limited, 'Minutes of the One Hundred and Fifty-Seventh Meeting of the Board of Directors' (16.09.1959); 'Minutes of the One Hundred and Sixty-Sixth Meeting of the Board of Directors' (15.06.1960).

[173] TNA BM 8/32, Remploy Limited, 'Managing Director's Report No. 86, Personnel Management: Appendix A' (11.04.1960).

[174] TNA BM 8/2, Remploy Limited, 'Minutes of the One Hundred and Fifty-Seventh Meeting of the Board of Directors' (16.09.1959); 'Minutes of the One Hundred and Sixty-Sixth Meeting of the Board of Directors' (15.06.1960); TNA BM 8/32, Remploy Limited, 'Managing Director's Report No. 86, Personnel Management: Appendix A' (11.04.1960).

[175] See for example, TNA LAB 20/399, Disabled Persons Employment Corporation Limited, 'Executive Director's Report No. 25, Appendix C' (19.11.1947); TNA BM 3/7, Remploy Limited, 'Personnel Department: Percentage of Able-Bodied Personnel employed on Production in Remploy Factories' (May, 1959).

[176] TNA BM 3/67, Remploy Limited, 'Report on Employment of Disabled People in Remploy, Appendix 2' (1979).

sheltered employment generally, as a place where disabled workers were, and indeed where sheltered employment still exists, are, isolated from the non-disabled is a powerful one. It was this which formed the basis of the desire to move away from sheltered employment in the United Kingdom in the name of 'inclusion' which grew in the 1980s and 90s, and which ultimately led to the closure of workshops and Remploy's transition to an employment services role. The concept of sheltered employment remains controversial, and it is not the intention of this study to challenge the conception of such places as inherently involving 'segregation' as disability activists have suggested.[177] Neither is it possible to determine if such workers enjoyed equality of status. What this does challenge however, is the understanding of Remploy as segregated in absolute terms, as it is clear that in numerous factories the severely disabled were working alongside non-disabled workers on the factory floor.

Conclusions

Remploy provided sheltered employment for thousands of severely disabled people during the period of the classic welfare state. However, it was never a catch-all scheme for all those designated as Section II. Remploy, in common with other aspects of the DPEA, did not live up to its initial lofty promise of providing sheltered employment for all those needing it.[178] Although the DPEA had a broad definition of disability, eligibility for a place in Remploy involved several barriers which put sheltered employment beyond the reach of many. Throughout the period, entry into Remploy and continued employment was subject to meeting a number of standards, maintaining a minimum level of productivity, continuous assessment and the vagaries of local factory particularities. As a result, the achievement of 'full employment', so central to the classic welfare state, was not extended to the Section II population, and for a significant number of disabled people, Remploy represented a further area of exclusion.

The analysis here has enabled a deeper understanding of who was employed by Remploy and how candidates were selected. It has been

[177] Barnes, *Disabled People in Britain and Discrimination*, p. 74.

[178] Roulstone and Prideaux, *Understanding Disability Policy*, pp. 27–8; Hampton, *Disability and the Welfare State in Britain*, p. 1; Borsay, *Disability and Social Policy in Britain Since 1750*, pp. 197–201.

demonstrated that Remploy was not the exclusive domain of disabled ex-service personnel, either in principle or in practice. Furthermore, the notion of preference for this group does not appear to have been a significant advantage in gaining employment and soon disappears from the records. Thus, we can see that in the case of Remploy, the long-held privilege in welfare and employment services for the war-disabled diminished quickly following the end of the Second World War, and Bevin's push for the end of differential treatment based upon the cause of disablement alone succeeded. Contrary then, to the notion that ex-servicemen continued to occupy a privileged position in the allocation of services after the war, this has been shown to not be the case here.[179]

Selection for Remploy was based on productivity, with policy dictating that only those with a minimum standard of productivity were recruited, and the realities of local factory recruitment prioritising this further still. Assessment of individual potential productivity was performed by medical experts, bureaucrats and factory management. Gulland has noted the privileged status afforded to medical evidence across incapacity benefit regimes over the period examined here, and indeed into the present day.[180] The kind of functional assessments performed to determine capability to gain and retain employment with Remploy, alongside the more subjective assessments made by DROs and factory managers, are clearly part of this enduring approach to assessing disabled people's capacity for work and eligibility for state provision in benefits and services.

This further supports the conclusions from Chapter 3, challenging any view of sheltered workshops having been slowly turned from places of charitable and humanitarian concern in the period here, to places of commercial enterprise in the 1980s.[181] As has been illustrated, productivity and economic concerns always played a key role in Remploy and nowhere more so than in recruitment. Remploy factories attempted to be places of productive industry and recruited according to this conception,

[179] See Anderson, *War, Disability and Rehabilitation in Britain*, pp. 187–9, 211; Elsey, 'The Rehabilitation and Employment of Disabled Ex-Servicemen after the Two World Wars', pp. 292–7; Hampton, *Disability and the Welfare State in Britain*, pp. 99, 199–209; Borsay, *Disability and Social Policy in Britain Since 1750*, pp. 160–62; Millward, 'Social Security Policy and the Early Disability Movement', p. 281; Fraser, *The Evolution of the British Welfare State*, p. 258.

[180] Gulland, *Gender, Work and Social Control*, pp. 53–76.

[181] Barnes, *Disabled People in Britain and Discrimination*, p. 73.

including taking on a percentage of non-disabled workers. For those who managed to get over the various hurdles, finally gaining employment with Remploy was no guarantee of a job with the company for life, with maintaining a level of productivity a pre-requisite for continued employment. Contrary to the suggestions of Borsay, Thane and Bolderson, Remploy was to be no place for 'ineffective' or non-productive workers.[182] Though the DPEA created two categories of disabled people, the application of its policies effectively created a third category deemed too unproductive even for sheltered employment.

This evidence has further shown the importance of understanding the realities of local administration of national schemes such as Remploy. In this case, there appears to have been a real gulf between Remploy's central policy and the local administration which was actually involved in recruiting. As such, we should not assume that central policy espoused by government and organisations reflected the reality for disabled people on the ground.[183] In the case of Remploy it is clear that candidates were subject to wide local variances in recruitment practice and standards, which would result in very different experience depending upon where they lived.

[182] Borsay, *Disability and Social Policy in Britain Since 1750*, p. 135; Bolderson, 'The Origins of the Disabled Persons Employment Quota and its Symbolic Significance', p. 178; Thane, *Foundations of the Welfare State*, p. 225.

[183] Topliss, *Provision for the Disabled*, p. 56.

CHAPTER 5

Women in Remploy: Access, Segregation and Status

Introduction

If the classic welfare state has been seen to have neglected disabled people from its provision, the same case has also been consistently made for women, with welfare and employment measures serving to reinforce the traditional roles of men as workers and women as domestic care-givers.[1] For disabled women this resulted in a particular neglect as both

[1] D. Fraser, *The Evolution of the British Welfare State*, 4th Edition (Basingstoke, Palgrave Macmillan, 2009), p. 258; K. Laybourn, *The Evolution of British Social Policy and the Welfare State, c.1800–1993* (Keele, Keele University Press, 1995), pp. 254–6; R. Lowe, *The Welfare State in Britain Since 1945* (Basingstoke, Palgrave Macmillan, 2005) pp. 40–3, 146; R. Page, *Revisiting the Welfare State* (Maidenhead, Open University Press, 2007), p. 40; D. Gladstone, 'The Welfare State and the State of Welfare', in D. Gladstone (ed.), *British Social Welfare: Past, Present and Future* (London, UCL Press, 1995), p. 23; N. Deakin, *The Politics of Welfare: Continuities and Change* (London, Harvester Wheatsheaf, 1994), pp. xiv, 4; D. Gladstone, *The Twentieth-Century Welfare State* (Basingstoke, Palgrave Macmillan, 1999), pp. 6–7; A. Digby, *British Welfare Policy: Workhouse to Workfare* (London, Faber and Faber, 1989), pp. 62–3; C. Pierson, *Beyond the Welfare State? The New Political Economy of Welfare* (Cambridge, Polity Press, 1991), pp. 69–79; C. Pierson, 'Theory in British Social Policy', in N. Ellison and C. Pierson (eds.), *Developments in British Social Policy* (London, Macmillan, 1998), pp. 19–21; H. Glennerster, *British Social Policy: 1945 to the Present*, 3rd Edition (Oxford, Blackwell Publishing, 2007), pp. 35–6; J. Brown, *The British Welfare State: A Critical History* (Oxford, Blackwell, 1995), p. 53; P. Thane, 'Visions of Gender in the Making of the British Welfare State', in

© The Author(s), under exclusive license to Springer Nature Switzerland AG 2025

A. Holroyde, *Sheltered Employment and Disability in the British Welfare State*, New Directions in Welfare History,
https://doi.org/10.1007/978-3-031-87876-3_5

women and disabled people, which Oliver deemed a 'double disability'.[2] In the case of Remploy there is a mixed conception of the place of disabled women, with simple references to the company employing severely disabled people in line with the DPEA raising the possibility that it was open to both disabled men and women equally.[3] The understanding within Remploy itself during the research for this study, was that the employment of an increasing number of women was a key aspect in the company's development. Yet it is the contention of scholars such as Anderson, Borsay, Hampton, Thane and Sainsbury that disabled women were disadvantaged in accessing the employment provisions of the welfare

G. Bock and P. Thane (eds.), *Maternity and Gender Policies: Women and the Rise of the European Welfare States, 1880s–1950s* (London, Routledge, 1991), p. 93; R. Crompton and K. Sanderson, *Gendered Jobs & Social Change* (London, Unwin Hyman, 1990), pp. 49–50; D.S. Wilson, 'Gender, Race and Ideal Labour Force', in L. Ryan and W. Webster (eds.), *Gendering Migration: Masculinity, Femininity and Ethnicity in Post-War Britain* (Aldershot, Ashgate, 2008), pp. 89–103; J. Gulland, *Gender, Work and Social Control: A Century of Disability Benefits* (Palgrave Macmillan, 2019).

[2] M. Oliver, *The Politics of Disablement* (Basingstoke, Macmillan, 1990), p. 70.

[3] J. Hampton, 'Discovering Disability: The General Classes of Disabled People and the Classic Welfare State, 1948–1964', *The Historian*, vol. 75, no. 1 (2013), p. 80; L. Bryder, *Below the Magic Mountain: A Social History of Tuberculosis in Twentieth-Century Britain* (Oxford, Clarendon Press, 1988), p. 237; S. Wheatcroft, *Worth Saving: Disabled Children During the Second World War* (Manchester, Manchester University Press, 2013), p. 168; M. Hyde, 'Sheltered and Supported Employment in the 1990s: The Experiences of Disabled Workers in the UK', *Disability & Society*, vol. 13, no. 2 (1998), p. 200; P. Bridgen and R. Lowe, *Welfare Policy Under the Conservatives 1951–1964* (London, PRO, 1998), pp. 262–3; H. Bolderson, *Social Security, Disability and Rehabilitation: Conflicts in the Development of Social Policy 1914–1946* (London, Jessica Kingsley Publishers, 1991), p. 109; E. Topliss, *Provision for the Disabled* (Oxford, Basil Blackwell, 1979), p. 56; M. Reiss, *Blind Workers Against Charity: The National League of the Blind of Great Britain and Ireland, 1893–1970* (London, Palgrave Macmillan, 2015), p. 139; E. Elsey, 'The Rehabilitation and Employment of Disabled Ex-Servicemen after the Two World Wars', unpublished PhD Thesis, University of Teesside (1994), pp. 276–7; C. Barnes, *Disabled People in Britainand Discrimination* (London, C. Hurst & Co., 2000), p. 71; M. Mantin, 'Coalmining and the National Scheme for Disabled Ex-Servicemen After the First World War', *Social History*, vol. 41, no. 2 (2016), p. 170; A. Borsay, *Disability and Social Policy in Britain Since 1750: A History of Exclusion* (Basingstoke, Palgrave Macmillan, 2005), p. 135; H. Bolderson, 'The Origins of the Disabled Persons Employment Quota and its Symbolic Significance', *Journal of Social Policy*, vol. 9, no. 2 (1980), p. 178; P. Thane, *Foundations of the Welfare State*, 2nd Edition (London, Longman, 1996), p. 225.

state, which were 'allocated overwhelmingly to men'.[4] Consideration of the case of Remploy in this has only been briefly referenced by Anderson who suggested that women were largely excluded from Remploy due to its nature as an industrial enterprise, as well as issues of accommodation and transport.[5] This chapter will therefore seek to clarify whether the experience of women in Remploy was one of exclusion.

As well as this issue of neglect in welfare provision, consideration of Remploy also provides an opportunity to examine further issues of employment for disabled women, which have thus far received relatively little attention. There is broad agreement from scholars that the position of women in employment generally during the period considered here was characterised by gender segregation, low pay, inferior status and a lack of opportunity for advancement.[6] This chapter will explore these areas for disabled women within Remploy to determine the degree to which these also applied in sheltered employment.

This chapter will begin by examining the numbers of female workers in Remploy over the period, to reveal the gender mix and to consider whether the organisation was indeed male-dominated. It will then

[4] J. Anderson, 'British Women, Disability and the Second World War', *Contemporary British History*, vol. 20, no. 1 (2006), p. 50; J. Anderson, *War, Disability and Rehabilitation in Britain: 'Soul of a Nation'* (Manchester, Manchester University Press, 2011), pp. 169–70; J. Hampton, *Disability and the Welfare State in Britain: Changes in Perception and Policy 1948–79* (Bristol, Policy Press, 2016), p. 119; Borsay, *Disability and Social Policy in Britain Since 1750*, p. 134; Thane, *Foundations of the Welfare State*, pp. 224–5; S. Sainsbury, 'Disabled People and the Personal Social Services', in D. Gladstone (ed.), *British Social Welfare: Past, Present and Future* (London, UCL Press, 1995), p.188.

[5] Anderson, *War, Disability and Rehabilitation in Britain*, p. 170; Anderson, 'British Women, Disability and the Second World War', p. 49.

[6] H. McCarthy, *Double Lives: A History of Working Motherhood* (London, Bloomsbury, 2020); Wilson, 'Gender, Race the Ideal Labour Force'; Lowe, *The Welfare State in Britain Since 1945*, pp. 42–3; K. Laybourn, *Unemployment and Employment Policies Concerning Women in Britain, 1900–1951* (Lampeter, Edwin Mellen Press, 2002), p. 187; S. Bruley, *Women in Britain Since 1900* (Basingstoke, Palgrave, 1999), pp. 99–119; P. Summerfield, *Women Workers in the Second World War: Production and Patriarchy in Conflict* (London, Routledge, 1984); M. Glucksmann, *Women Assemble: Women Workers and the New Industries in Inter-War Britain* (London, Routledge, 1990), p. 281; Gladstone, *The Twentieth-Century Welfare State*, pp. 119–122; G. Holloway, *Women and Work in Britain Since 1840* (London, Routledge, 2005), p. 186; P. Thane, 'Towards Equal Opportunities? Women in Britain Since 1945', in T. Gourvish and A. O'Day (eds.), *Britain Since 1945* (Basingstoke, Macmillan, 1991), pp. 183–208; J. Lewis, *Women in Britain Since 1945: Women, Family, Work and the State in the Post-War Years* (Oxford, Blackwell, 1992), pp. 78–91.

consider the points made by Anderson to determine the factors which may have prevented women from gaining employment with the company. Following this, the chapter will explore the experiences of women within Remploy and whether the same issues of segregation, lower pay and lower status applied as they did in open employment. This will begin with the question of whether Remploy was gender segregated, both in terms of work and social activities, followed by consideration of the status of women in terms of pay, promotion and representation.

Gender Composition

Unfortunately, there is no document extant which provides a complete breakdown of Remploy's disabled employees by gender for the entirety of the period considered here. Those figures which have been located are also problematic, being frequently contradictory, incomplete, for different times of year, or averages for a set period. Table 5.1 has been compiled from a range of Remploy and MOL/DE sources including Remploy's Executive Director reports, and is intended to be indicative of the general trend. As can be seen, disabled women were always a minority in Remploy during the period considered here. Few women joined the company in its infancy, and it took 6 years of factory operation to reach a proportion of even 5% of the overall disabled workforce being women. There was an overall trend of steady growth in the number of female workers, which corresponds to the trend in employment more generally in the postwar period.[7] In open employment, figures show that in 1951 women represented 31% of the total workforce, 10 years later, this had increased to 33%, by 1971 this had grown to 37%, and by 1980 had reached 40%.[8] Though numbers of women in Remploy did increase steadily over the period, the proportion was far lower than that in open employment generally, as it still remained below 20% of the overall Remploy workforce by 1979.[9]

[7] Gladstone, *The Twentieth-Century Welfare State*, p. 119.

[8] H. Pemberton, 'The Transformation of the Economy', in P. Addison and H. Jones (eds.), *A Companion to Contemporary Britain 1939–2000* (Oxford, Blackwell, 2005), pp. 190–1; Lewis, *Women in Britain since 1945*, p. 65.

[9] Pemberton, 'The Transformation of the Economy', pp. 190–1; M. Pugh, *Women and the Women's movement in Britain 1914–1959* (London, Macmillan, 1992); Gladstone, *The Twentieth-Century Welfare State*, p. 119.

Table 5.1 Numbers of disabled men and women employed in Remploy, 1946–1979

Year	*Men*	*Women*	*% Women workers*
1946	160	4	2.43%
1947	587	12	2%
1948	1749	40	2.24%
1949	3868	111	2.79%
1950	4781	158	3.20%
1951	4797	161	3.24%
1952	5547	291	5%
1953	–	–	–
1954	6018	415	6.45%
1955	–	–	–
1956	5461	402	6.86%
1957	–	–	–
1958	5500	500	8.33%
1959	–	–	–
1960	5637	747	11.70%
1961	5495	756	12.09%
1962–1964	–	–	–
1965	5789	872	13.09%
1966–1968	–	–	–
1969	6387	1092	14.6%
1970	6501	1165	15.2%
1971–1972	–	–	–
1973	6534	1323	16.83%
1974	6664	1349	16.83%
1975	6770	1475	17.88%
1976	6840	1535	18.32%
1977	6466	1511	18.94%
1978	–	–	–
1979	6450	1558	19.45%

Sources Compiled from range of documents e.g. Remploy Executive Director Reports in TNA LAB 20/187, LAB 20/399, LAB 20/444, LAB 20/35, LAB 20/43, LAB 20/1035, LAB 13/1029, BM 8/13, BM 8/18, BM 8/81, BM 3/67, BM 10/12, BM 8/84[10]

[10] Note on discrepancies with other tables: figures are from a range of documents with variations in type of document, time of publication, and qualifications on statistics, for example the numbers for 1947–1949 are for the end of the respective years.

Remploy as a whole was always therefore a male-dominated organisation in terms of its disabled workforce. These statistics confirm that just as has been suggested of the provisions of the welfare state generally and in terms of employment services specifically, sheltered employment in the form of Remploy was indeed 'allocated overwhelmingly to men'.[11] This chapter will now consider why this was the case.

Issues of Access and Entry

The DPEA itself made no distinction between men and women, and, therefore, according to this legislation, Remploy was intended to be open equally to both.[12] However, in considering the employment prospects for disabled women immediately following the Second World War, Anderson suggested that when it came to Remploy, women 'may not have been able to avail themselves of this service'.[13] This was due to barriers relating to accommodation and transport, and, more fundamentally, the industrial nature of Remploy as 'an area where women were less likely to be employed'.[14]

In terms of accommodation, this reflects Anderson's wider argument that following the Second World War, disabled women struggled to gain suitable housing, resulting in many being forced into institutional settings or remaining with family.[15] This may indeed have proved to be a barrier, with the provision of accommodation usually lying beyond the remit of Remploy.[16] Only one Remploy factory had hostel accommodation attached, the Radcliffe factory, which represented an exceptional case with a need to provide accommodation for disabled Polish ex-servicemen who had fought for Britain during the Second World War, though it was noted that beyond this 'there have been isolated instances where accommodation has been found either in nearby hostels or in billets'.[17]

[11] Sainsbury, 'Disabled People and the Personal Social Services', p. 188.

[12] DPEA.

[13] Anderson, *War, Disability and Rehabilitation in Britain*, p. 170.

[14] Anderson, 'British Women, Disability and the Second World War', p. 49.

[15] Anderson, *Disability and Rehabilitation in Britain*, pp. 154–69.

[16] The National Archives (TNA) BM 10/1, Remploy Limited, 'A Review of the working of the Company during its first seven years' (March, 1953), p. 37.

[17] Ibid.

Generally however, Remploy was not made responsible for providing accommodation for its workers.

In terms of problems with transport, again this reflects Anderson's argument that in the allocation of disabled 'motor cars' by the Ministry of Pensions for the most severely disabled people, men received them quicker than women.[18] It is not clear how much this would affect the recruitment of women into Remploy specifically. As was noted in Chapter 4, Remploy factories were situated to allow access via public transport with some financial assistance available for travel expenses. It may be that disabled women had specific troubles with these areas, but there is nothing in the records examined here which suggests that either Remploy or the MOL and its successors, felt that this was a particular reason for the low numbers of women joining the company.

A more detailed examination is required to consider whether Remploy's position as part of 'industry' was fundamentally problematic for disabled women, as this was an area where women were generally less likely to be employed. This suggests that either women were not interested in joining Remploy, or that Remploy was not interested in employing women. In terms of the latter, the company's central recruitment policy itself does not appear to have explicitly privileged men over women. There is no evidence in any of the records examined on recruitment of a notion of women being considered less desirable as workers or recommendations that they be excluded from recruitment. There was similarly no mention of such an attitude in the examination undertaken by the NACED on the issue of unemployment 'among registered disabled women' in 1951.[19] As part of this investigation, findings from questions asked of MOL Regional Officers suggested that there was an issue with those disabled women designated as Section I in finding work, with some employers apparently 'cautious' in taking them on, but there was no mention of any similar issue with those designated as Section II who were eligible for Remploy.[20]

[18] Anderson, 'British Women, Disability and the Second World War', pp. 47–8.

[19] TNA LAB 20/591, NACED, 'Training and Employment Committee T.E.C.45' (31.10.1951).

[20] Ibid; TNA LAB 20/591, 'Letter from MOL Wales Office' (19.05.1951); 'Letter from MOL Southern Regional Office' (17.05.1951); 'Letter from MOL Manchester Regional Office' (23.05.1951); 'Letter from MOL East and West Ridings Regional Office' (23.05.1951); 'Letter from MOL Eastern Regional Office' (28.05.1951); 'Letter from

There is also evidence that as Remploy began to operate, the Board of Directors was expecting to recruit female workers and did not see them as a less-appealing workforce. In his report for June 1946 the Executive Director of Remploy revealed the expectation of the inclusion of women when he commented on the numbers employed at the Bridgend factory since its opening.[21] Of the Longton Disabled Soldiers' and Sailors' Cardboard factory which had been taken over that month, he again noted the intention of replacing the several non-disabled workers in the factory with disabled 'men and women'.[22] The first woman to join Remploy was employed in 1946 as 'a telephone operator' and a further intake of three disabled women were taken on at Longton soon after.[23] In addition to this, six disabled women were called to interview as possible employees for the Bridgend factory.[24] There is thus no archival evidence that the Remploy Board itself was seeking to exclude the recruitment of women as policy.

However, while these cases may have reflected the attitude of the Remploy Board, and while official company policy may not have discriminated against female applicants, as has been shown in previous chapters, there could often be a wide divide between central policy and the reality at the local factory level. Chapter 4 also illustrated that recruitment focused on the assessment of an applicant's productivity for the role available, and this was ultimately decided at the factory level. It is entirely possible therefore that women were considered less productive or desirable for the work available based upon the attitude of the individual factory manager. There is no direct evidence available to either support or discredit this notion, but it must be considered that applicants would be assessed for a place at the factory by a panel of men who would inevitably bring their

MOL Bristol Regional Office' (28.05.1951); 'Letter from MOL North Midlands Regional Office' (31.05.1951); 'Letter from MOL Scottish Headquarters' (19.05.1951).

[21] TNA LAB 20/187, Disabled Persons Employment Corporation Limited, 'Executive Director Report No. 11: Appendix F' (18.06.1946).

[22] TNA LAB 20/187, Disabled Persons Employment Corporation Limited, 'Executive Director Report No. 11: Appendix F' (18.06.1946).

[23] TNA LAB 20/187, Disabled Persons Employment Corporation Limited, 'Executive Director Report No. 12: Appendix F' (23.07.1946); *Remploy News*, 5 (April, 1953); TNA LAB 20/187, Disabled Persons Employment Corporation Limited, 'Executive Director Report No. 13: Appendix F' (19.09.1946).

[24] TNA LAB 20/187, Disabled Persons Employment Corporation Limited, 'Executive Director Report No. 15: Appendix C' (19.11.1946).

own attitudes and views into making their decision. The lack of archival evidence of discrimination in recruitment does not mean that it did not occur. Scholars have highlighted the stubborn prevalence of traditional views that women's primary responsibility was to home and family over work across this period and indeed beyond.[25] There is also the question of whether particular types of work done in Remploy were considered as particularly suitable for men or women, in which case gender might also play a more explicit, yet undocumented, role in recruitment which has not been preserved in the archives. This issue will be considered further in the following section.

In terms of how attractive Remploy, as part of 'industry', was for disabled women themselves, this does seem to be an important factor. This also appears to be a wider problem, reflected in the low numbers of women willing even to register as Section II on the Disabled Persons' Employment Register, and thereby become eligible for sheltered employment such as Remploy. As of February 1946 only 469 women were registered as Section II, compared to 7714 men.[26] It was noted by the MOL in its initial guidance for DROs that 'since the inception of the register of disabled persons, it has become increasingly clear that the number of registered disabled women requiring employment is only a small proportion of the total and proportionately very much smaller over the whole employment field than the number of registered men'.[27] It was immediately apparent therefore that proportionally far fewer women were registering as disabled, and thereby making themselves eligible for the provisions contained in the DPEA. This was further discussed in the Remploy Regional Executive Officers' Conference in June 1946, which concluded with the expectation that as provisions became established, 'many more will register'.[28]

[25] Lewis, *Women in Britain since 1945*, pp. 68, 85; Bruley, *Women in Britain Since 1900*, p. 122; J. Lewis, *Women in England 1870–1950: Sexual Divisions and Social Change* (Brighton, Wheatsheaf Books Ltd, 1984), p. 184; Thane, 'Towards Equal Opportunities', pp. 198–201; McCarthy, *Double Lives*; Gulland, *Gender, Work and Social Control*; Holloway, *Women and Work in Britain Since 1840*, pp. 208–221.

[26] TNA LAB 20/187, Disabled Persons Employment Corporation Limited, 'Executive Director Report No. 8: Appendix E' (18.03.1946).

[27] TNA LAB 20/328, MOL, 'Guide to the Quota and Designated Employment Schemes for the use of Disablement Resettlement Officers'.

[28] TNA LAB 20/187, Disabled Persons Employment Corporation Limited, 'Executive Director Report No. 12: Appendix B' (23.07.1946).

This was not to be the case, however, with the 1951 report from the NACED on 'unemployment among disabled women' noting that the 'number of women who have registered as disabled is much less than the number who would qualify for registration'.[29] The Piercy Report in 1956, included a breakdown of the numbers of unemployed registered disabled persons (Table 5.2), which proves illustrative of this continuing trend. Here we can see the numbers of registered Section II women seeking employment standing at 427 by 1956, compared to 3523 men. It is apparent therefore that there was a general issue of women choosing not to register as disabled and thereby gain access to provision such as Remploy.[30] The result was that the company was left with a pool of relatively few women recruits to choose from. This can be seen most clearly at the local level. For example, queries in Parliament about Remploy factories in the Stoke-on-Trent area in 1950 and again the following year, suggest that following the employment of 11 disabled women, there were no further applicants available.[31]

The number of women in Remploy did steadily increase during the period, and so too did the number of women registering as Section II. In 1969, the number of unemployed disabled women on the Section II

Table 5.2 Number of registered disabled persons unemployed, 1953–1956

Year	*Section I*		*Section II*	
	Men	*Women*	*Men*	*Women*
1953	48,981	7228	6525	628
1954	43,189	6476	5069	523
1955	36,019	4603	4122	453
1956	32,438	5466	3523	427

Source *Report of the Committee of Inquiry on The Rehabilitation, Training and Resettlement of Disabled Persons*, 9883, *Appendix G* (1956)

29 TNA LAB 20/591, NACED, 'Unemployment Among Registered Disabled Women, N.A.C. 171',

30 H. Malisoff, 'The British Disabled Persons (Employment) Act', *Industrial and Labor Relations Review*, vol. 5, no. 2 (1952), p. 252.

31 Mr. George Isaacs, *Hansard* (27.06.1950), vol. 476 cc. 2069; Sir Monckton, *Hansard* (20.11.1951), vol. 494 cc.33w.

register was 1095, and by the end of 1979, this had grown to 1434.[32] The reasons behind this increase were considered by a working party setup by Remploy looking into the 'mix of disabilities employed by Remploy' in March 1981. The resulting report suggested this was largely down to wider factors which applied to all women in terms of changes in expectations, sexual discrimination legislation, changing attitudes and an evolving labour market.[33] These factors have also been highlighted by scholars such as Lewis, Bruley, Wilson and Deirdre McCloskey in supporting the trend in general employment of increasing numbers of women, particularly married women including mothers, choosing to enter work over the period.[34] However, as Table 5.3 shows, the numbers of registered Section II women always remained only a fraction of the numbers of men.[35]

It is apparent therefore that disabled women continued to be less likely to register as Section II than men throughout the period. Several reasons were suggested as to why this was the case. The attractiveness of Remploy itself as an industrial concern was clearly recognised at the time as an important factor. The Remploy chairman, Sir Robert Burrows, when giving evidence to the Select Committee on Estimates in 1952, suggested that the scarcity of women in Remploy was indeed because 'most of them apparently do not want to come out into industry'.[36] In the same year, the MOL asked a selection of those eligible to register at local employment exchanges why they would not do so. There is no breakdown of whether these respondents were from people designated as Section I or Section II, but the chief reason given, both for men and for women, was that they saw 'no apparent benefit to do so' in terms

[32] TNA BM 8/51, Remploy Limited, 'Managing Director's Report No. 191, Appendix Pers. 1: Section II Disabled Employees' (November, 1969); BM 3/70, Remploy Limited, 'Report of the Working Party on the Mix of Disabilities Employed by Remploy' (March, 1981), p. 13.

[33] Ibid, pp. 25–7.

[34] Lewis, *Women in Britain since 1945*, pp. 65–85; Bruley, *Women in Britain Since 1900*, p. 122; D. McCloskey, 'Paid Work', in I. Zweiniger-Bargielowska (ed.), *Women in Twentieth-Century Britain* (London, Routledge, 2014), pp. 169–70; McCarthy, *Double Lives*.

[35] TNA BM 8/51, Remploy Limited, 'Managing Director's Report No. 191, Appendix Pers. 1: Section II Disabled Employees' (November, 1969); TNA BM 3/70, Remploy Limited, 'Report of the Working Party on the Mix of Disabilities Employed by Remploy' (March, 1981), p. 13.

[36] *Fourth Report from the Select Committee on Estimates*, 162 (1952), para. 281, p. 21.

Table 5.3 Number of section II registered unemployed, 1963–1973

Year	*Men*	*Women*	*Total*	*% Women*
1963	4889	622	5511	11.3%
1964	5291	687	5978	11.5%
1965	5410	731	6141	11.9%
1966	5603	779	6382	12.2%
1967	6636	897	7533	11.9%
1968	7650	980	8630	11.4%
1969	8570	1032	9602	10.7%
1970	8900	1113	10,013	11.1%
1971	9811	1309	11,120	11.8%
1972	10,563	1542	12,105	12.7%
1973	9681	1483	11,164	13.3%

Source TNA LAB 20/1429, DE, 'Sheltered Employment: A Draft Consultative Document: Table VIII' (October, 1973)

of the provision that would become available.[37] This kind of apathy for what was offered through Remploy was also apparent in the interviews of the six women for the first Remploy factory at Bridgend in 1946. Of these applicants, two 'failed to turn up' for the interview and one 'refused the work' offered.[38] This attitude aligns with that for employment more generally, as although factory work, generally limited to light and unskilled work, remained an area where women were employed after the Second World War, there was a growing preference in the period for 'clean, respectable work with a reasonable wage', with clerical work and roles associated with the expanded welfare state such as social care proving popular areas, though options depended on factors such as education.[39] Similarly, the limited opportunities for part-time work could also make entering employment challenging for women, especially for mothers for whom childcare could prove a further barrier.[40] The question of wages

[37] TNA LAB 20/350, NACED, 'Joint Meeting of the Medical Committee and the Training and Employment Committee, M.C 33 T.E.C 64' (1952).

[38] TNA LAB 20/187, Disabled Persons Employment Corporation Limited, 'Executive Director Report No. 15: Appendix C' (19.11.1946).

[39] Holloway, *Women and Work in Britain Since 1840*, p. 191; McCarthy, *Double Lives*, pp. 261–76.

[40] McCarthy, *Double Lives;* Wilson, 'Gender, Race and the Ideal Labour Force'.

will be considered in a subsequent section, but this could also have dissuaded disabled women from joining Remploy. Considering the issue in 1981, an internal Remploy report concluded that one of the chief reasons for the lack of women registering over the preceding decades was the industrial nature of sheltered employment which was viewed as continuing to appeal more to men.[41]

We can also see this reflected in the Remploy factory environments themselves. As Chapter 3 has shown, the establishment of many of the initial factories involved the company adopting existing premises of various kinds, which left little room for adaptation to suit the needs of the employees. However, as custom-built Remploy factories, designed and built by the Ministry of Works, began to replace these, there was an opportunity to tailor the environment to suit the needs of the entire workforce, including women. There appears to have been little consideration of suiting the factory environment to the needs or desires of women however, which both Braybon and Summerfield suggest was a common problem in open industry as well.[42] In terms of the basic requirements of lavatory facilities, the original 1946 Remploy factory plans show that while women's lavatories were included, they were much smaller than those for men, with one or two toilets only, and despite the increase in female employees, the plans from 1975 show only a modest adjustment to three toilets.[43] This began to be recognised in Remploy as a pressing issue at the end of the period, with an internal report suggesting the lack of toilet facilities had likely led to the 'preclusion of females for employment', and the Board acknowledging the urgent need for improvement.[44] A further internal report produced in 1981 on Remploy's workforce, went further still and suggested that the company required a fundamental re-think of the factory environment in the face of the increasing numbers

[41] TNA BM 3/70, Remploy Limited, 'Report of the Working Party on the Mix of Disabilities Employed by Remploy' (March, 1981), p. 25.

[42] G. Braybon and P. Summerfield, *Out of the Cage: Women's Experiences in Two World Wars* (Abingdon, Routledge, 2013), p. 285.

[43] TNA BM 10/7, Ministry of Works, 'British Factories for Disabled Persons Employment Corporation Ltd.: Model Plans'; BM 10/26, Remploy Limited, 'Standard Factory Plan' (13.02.1975).

[44] TNA BM 10/48, Remploy Limited, 'Objectives and Criteria of Success' (July, 1980), p. 24; BM 8/85, Remploy Limited, 'Company Estimates for the Year Ended 31st March 1981' (1979).

of women employees, stating 'first, it would be advisable to ensure that welfare facilities such as canteens, rest rooms, lavatories etc. are furnished in such a way as to be attractive to women'.[45] Such statements make it apparent that during the period considered here, women workers in Remploy were employed in an environment designed primarily around men.

There is therefore clearly some validity to the notion that Remploy's nature as an industrial concern failed to adequately entice disabled women to take the steps necessary to gain employment with the company. However, the traditional ties of women to the home were also important. Many women who had entered into industry during the Second World War had decided to return to domestic life, or had been forced to make way for returning men, and this could equally have been the case for disabled women as well.[46] Similarly, the Executive Director of Remploy noted in 1952 that significant numbers of women continued to leave the company and employment upon getting married.[47] Women leaving work for marriage or to start a family was again a common feature of postwar employment generally.[48] Though this had started to change following the war, and over subsequent decades increasing numbers of married women and mothers joined the labour market, this did not entail freedom from holding the prime responsibility for home and care.[49] Limited availability of part-time or flexible work could make managing employment impossible. A more sinister explanation in this vein was proposed at the time by Dame Georgiana Buller, an early champion of disability rights and founder of St Loyes Training College for Cripples, who expressed her suspicions that the low numbers of registered disabled women was mainly due to 'many cases where people liked to keep their disabled relatives at

[45] TNA BM 10/34, Remploy Limited, 'Report of the Working Party on the Mix of Disabilities Employed by Remploy, Table II' (June, 1981), pp. 38–9.

[46] Thane, 'Towards Equal Opportunities?', pp. 192–4; E. Wilson, *Women and the Welfare State* (London, Tavistock Publications, 1977), p. 155; Holloway, *Women and Work in Britain Since 1840*, pp. 191–2.

[47] *Fourth Report from the Select Committee on Estimates*, 162 (1952), para. 339, p. 26.

[48] Holloway, *Women and Work in Britain Since 1840*, pp. 196–8; Lewis, *Women in Britain since 1945*, pp. 68, 76; McCloskey, 'Paid Work', pp. 169–70.

[49] McCarthy, *Double Lives*.

home for cheap labour'.[50] This was also a further reason proposed by Remploy in its 1981 report which suggested many disabled women had been 'hidden by their families'.[51] Thus the persistence of traditional ties to the domestic sphere, and challenges of securing work to align with them, could have proven to be even stronger for disabled women.

Gender Segregation

An understood key feature of employment for women in the postwar period considered here is the continued segregation of work along gendered lines. Despite the increasing numbers of women entering employment, the prevalence of a labour market 'strictly divided by gender' has been highlighted by a number of historians such as Thane, Bruley, Glucksmann, Gladstone, Holloway and Summerfield.[52] In this division, it was 'women's work' which was viewed as lower skilled.[53] As both Thane and Lewis have explained, this was predicated on the understanding that men were more productive than women owing to their physical attributes.[54] In considering severely disabled people however, this simple assumption of male physical 'superiority' cannot hold, with the reduced productivity and assumed lower skill of work in sheltered employment reflecting some of the same characteristics as those seen to apply to 'women's work'.[55] While Anderson has suggested that gender

[50] 'No "Remploy" Factory', *Exeter and Plymouth Gazette* (03.06.1949); Wheatcroft, *Worth Saving*, pp. 101–2; C. Haines, 'Buller, Dame (Audrey Charlotte) Georgiana (1883–1953), Worker for the Disabled', *Oxford Dictionary of National Biography* (25.05.2006). https://www.oxforddnb.com/. Accessed 26 August 2019.

[51] TNA BM 3/70, Remploy Limited, 'Report of the Working Party on the Mix of Disabilities Employed by Remploy' (March, 1981), p. 25.

[52] Bruley, *Women in Britain Since 1900*, pp. 99, 119; Thane, 'Towards Equal Opportunities?', p. 188; Glucksmann, *Women Assemble*, p. 281; Gladstone, *The Twentieth Century Welfare State*, pp. 119–22; Holloway, *Women and Work in Britain Since 1840*, p. 186.

[53] Bruley, *Women in Britain Since 1900*, pp. 99, 119; Lewis, *Women in Britain Since 1945*, pp. 65–91.

[54] Lewis, *Women in Britain since 1945*, p. 79; Thane, 'Towards Equal Opportunities?', p. 188.

[55] D.S. Wilson, 'Gender: Change and Continuity', in P. Addison and H. Jones (eds.), *A Companion to Contemporary Britain 1939–2000* (Oxford, Blackwell, 2005), pp. 247–8; H. Bradley, *Men's Work, Women's Work* (Cambridge, Polity Press, 1989), p. 171.

segregation also applied to disabled women in the immediate postwar period, there has been little detailed examination of this.[56]

There initially appears to have been no gender segregation in the early period of Remploy, though of course there were only very few women workers.[57] In the case of the initial six women who interviewed for the Bridgend factory, there was no indication that they would be doing different work, and this was implied more generally in discussions of wage rates among the Remploy Board at this time.[58] Indeed, given the situation in many of the factories outlined in Chapter 3 during the early years of Remploy, with factories desperately struggling to find work to do, it would have been extremely difficult to demarcate the limited and ad hoc jobs which were found. This changed as Remploy became more established and reorganised into trade groups during the 1950s, from which point onwards there is clear evidence of some segregation in terms of types of work being considered suitable for men or for women. For men, it was considered that work in factories in the Engineering Group and the Furniture Group was particularly suitable, reflecting the traditional focus of male employment and education in the period more generally.[59] Table 5.4 reveals that by 1969 factories in these two groups had the lowest proportion of women. For the Engineering Group this was 1 woman to every 9 men, and in the Furniture Group 1 woman to 25 men. Table 5.5, though unfortunately missing the information for the Engineering Group, shows that by 1977 the Furniture Group remained chiefly the domain of male workers, with a ratio of 1 woman to every 24.5 men. An internal Remploy report compiled in 1980 noted that furniture manufacturing and engineering were 'still regarded traditionally as male trades'.[60]

[56] Anderson, 'British Women, Disability and the Second World War', p. 50; Anderson, *War, Disability and Rehabilitation in Britain*, pp. 169–70.

[57] TNA LAB 20/187, Disabled Persons Employment Corporation Limited, 'Executive Director Report No. 1' (23.07.1945).

[58] TNA BM 8/1, Remploy Limited, 'Minutes of the Eighteenth Meeting of the Board of Directors' (28.01.1947); 'Minutes of the Twenty-First Meeting of the Board of Directors' (29.04.1947).

[59] TNA BM 10/2, Remploy Limited, 'A Brief Outline of the Birth and Early Development of Remploy Limited' (May, 1979); Crompton and Sanderson, *Gendered Jobs & Social Change*, p. 54.

[60] TNA BM 10/34, Remploy Limited, 'Report of the Working Party on the Mix of Disabilities Employed by Remploy, Table II' (June, 1981), pp. 38–9.

Table 5.4 Distribution of female disabled employees across Remploy trade groups, 1969

Trade group	*No. of disabled women*	*Ratio of female to male*
Furniture	66	1:25
Engineering	163	1:9
Leather and textiles	255	1:4
Packaging and assembly	495	1:3.25
Knitwear	135	1:2.5

Source TNA BM 8/51, Remploy Limited, 'Managing Director Report' (November, 1969)

Table 5.5 Distribution of female disabled employees across Remploy trade groups, 1977

Trade group	*No. of disabled women*	*Ratio of female to male*
Furniture	97	1:24.5
Packaging and assembly	839	1:3.1
Leather and textiles	548	1:2.7

Source TNA BM 8/84, Remploy Limited, 'National Joint Consultative Committee Meeting, Personnel Statistics' (April, 1977)

In her sociological survey of historical developments in work segregation, Harriet Bradley suggested that in employment generally there was always strong resistance from men to doing jobs deemed as 'women's work'.[61] Something of this can be seen in Remploy, as in discussion among the Board in 1978 on the issue of changing trades in some of these factories, it was noted that many men would object to being put onto 'women's work'.[62] Similarly the report compiled in 1980 suggested that, in order to accommodate the increasing numbers entering the company, women would have to be given more work in the engineering and furniture factories, but warned that this could result in 'resistance from men'.[63]

[61] Bradley, *Men's Work, Women's Work*, p. 145.

[62] TNA BM 8/79, Remploy Limited, 'Minutes of the Three Hundred and Sixty-First Meeting of the Board of Directors' (16.03.1978).

[63] TNA BM 10/34, Remploy Limited, 'Report of the Working Party on the Mix of Disabilities Employed by Remploy, Table II' (June, 1981), pp. 38–9.

Lewis has suggested that male workers in general could fear female substitution and wished to preserve the demarcation of jobs, though stressed this was not uniform.[64] In the examples here, it is not possible to determine if the Board's concerns were valid, but they clearly believed such resistance was possible. The Board was therefore concerned about potential problems both in terms of moving men onto 'women's work' and of moving women into 'men's work', concerns which were consistent with issues across employment in the period.[65]

As a corollary, there were areas considered particularly suitable for women. Returning to Tables 5.4 and 5.5, we can see this reflected at a Trade Group level. The vast majority of women were employed in the Packaging and Assembly, and Leather and Textile Groups, and a high proportion in 1969 in the separate Knitwear group. Textiles and clothing were also areas in open employment with 'a long tradition of "women's work"'.[66] This was also the case for Remploy's Homework Scheme, where a local factory could take on a small number of 'homeworkers' who, unable to come to the factory, would do specific tasks in their own home. The fundamental view throughout the period remained that homeworking was 'a woman's job'.[67] As Holloway and Lewis have noted this understanding was widely shared across homeworking schemes in open employment, tied to traditional views that men belonged in the factory and women in the home.[68]

As well as the negative connotations associated with 'women's work' across employment there was a 'significant exception' in that women were expected to be able to demonstrate superior dexterity 'because of their smaller "nimble fingers"'.[69] Such sentiments can also be found in relation to Remploy. It was noted, for example, in the report of the Organisation and Methods Division of the Treasury on Remploy in 1955 that the 'lighter packing work' in the Packaging Group of the company was 'very

[64] Lewis, *Women in Britain Since 1945*, p. 84.

[65] *Remploy News*, 112 (November, 1976); Bradley, *Men's Work, Women's Work*, p. 116.

[66] Crompton and Sanderson, *Gendered Jobs & Social Change*, p. 59.

[67] TNA BM 8/1, Remploy Limited, 'Minutes of the Twentieth Meeting of the Board of Directors' (25.03.1947); TNA BM 3/72, 'Note from Mr Owen to Sir Barnes' (27.11.1979).

[68] Holloway, *Women and Work in Britain Since 1840*, p. 186; Lewis, *Women in England 1870–1950*, p. 186.

[69] Wilson, 'Gender: Change and Continuity', pp. 247–8.

suitable for disabled women'.[70] Disabled men, it was explained, 'seldom have the dexterity to reach speeds comparable with those of women'.[71] A resulting issue across postwar employment was that certain 'female roles' were difficult to fill.[72] In the case of Remploy, it was noted by the Park Royal factory in 1955 that despite the work undertaken in the factory being considered particularly suitable for women, the factory had none employed because there were no suitable disabled women to recruit.[73] A similar problem later placed a knitwear sponsorship scheme in jeopardy as 'more women were needed' yet 'difficulty was being experienced in finding suitable new female labour'.[74]

Throughout the period therefore, there remained a clear association with particular trades and roles as being either particularly suitable for men or for women. Such segregation was never absolute, however. As Tables 5.4 and 5.5 show, there were always more men than women working in each Trade Group, including those traditionally associated with 'women's work'.[75] Even in the case of those trades considered 'man's work', there were exceptions which appear to have been unavoidable due to the particular nature of Remploy. Tables 5.4 and 5.5 show both the Furniture Group and the Engineering Group did include female workers, even though these numbers were small. There are a number of specific examples of this at the factory level. In 1964, for example, the engineering factory in Birmingham performed work for the motor industry and had 172 disabled employees, a quarter of whom were women.[76] Similarly, it was reported in 1976 that the Neath engineering factory had 6 female employees engaged in its 'metal welding and cutting' work.[77]

[70] TNA BM 10/12, 'Report of a Survey Undertaken by the Organisation and Methods Division of H.M. Treasury' (1955).

[71] Ibid.

[72] Bradley, *Men's Work, Women's Work*, p. 142.

[73] TNA BM 10/12, 'Report of a Survey Undertaken by the Organisation and Methods Division of H.M. Treasury' (1955).

[74] TNA BM 8/2, Remploy Limited, 'Minutes of the One Hundred and Thirty-Eighth Meeting of the Board of Directors' (18.12.1957).

[75] TNA BM 10/12, 'Report of a Survey undertaken by the Organisation and Methods Division of H.M. Treasury' (1955).

[76] TNA BM 6/10, *Remploy News*, 62 (Summer, 1964).

[77] *Remploy News*, 112 (November, 1976).

It is likely a case of it proving unavoidable to completely segregate the kind of work Remploy was involved in. As Chapter 4 has shown, Remploy's recruitment was based upon sourcing workers in the factory locality and was primarily decided upon assessment of potential productivity. While factory managers could select employees, and therefore could in theory select only men, the presence of some female workers suggests that this was either not desirable or not practical. While men may have been considered the most suitable for certain trades, the question of an individual's potential productivity could perhaps trump such concerns. Given the choice between a less productive male employee and a more productive female one, managers could be prepared to bend the notion of traditional male and female trades. In this way it is possible that the question of disability proved more important than traditional gender roles as the assumption of male physical superiority in production broke down. It is also a question of how Remploy operated, with factories occasionally having to change trade to provide a steady flow of work. In such cases women could not be laid-off or transferred to another factory if the adopted trade was considered 'man's work'. One such example is provided in the employee profile of a female worker from the Kidbrooke Factory in the annual company review of 1965.[78] This described how the worker started when the factory was part of the Knitwear Group but since that time the factory had changed production and now manufactured spectacle frames instead.[79] The Homework Scheme also proved different in reality from the perception that it was primarily a scheme for women. It was noted in 1955 that demand for a place on the scheme was outpacing what was available and therefore preference was being given to those termed 'breadwinners', who supported a family with their wage, and 'to men over women'.[80] By 1961 therefore, there were, in reality, more men than women in the scheme.[81]

Furthermore, while some segregation existed in the Furniture and Engineering Groups, this still left the majority of factories with a mixture of male and female employees. Tables 5.4 and 5.5 show a significant

[78] TNA T224/1891, 'Remploy Annual Review for 1965'.

[79] Ibid.

[80] TNA BM 10/12, 'Report of a Survey Undertaken by the Organisation and Methods Division of H.M. Treasury' (1955).

[81] TNA LAB 20/1035, Remploy Limited, 'Strength State—Section II Disabled Period Ended 3rd January 1961' (27.01.1961).

gender mix in the Packaging and Assembly Group, the largest group in terms of employee numbers, the Leather and Textiles Group, and the Knitwear Group.[82] As with much of Remploy, the numbers within a factory would vary greatly across localities. Though there is no extant breakdown of the numbers of women employed on a factory-by-factory basis for the whole company, there is a useful indication of the kind of variance that existed across the factories in Wales presented in Table 5.6. This shows that out of 14 factories, half were exclusively male. The factory at Bridgend included only 11 female workers, less than 10% of its workforce, whereas the Ystradgynlais factory included 32 women, representing a little over 40% of workers.

Where men and women worked in the same Remploy factory there is no evidence of segregation, and indications that this did not occur. An article in the *Sunday Dispatch* in February 1959 reporting on Remploy, described how men and women 'all work together'.[83] This is also

Table 5.6 Numbers of men and women employed in Remploy factories in Wales, 1972

Remploy factories in Wales	*Employees*	
	Men	*Women*
Abertillery	57	15
Blackwood	48	7
Bridgend	118	11
Brynamman	58	0
Merthyr (engineering)	73	0
Merthyr (leather/textile)	31	2
Neath	66	0
Pentre	56	0
Porth	80	18
Swansea	104	0
Tonyrefail	62	0
Treforest	142	4
Wrexham	76	0
Ystradgynlais	47	32
Total	1,018	89

Source Government Answer, *Hansard* (12.05.1972), vol. 836, cc. 446-7W

[82] TNA BM 10/2, Remploy Limited, 'A Brief Outline of the Birth and Early Development of Remploy Limited' (May, 1979).

[83] TNA BM 8/9, 'They Said Bill Would Never Walk', *Sunday Dispatch* (15.02.1959).

apparent in reports in the company newsletter *Remploy News* which was produced regularly from 1952. In many issues there were numerous photographs and reports of factories with men and women working side-by-side on the factory floor and seemingly on the same kind of job.[84] We can also find similar examples in the published end-of-year reports for the company which regularly featured photographs of men and women working together.[85] This appears to have been unusual compared to open industry where, as well as the segregation in terms of jobs for men and women, there was also segregation in terms of processes and spaces within jobs.[86] That the evidence suggests both male and female disabled workers were involved in the same work in the same space is therefore notable as a feature of sheltered employment.

There is a further question, however, regarding segregation outside of work. Anderson highlighted the importance of the development of social activities in rehabilitation centres such as Stoke Mandeville, noting these were specifically organised 'in such a way as to put meaning and purpose into life'.[87] Recreation and sporting activities organised for the benefit of workers were also a feature in some factories in open industry.[88] In Remploy this was not officially organised, but it was endorsed through the formation of 'Social and Welfare Clubs' managed by the workers themselves at the factory level. The social function of the factory, while secondary to its primary role, was considered important by Remploy's senior management in helping to foster a 'community spirit' in the company.[89] The setting up of these clubs designed primarily 'to

[84] Numerous reports in *Remploy News* throughout period, for example: TNA BM 6/2, *Remploy News*, 30 (January, 1956); BM 6/7, *Remploy News*, 49 (Spring, 1961); BM 6/16, *Remploy News*, 84 (Summer, 1970); BM 6/20, *Remploy News*, 125 (December, 1978).

[85] TNA T227/1106, 'Remploy Annual Review for 1959'; TNA T222/1085, 'Remploy Annual Review for 1956'; TNA T224/1891, 'Remploy Annual Review for 1964'; 'Remploy Annual Review for 1966'; 'Remploy Annual Review for 1967'; 'Remploy Annual Review for 1968'.

[86] Lewis, *Women in Britain since 1945*, p. 78; Bradley, *Men's Work, Women's Work*, p. 116.

[87] Anderson, *War, Disability and Rehabilitation in Britain*, p. 138.

[88] V. Long, *The Rise and Fall of the Healthy Factory: The Politics of Industrial Health in Britain, 1914–60* (Basingstoke, Palgrave Macmillan, 2011), p. 68.

[89] TNA BM 10/19, MOL, 'Fact Finding of Typical Remploy Factories' (1955), p. 10.

provide all employees with social benefits and entertainment', was therefore encouraged.[90] Most factories appear to have had such clubs and held various social events, such as parties, dances, outings and even holidays, throughout the year.[91]

In terms of sports and games, there are numerous references in *Remploy News* to various clubs and leagues with friendly competitions between different factories.[92] The majority of references revolve around popular games such as snooker, darts, table tennis and dominoes.[93] There are also occasional references to other sports such as the mention of a cricket tournament between factories in 1953, and features on archery, football and fishing clubs.[94] The postwar period saw the growth of organised sports for disabled people and it is apparent that Remploy was part of this trend.[95] It is noticeable that in the vast majority of reports on these activities, whether in terms of which employees were organising them, or of winners of the various inter-factory tournaments, there is no mention of any women employees taking part until the Summer issue of 1963 which reported on the first large-scale 'Remploy Rally' where over 2000 people from 30 factories gathered for a day of sport and games.[96] This report referred to women employees taking part in an invalid tricycle rally race.[97] The following issue noted that a further race had been held by the Wakefield factory, again with women employees highlighted in the results.[98] The end of the year brought mention of women as winners in the Aberdeen factory games day and as winners in a table tennis contest.[99] These are the only references made. Such evidence is, of course, hardly

[90] *Remploy News*, 1 (December, 1952).

[91] TNA BM 10/19, MOL, 'Fact Finding of Typical Remploy Factories' (1955), p. 10.

[92] See *Remploy News* issues in TNA BM 6.

[93] Ibid.

[94] *Remploy News*, 9 (August, 1953); *Remploy News*, 12 (November, 1953); *Remploy News*, 21 (August, 1954); *Remploy News*, 22 (September, 1954); *Remploy News*, 24 (November, 1954); TNA BM 6/4, *Remploy News*, 40 (Winter, 1958).

[95] R. Holt and T. Mason, *Sport in Britain 1945–2000* (Oxford, Blackwell, 2000), pp. 15–7.

[96] TNA BM 6/9, *Remploy News*, 58 (Summer, 1963).

[97] Ibid.

[98] TNA BM 6/9, *Remploy News*, 59 (Autumn, 1963).

[99] TNA BM 6/9, *Remploy News*, 60 (Winter, 1963–64).

conclusive. It may be that the emphasis on 'pub games' in social clubs excluded some women, with gender segregation in pubs remaining relatively common for most of the period.[100] Similarly, it may be that the general trend noted by Martin Francis and Richard Holt of low female participation in sport in the 1940s and 1950s, which slowly changed during the 1960s, may also have been reflected in Remploy.[101] As Francis argues such generalisations tend to obscure a range of experiences for women.[102] What is readily apparent however, is that many of the other social events organised by the factories had always involved both men and women. Reports and accompanying photographs indicate that events such as parties, dances and outings provided a valuable opportunity for male and female employees to participate and socialise together.[103]

A further testament to this was the frequency of marriages between disabled employees. Again, these were a notably common feature in issues of *Remploy News* throughout the period.[104] The first report of a wedding occurred in the July 1953 issue (the first issue was published in December 1952), with two disabled employees of the Coventry factory having been married the previous month.[105] The Winter issue for 1958 claimed that the Southampton factory had the highest proportion of women to men

[100] M. Francis, 'Leisure and Popular Culture', in I. Zweiniger-Bargielowska (ed.), *Women in Twentieth-Century Britain* (London, Routledge, 2014), p. 236.

[101] Ibid., pp. 230–7; R. Holt, 'Sport and Recreation', in P. Addison and H. Jones (eds.), *A Companion to Contemporary Britain 1939–2000* (Oxford, Blackwell, 2005), p. 113.

[102] Francis, 'Leisure and Popular Culture', p. 236.

[103] Numerous reports in *Remploy News* throughout period, for example: *Remploy News*, 1 (December, 1952); *Remploy News*, 9 (August, 1953). TNA BM 6/7, *Remploy News*, 51 (Autumn, 1961); TNA BM 6/11, *Remploy News*, 66 (Summer, 1965); *Remploy News*, 67 (Autumn, 1965); TNA BM 6/12, *Remploy News*, 71 (Winter 1966–7); TNA BM 6/ 15, *Remploy News*, 80 (Winter, 1968–9); TNA BM 6/16, *Remploy News*, 84 (Summer, 1970); TNA BM 6/19, *Remploy News*, 93 (August, 1973). *Remploy News*, 108 (March, 1976).

[104] Numerous reports in *Remploy News* throughout period, for example: TNA BM 6/5, *Remploy News*, 42 (Summer, 1959); TNA BM 6/7, *Remploy News*, 51 (Autumn, 1961); TNA BM 6/16, *Remploy News*, 84 (Summer, 1970); TNA BM 6/20, *Remploy News*, 130 (October, 1979).

[105] *Remploy News*, 8 (July, 1953).

of any Remploy factory and thus 'it is not surprising to learn that the incidence of marriages between employees is also high'.[106] This also included an article which posed the question 'Who is leading in the Remploy Marriages Stakes?', noting that the Bristol factory had laid claim to 'the record for the greatest number of marriages between employees'.[107] The factory had recently had 'a wedding a month' for three months and 'in the past seven years we have had a total of eight marriages'.[108] Significantly, in a number of cases it was noted that the couple met working side-by-side on the factory floor and occasionally reports included photographs showing the couple working together.[109] Thus, for example, the report of a wedding at the Abertillery factory in 1974 noted that the bride 'started work at a sewing machine in the next row to his – and they fell in love'.[110]

Overall, in terms of segregation in Remploy, we see something of a mixed picture. There was clearly an association with certain trades being particularly suitable for men or for women. This was never absolute, however, with instances of women on 'men's work' and men on 'women's work'. As with so much of Remploy, the gender mix would vary from factory to factory—one might find oneself working in an entirely male environment in one factory, and in a much closer gender mix in another. In the case of the latter, which represented a significant proportion, there is little evidence of segregation on the factory floor. In this way the nature of sheltered employment may have blurred the traditional gender roles to a certain degree. This does not, of course, mean that true gender equality existed, and it is to this question of status that this chapter will now turn.

[106] TNA BM 6/4, *Remploy News*, 40 (Winter, 1958).

[107] Ibid.

[108] Ibid.

[109] TNA BM 6/13, *Remploy News*, 75 (Winter, 1967–8), notes a wedding at York where both worked on the knitting machines. *Remploy News,* 130 (October, 1979) notes there was a wedding at the Abertillery factory where both bride and groom were machinists. For pictures see TNA BM 6/10, *Remploy News,* 61 (Spring, 1964); TNA BM 6/18, *Remploy News*, 88 (Autumn, 1971); TNA BM 6/20, *Remploy News,* 98 (September, 1974).

[110] TNA BM 6/20, *Remploy News*, 96 (April, 1974).

Status of Women: Pay

There is broad agreement from historians that the position of women in employment during the postwar period considered here was characterised by its inferior status to that of men.[111] This manifested most notably in terms of wages, with women paid significantly less.[112] The question of equal pay for men and women had long been considered in Britain, with the Second World War adding a fresh urgency.[113] The resulting Report of the Royal Commission on Equal Pay, published in 1946, highlighted the scope of the problem of differing wage levels while offering little in the form of solutions.[114] Thane has suggested that by 1946 there was already 'a broad consensus that equal pay was desirable', but disagreements over its precise terms meant 'no one in a position of power was in any hurry to do anything about it'.[115] Despite the postwar labour shortage leaving some industries with no choice but to offer higher wages to attract women, separate wage rates remained intact.[116] It would take until the 1970s and the passing of the Equal Pay Act for equality in pay for men and women to begin to develop in industry.

In the case of Remploy, differing wages for men and women were also the norm until the passing of the Equal Pay Act. Initially, wages for women followed the same formula as those for men, with wage bandings related to trade rates in 'outside' industry, modified to reflect the

[111] Lowe, *The Welfare State in Britain Since 1945*, pp. 42–3; Laybourn, *Unemployment and Employment Policies Concerning Women in Britain*, p. 187; Bruley, *Women in Britain Since 1900*, pp. 99–119; Summerfield, *Women Workers in the Second World War;* Glucksmann, *Women Assemble,* p. 281; Gladstone, *The Twentieth-Century Welfare State*, pp. 119–122; Holloway, *Women and Work in Britain Since 1840*, p. 186; Thane, 'Towards Equal Opportunities?', p. 184.

[112] Laybourn, *Unemployment and Employment Policies Concerning Women in Britain*, p. 187; Bruley, *Women in Britain Since 1900*, pp. 99, 119; Glucksmann, *Women Assemble*, p. 281; Holloway, *Women and Work in Britain Since 1840*, pp. 162–78; Thane, 'Towards Equal Opportunities?', p. 184.

[113] Thane, 'Towards Equal Opportunities?', p. 184; Wilson, *Women and the Welfare State*, pp. 131–2.

[114] Bruley, *Women in Britain Since 1900*, pp. 119–20; Thane, 'Towards Equal Opportunities?', pp. 185–6.

[115] Thane, 'Towards Equal Opportunities?', p. 191.

[116] C. Wightman, *More than Munitions: Women, Work and the Engineering Industries 1900–1950* (Harlow, Longman, 1999), pp. 173–85.

reduced productivity of the disabled workforce.[117] This involved three wage bandings: an 'A' rate for those deemed fully competent at the full trade rate, a 'B' rate for those who had completed training but not yet become productive enough to earn the higher rate, set at 80% of the full trade rate, and a 'C' rate during the period of training set at 70%.[118] As such, for female employees the wage formula was to be the same matched to the trade rate for women where this existed.[119] This formula itself was soon to change, both as a result of pressure from trade unions to increase wages for Remploy workers, and from the difficulty in paying wages based on a trade rate when most factories were engaged in multiple trades.[120] The result was the adoption of a standard 'Remploy wage rate' in 1951.[121] During the discussions which led to this, the possibility of 'a common rate' for both men and women was briefly raised by the MOL for the Remploy Board to consider.[122] The minutes of the relevant meeting made reference to discussions having taken place regarding the MOL's suggestions, but made no specific mention of gender differentiation being abolished.[123] In any case it was decided that the women's rate would be set at 80% of the men's.[124] In addition, a minimum level of pay for women was set at '1/7d. per hour', rising to '1/10d. per hour' after 2 years of service, which similarly reflected 80% of the minimum level for

[117] TNA LAB 20/200, 'Note to Mr Hughes' (31.05.1946).

[118] TNA LAB 20/200, 'Note to Mr Goldberg' (09.04.1946).

[119] TNA LAB 20/200, 'Note to Mr Hughes' (31.05.1946).

[120] TNA LAB 20/200, 'Note to Mr Mitchell' (13.02.1951); TNA BM 10/1, Remploy Limited, 'A Review of the Working of the Company During Its First Seven Years' (March, 1953), p. 37.

[121] TNA BM 10/1, Remploy Limited, 'A Review of the working of the Company During its First Seven Years' (March, 1953), p. 37.

[122] TNA LAB 20/200, 'Note to Mr Hinton' (24.01.1951).

[123] TNA BM 8/2, Remploy Limited, 'Minutes of the Sixty-first Meeting of the Board of Directors' (31.01.1951).

[124] TNA LAB 20/200, 'Note to Mr Mitchell' (13.02.1951); TNA BM 8/2, Remploy Limited, 'Minutes of the Sixty-third Meeting of the Board of Directors' (28.03.1951).

men.[125] Wage rates continued to rise over the 1950s, but always within this same overall formula.[126]

A further agreement between the trade unions and Remploy in 1960 saw a new wage settlement reached which retained the same approach.[127] However, this settlement included a wage increase for men after a period of six months, another after one year and further increase after two years, whereas for women it was increased only after a period of one year and then again after two years.[128] Further wage increases and settlements throughout the 1960s then adopted this same formula. Women workers in Remploy were therefore paid less for their work in terms of the standard wage and this gap was further extended in terms of estimated average gross earnings when bonuses and overtime, also set differently for women, were taken into account.[129]

In determining these rates, the overall guiding principles were to keep Remploy as close as possible to conditions in 'outside industry' and avoid any instance of wage rates within the company being higher. This was the case from the very beginning, with the MOL emphasising to Remploy in 1947, during discussion of how to set the wages for women, that it was 'undesirable to exceed in any case the agreed trade rates'.[130] So while there can be no doubt that women received lower wages than men, this was, at this point, related to a belief that is was not appropriate to have wages be more than in open industry. We see this again in discussion of the 1951 standard rate. In raising the possibility of common rate for men

[125] TNA BM 8/18, Remploy Limited, 'Executive Director Report no. 116: Appendix D: Disabled Employees Wage Rates' (11.04.1956).

[126] TNA LAB 13/1029, J. L. Edwards, 'Remploy: An Experiment in Sheltered Employment for the Severely Disabled in Great Britain', *International Labour Review*, vol. LXXVII, no. 2 (February, 1958), p. 10; TNA BM 10/1, Remploy Limited, 'A Review of the Working of the Company During Its First Seven Years' (March, 1953), p. 37; TNA BM 8/18, Remploy Limited, 'Executive Director Report No. 116: Appendix D: Disabled Employees Wage Rates' (11.04.1956); TNA LAB 20/1054, Remploy Limited, 'Managing Director Report 85: Appendix G: Disabled Employees Wage Rate' (09.03.1960).

[127] TNA LAB 20/1054, 'Remploy Limited: Remploy Wages Agreement' (03.02.1960).

[128] Ibid.

[129] TNA BM 5/1, 'Remploy Wages Agreement' (1974); TNA LAB 20/1173, 'Managing Director Report 165: Personnel Director Report' (June, 1967); TNA BM 8/51, 'Managing Director Report 190: Personnel Director Report' (October, 1969).

[130] TNA LAB 20/200, 'Note to Mr Hughes' (25.03.1947). See also discussion among MOL officials, TNA LAB 20/200, 'Note by Mr Lodge' (30.01.1947).

and women, the MOL noted that differentials were 'the general practice of industry'.[131] In terms of the level of wage differential, the original trade union proposals had called for a women's rate of 90% of the male rate.[132] This was considered 'too high' by both Remploy and the MOL which seems to have been again based on it being too different from standard employment practices.[133] The MOL suggested that a figure of 70% of the male rate would actually reflect the open industry situation better.[134] In the end the Remploy Board settled on a compromise of 80%.[135]

This principle again guided the 1960 settlement and played a key role soon after, when an increase in the Index of Retail Prices and in the National Index of Wage Rates, led the unions involved to call for a general wage increase in Remploy.[136] At a meeting between representatives of the company and the unions, the latter asked for a 5% increase to wages.[137] Remploy countered with an increase of 4%, which would represent 'an increase of 1½d. per hour for men and 1½d. per hour for women'.[138] The union representatives replied that 'the rates paid to disabled women employed by Remploy were already much nearer to the normal trade rates than those paid to disabled men and asked as an alternative that consideration be given to an increase of 2d. for men and 1d. for women'.[139] This was put to the Board to approve, with only Dame Florence Hancock, the lone female Board member at this time and former trade union leader who had long campaigned for improvements in working conditions for women, dissenting, saying 'that she felt that she could not agree to the proposed award as it inferred that the women were to receive only 50% of the increase awarded to the men and her disagreement was a matter

[131] TNA LAB 20/200, 'Note to Mr Hinton' (24.01.1951).

[132] TNA LAB20/200, 'Note by Mr Slater' (29.12.1950).

[133] Ibid; TNA LAB 20/200, 'Note to Mr Mitchell' (13.02.1951).

[134] TNA LAB 20/200, 'Note by Mr Maher' (15.01.1951).

[135] TNA LAB 20/200, 'Note to Mr Mitchell' (13.02.1951); TNA BM 8/2, Remploy Limited, 'Minutes of the Sixty-third Meeting of the Board of Directors' (28.03.1951).

[136] TNA LAB 20/1054, Remploy Limited, 'Remploy Wages Agreement' (03.02.1960); TNA LAB 20/1054, Remploy Limited, 'Wage Rate—Disabled Employees' (07.03.1961).

[137] TNA LAB 20/1054, Remploy Limited, 'Notes of Meeting Concerning Claim for Increase in the Basic Wage Rates of Disabled Employees' (07.03.1961).

[138] Ibid.

[139] TNA LAB 20/1054, Remploy Limited, 'Notes of Meeting Concerning Claim for Increase in the Basic Wage Rates of Disabled Employees' (07.03.1961).

of principle'.[140] In discussions between the MOL and the Treasury on the proposed increase, the issue of how the wages matched with those in outside industry was again the focus.[141] It was agreed by the MOL, the Treasury and Remploy to grant the increase on the lines proposed, with a 2d. increase for men and 1d. increase for women.[142] Here we see again that the link to 'normal' trade rates was the goal and in this case it led to a lower rate for women than had been initially proposed by Remploy.

It is worth noting that the rate of pay for women does indeed at this point appear to have been closer to the average in open industry than that of men. For October 1964, for example, the average weekly earnings in Remploy for men were '£10.2.6', and the average for all manufacturing industries was '£18.13.4', whereas for women the Remploy average was '£7.5.0' compared to '£8.18.11' in outside industry.[143] This point was later raised in 1967 by the Financial Director of Remploy when Dame Florence's successor on the Board, Mrs Marie Patterson, who also had a background as a trade unionist, queried the differentiation in pay, as he noted 'our wage rates for females were very close to those in outside industry'.[144]

Given the specific circumstances of Remploy, however, this wish to emulate outside industry was not always possible, resulting in a number of anomalies in the wage rates for women when put into practice. The question of what wages to pay female workers does not appear to have considered in the planning of Remploy until the first factory was on the verge of opening.[145] With the Bridgend factory set to open at the end of April 1946, Remploy contacted the MOL on 9 April in some urgency

[140] TNA BM 8/3, Remploy Limited: 'Minutes of the One Hundred and Seventy-Fourth Meeting of the Board of Directors' (15.03.1961). J. Hannam, 'Hancock [Married Name Donovan], Dame Florence May (1893–1974), Trade Union Leader', *Oxford Dictionary of National Biography* (06.01.2011). https://www.oxforddnb.com/. Accessed 17 August 2018.

[141] TNA LAB 20/1054, 'Note to D'encer' (22.03.1961).

[142] TNA LAB 20/1054, 'Note to Wright' (20.03.1961); 'Note to D'encer' (22.03.1961); 'Note to Mr Pointon' (27.03.1961); Remploy Limited, 'Remploy Wages Agreement' (24.03.1961).

[143] Mr Marsh, *Hansard* (24.05.1965), vol.713 cc.14w.

[144] TNA BM 8/3, Remploy Limited, 'Minutes of the Two Hundredth and Forty-Fifth Meeting of the Board of Directors' (21.09.1967).

[145] Discussion was exclusively on wage rates for men, see TNA LAB 20/200.

to confirm the wage rates for women.[146] The MOL response did not come until 31 May, when the factory had been in operation for a month, though with only male employees.[147] Here, the MOL advised Remploy that the wage structure for women should be the same as for men, based on average trade rates for women.[148] However, where such a trade rate did not exist for women there was uncertainty and even where it did exist the wage formula proved problematic as the realities of using it for employing women became apparent. When interviewing the six women in November 1946 for the leatherwork section of the Bridgend factory, it was noted that two 'were reluctant' to work at the wages proposed.[149] Using the same formula as male wage rates, it was noted by Remploy themselves that the women would be scarcely better off through employment.[150] As a result, 'it was decided to defer their engagement until it could be seen whether they could not be employed in work for which they would receive a higher wage'.[151]

This particular local situation provoked an urgent national reconsideration of wage rates in the company.[152] Remploy explained to the MOL in 1947, that there were then two women employed at Bridgend on leatherwork, possibly the same two who had previously deferred, with a wage rate that the company felt was too low.[153] Remploy proposed instead that a new rate for women workers should be set 'for all trades'.[154] This was to be an 'A' rate of 'about 1/10d. an hour', a 'B' rate of '1/5d.' and a 'C' rate of '1/2d.'.[155] The MOL replied that the A rate was too high and suggested an alternative rate of 'about 1s. 4½d' in the case of Bridgend, and that in future 'in cases where the A rate fixed by the trade is low it

146 TNA LAB 20/200, 'Note to Mr Goldberg' (09.04.1946).

147 TNA LAB 20/200, 'Note to Mr Hughes' (31.05.1946).

148 Ibid.

149 TNA LAB 20/187, Disabled Persons Employment Corporation Limited, 'Monthly Report on Remploy Factory: Appendix "C" to E.D.R. NO.15' (19.11.1946).

150 Ibid.

151 Ibid.

152 Ibid.

153 Ibid; TNA LAB 20/200, 'Note to Colonel Robertson' (06.01.1947).

154 Ibid.

155 Ibid.

may be desirable to fix the B and C rates at rather higher percentages than 80 and 70 respectively'.[156]

Instructions along these lines were circulated within Remploy, however, whereas for men there was a minimum rate set at '1/9d', this was not the case for women.[157] Here instead, the instruction was that where no separate trade rate existed, or where the rate was 'low', 'full details should be submitted to Head Office in order that consideration may be given to the possibility of fixing 'Rate "C" at a rather higher percentage than 70'.[158] The principle of relating wages to outside industry was therefore adjusted to mitigate for a wage rate which was considered too low for women workers. This was also the case in the settlement of the standard wage in 1951, with the Board settling for a compromise figure of 80% despite the notification of the MOL that 70% would reflect outside industry better.[159] So while Remploy was trying to mimic open industry, and adjust for reduced productivity, the realities proved different in a number of ways, including instances which could prove relatively advantageous for their female employees.

The Equal Pay Act of 1970—the result of long-term pressure from advocate groups, supportive trade unions and politicians and short-term pressure by the Minister of Labour, Barbara Castle, in pushing the measure through before the change of government, allowed for 'equal pay for the same or similar work'.[160] Scholars such as Glennerster and Marwick have pointed out the various loopholes firms could utilise to avoid abiding by the terms of the Act and the limitations of the legislation to really improve women's wages.[161] Similarly, Thane believed the Act had only a limited effect beyond serving as a symbol of

[156] TNA LAB 20/200, 'Note to Mr Hughes' (25.03.1947).

[157] TNA LAB 20/200, Disabled Persons Employment Corporation Limited, 'General Circular No. 39: Disabled Employees—Rates of Wages' (08.05.1947).

[158] Ibid.

[159] TNA LAB 20/200, 'Note by Mr Maher' (15.01.1951); 'Note to Mr. Mitchell' (13.02.1951); TNA BM 8/2, Remploy Limited, 'Minutes of the Sixty-Third Meeting of the Board of Directors' (28.03.1951).

[160] Thane, 'Towards Equal Opportunities?', pp. 205–7; Bruley, *Women in Britain Since 1900*, p. 158; K. Jones, *The Making of Social Policy in Britain, 1830–1990*, 2nd Edition (London, Athlone Press, 1994), p. 168.

[161] Glennerster, *British Social Policy*, pp. 150–1; A. Marwick, *A History of the Modern British Isles 1914–1999* (Oxford: Blackwell, 2000), pp. 218–9.

intent.[162] Remploy however, likely because of its place as a 'government company'—a feature referred to in discussion of the issue in Parliament—did initiate equal pay in line with the terms of the Act.[163] This was phased in over several years with a series of pay increases for women designed for 'bridging the gap'.[164] By June 1975 the equal wage rate was set.[165] In this way Remploy was used as an example by the Government, with the then Secretary of State for Employment, Michael Foot, who would later become leader of the Labour Party, congratulating Remploy on having administered the policy effectively.[166] The adoption of equal pay in Remploy ultimately led to wages exceeding the average rate for women in outside industry, something Remploy had always wanted to avoid. As a result of trade union pressure to match wage rises in 'Blind Workshops', an increase was grudgingly awarded which, as was noted at a meeting of the Board, alongside bonus pay meant that the pay for women was then 'above fit rates'.[167] The DE representative at the meeting suggested that 'care should be taken to avoid undue publicity of this fact'.[168] The result was that disabled women in Remploy at this time enjoyed a wage rate higher than the average of their non-disabled counterparts. However, while the rates of pay for men and women were established in Remploy

[162] Thane, 'Towards Equal Opportunities?', p. 206.

[163] Dame Joan Vickers, *Hansard* (21.10.1968), vol. 770, cc. 863–4; Mr Ashley, *Hansard* (01.08.1972), vol. 842, cc. 75-6w. See also TNA BM 3/54, 'An Anniversary message from Secretary of State for Employment—The Rt. Hon. Michael Foot', *Remploy News* (November, 1975).

[164] TNA BM 5/1, Remploy Limited, 'Remploy Wages Agreement' (1973); TNA BM 5/1, Remploy Limited, 'Personnel Department Circular No. 1271: Equal Pay Act and Fit Female Industrial Staff' (28.03.1973); TNA BM 8/49, Remploy Limited, 'Minutes of the Three-Hundred and Fifth Meeting of the Board of Directors' (22.02.1973).

[165] TNA BM 5/1, 'Remploy Wages Agreement' (1974). Mr. Harold Walker, *Hansard* (30.06.1975), vol. 894, cc. 302-3w.

[166] TNA BM 3/54, 'An Anniversary Message from Secretary of State for Employment—The Rt. Hon. Michael Foot', *Remploy News* (November, 1975).

[167] TNA BM 8/79, Remploy Limited, 'Minutes of the Three Hundred and Twenty-Sixth Meeting of the Board of Directors' (15.01.1975). For further discussion, TNA BM 8/79, Remploy Limited, 'Minutes of the Three Hundred and Thirty-Fourth Meeting of the Board of Directors' (16.10.1975); 'Minutes of the Three Hundred and Thirty-Sixth Meeting of the Board of Directors' (18.12.1975). For pressure from Blind Workshop rates see meetings of 1974 in TNA BM 8/49.

[168] TNA BM 8/79, Remploy Limited, 'Minutes of the Three Hundred and Twenty-Sixth Meeting of the Board of Directors' (15.01.1975).

as the same, average actual weekly earnings, factoring in bonuses and overtime, continued to be different, with, for example, these reported in November 1976 to be £43.18 for men and £41.62 for women.[169] Though this was not a large difference, it nevertheless demonstrates that despite Remploy adopting equal pay in line with the 1970 Act, disabled men in Remploy still tended to earn more than their female colleagues.

Status of Women: Promotion and Representation

It has been noted by historians such as Bruley, Summerfield, Holloway and Thane that women during the period were less likely to hold senior positions, with a so-called 'glass ceiling', referring to the invisible barriers faced by women in advancement 'up' the promotion ladder, resulting in women occupying an inferior position in the workplace.[170] The Executive Director claimed in his overview of Remploy in 1953 that 'it has always been the policy of the Company to advance disabled employees to supervisory posts where they were considered to be capable of the work'.[171] Again there is no clear breakdown but it does appear that this applied to women as well as to men, at least to a certain level. The same document noted that in all the Packaging factories the inspectors and leading hands were comprised of 'both male and female' employees.[172] It is possible to get a better sense of this from the 1960s onwards in the pages of *Remploy News*. Here we see in the regular reports of different factories, mentions of women as 'charge-hands', 'supervisors' or 'inspectors', and it appears that this is not something out of the ordinary.[173]

[169] TNA BM 8/84, Remploy Limited, 'National Consultative Committee Meeting: Personnel Statistics, Company Personnel Strengths' (14.04.1977).

[170] Laybourn, *Unemployment and Employment Policies Concerning Women in Britain*, p. 187; Bruley, *Women in Britain Since 1900*, p. 99; Summerfield, *Women Workers in the Second World War*; Holloway, *Women and Work in Britain Since 1840*, p. 209; Thane, 'Towards Equal Opportunities?', p. 184.

[171] TNA BM 10/1, Remploy Limited, 'A Review of the Working of the Company During Its First Seven Years' (March, 1953), p. 38.

[172] Ibid, p. 55.

[173] See for example, TNA BM 6/8, *Remploy News*, 55 (Autumn, 1962); TNA BM 6/10, *Remploy News*, 61 (Spring, 1964); *Remploy News*, 62 (Summer, 1964); TNA BM 6/13, *Remploy News*, 73 (Summer, 1967); TNA BM 6/15, *Remploy News*, 82 (Autumn, 1969); *Remploy News*, 83 (Winter, 1969–70); TNA BM 6/18, *Remploy News*, 88 (Autumn, 1971); *Remploy News*, 88 (February,1972); *Remploy News*, 89 (August,

More senior positions rarely opened up for women however, whether disabled or not. Two articles in *Remploy News* in 1972 claimed there were only 'two lady foremen', both of whom were in factories in the Knitwear Group.[174] The first article was a profile of one of these women who worked at the Abertillery factory, under the headline 'Mother Superior', a nickname apparently used to refer to her in the factory.[175] It was explained that she had been with the company for 11 years 'and worked her way up from sewing machinist to her present position'.[176] The article noted that the factory 'leading hand' was also a woman and that this had left them in 'sole charge of the factory floor' and 70 male employees when the manager had recently been ill.[177] The article's focus was on the peculiarity of this situation.

In 1976 there was a further article on the Abertillery factory which was apparently unique in that 'apart from the manager, all the top jobs are held by women'.[178] Specifically these were the forewoman previously profiled, alongside two charge-hands and the factory accountant.[179] All these women had been employed for some years within the company and appear to have worked their way up to their position.[180] Promotion to the position of 'foreman' for women remained rare as the article claimed that it was 'a position achieved by only a handful of women throughout our factories'.[181] The promotion of women to management was rarer still. *Remploy News* reported in 1971 that for the first time a woman had been made 'manageress of the Bristol showroom'.[182] The first woman factory manager would have to wait until 1975.[183] This occasion was marked by

1972); *Remploy News*, 90 (11.1972). *Remploy News*, 108 (March, 1976); *Remploy News*, 110 (July, 1976); *Remploy News*, 121 (April, 1978).

[174] TNA BM 6/18, *Remploy News*, 89 (August, 1972); *Remploy News*, 90 (November, 1972).

[175] TNA BM 6/18, *Remploy News*, 89 (August, 1972).

[176] Ibid.

[177] Ibid.

[178] *Remploy News*, 110 (July, 1976).

[179] Ibid.

[180] Ibid.

[181] Ibid.

[182] TNA BM 6/17, *Remploy News*, 86 (Spring, 1971).

[183] *Remploy News*, 105 (October, 1975).

an article under the headline 'A Woman Becomes Factory Manager' as the person in question took charge of the Salford factory.[184] By 1979 she remained the only female factory manager in Remploy.[185]

From the beginning of the company there was a single female on the Board of Directors, Miss (later Dame) Caroline Haslett, founder of the Electrical Association for Women in 1924 and the first woman to become a member of the British Electricity Authority, who resigned from Remploy in 1948.[186] In choosing a successor to the position, the MOL informed the Board that pressure was coming from the Women's Advisory Committee to replace her with another woman.[187] This was something that the MOL was already considering with one official remarking 'there is no particular necessity that the Board should contain a woman, but I think this is desirable if it can be done'.[188] MOL officials raised a number of suggestions with one document listing potential candidates with comments on their experience and personality.[189] The eventual choice was Countess Roseberry who first attended a Board meeting in May 1949.[190] She was to resign a little over a year later and was replaced in November 1950 by a man, leaving no woman member on the Board

184 Ibid.

185 *Remploy News*, 125 (December, 1978).

186 TNA BM 8/1, Remploy Limited, 'Minutes of the First Meeting of the Board of Directors' (30.05.1945). She became Dame Haslett in 1947, TNA BM 8/1, Remploy Limited, 'Minutes of the Twenty-Fourth Meeting of the Board of Directors' (29.07.1947); TNA BM 10/1, Remploy Limited, 'A Review of the Working of the Company During Its First Seven Years: Appendix H' (March, 1953). Citrine revised by E. Symons, 'Haslett, Dame Caroline Harriet (1895–1957), Electrical Engineer and Electricity Industry Administrator', *Oxford Dictionary of National Biography* (06.01.2011). https://www.oxforddnb.com/. Accessed 30 July 2019.

187 TNA BM 8/1, Remploy Limited, 'Minutes of the Thirty-Eighth Meeting of the Board of Directors' (24.11.1948).

188 TNA LAB 20/120, 'Note from Sir Wiles' (26.04.1948).

189 TNA LAB 20/120, 'Note to Sir Wiles' (24.04.1948).

190 TNA BM 8/1, Remploy Limited, 'Minutes of the Forty-First Meeting of the Board of Directors' (23.02.1949); 'Minutes of the Forty-Fourth Meeting of the Board of Directors' (25.05.1949).

until the appointment of Dame Hancock in 1958.[191] Upon her retirement in April 1966, the Board was informed that the MOL had decided upon her replacement, Mrs Patterson, who remained on the Board as the only female member for the remainder of the period.[192] Such positions were not part of the normal promotion structure, but this is important in terms of the representation at Board level of the interests of Remploy's female workers. This chapter has already noted that the factories themselves were not geared towards the needs of the women. It is readily apparent from examination of the minutes of Board Meetings that it was these female Board members who raised the needs of women employees. Dame Haslett for example, queried the separate rates of pay and campaigned, unsuccessfully, for Remploy to adopt the same rates for men and women.[193] Dame Hancock registered her opposition to the 1961 wage settlement which disadvantaged women employees.[194] Mrs Patterson was perhaps the most active in this regard. During the period of her appointment she campaigned, again unsuccessfully, for female employees to have facilities for cervical cancer tests in Remploy, raised again the question of wage differentiation between men and women, and suggested a raised minimum wage rate for women.[195]

In Remploy therefore, while there was clearly some promotion of female employees to mid-level supervisory positions, there were only a handful of instances of women being promoted beyond this. We can see therefore a 'glass ceiling', with promotion beyond the supervisory level

[191] TNA BM 8/2, Remploy Limited, 'Minutes of the Fifty-Seventh Meeting of the Board of Directors' (27.09.1950); 'Minutes of the Fifty-Ninth Meeting of the Board of Directors' (22.11.1950); BM 8/2, Remploy Limited, 'Minutes of the One Hundred and Thirty-Ninth Meeting of the Board of Directors' (15.01.1958).

[192] TNA BM 8/3, Remploy Limited, 'Minutes of the Two Hundredth and Thirtieth Meeting of the Board of Directors' (21.04.1966). For end of period see TNA BM 8/80.

[193] TNA BM 8/1, Remploy Limited, 'Minutes of the Eighteenth Meeting of the Board of Directors' (28.01.1947); 'Minutes of the Twenty-First Meeting of the Board of Directors' (21.04.1947).

[194] TNA BM 8/3, Remploy Limited, 'Minutes of the One Hundred and Seventy-Fourth Meeting of the Board of Directors' (15.03.1961).

[195] TNA BM 8/3, Remploy Limited, 'Minutes of the Two Hundred and Forty-First Meeting of the Board of Directors' (20.04.1967); 'Minutes of the Two Hundred and Forty-Second Meeting of the Board of Directors' (18.05.1967); 'Minutes of the Two Hundred and Forty-Fifth Meeting of the Board of Directors' (21.09.1967); TNA BM 8/49, 'Minutes of the Two Hundred and Eighty-First Meeting of the Board of Directors' (17.12.1970).

a rarity and only a single instance of a female factory manager which would have to wait until 1975. Representation at Board level was likewise extremely limited and as a result the needs of women employees were not always highlighted or given priority within the company.

Conclusions

Through the period considered here, women in Remploy were always a minority. As with employment generally, the number of women workers increased steadily but this was only to reach slightly less than 20% of the overall workforce by 1979. In this way, Remploy represents a further area of welfare and employment provision which was indeed allocated, as Sainsbury and others have argued, 'overwhelmingly to men' in the period.[196] This raises questions of access to Remploy for women, and this chapter has revealed that there were a number of factors which may have prevented disabled women from registering as Section II on the Disabled Persons Register and attempting to enter sheltered employment which include, but are not limited to, those highlighted by Anderson. The suggestion that industry was an area in which women were unlikely to get involved has been shown to have merit, as this was one of the primary issues considered at the time. It is apparent that little thought was given as to how to target sheltered employment to meet the desires and needs of severely disabled women. Alongside this, the traditional ties to the home, understood to have prevented many women seeking employment in the period generally, have also been shown to have been equally applicable for disabled women as well, with the additional possibility of disabled women being 'hidden' by their families.

Furthermore, we cannot discount discrimination in recruitment practice, if not in policy, as the understanding of particular trades as inherently suitable for either men or women could mean that applicants for Remploy may have been discounted because of their gender. Attempts in Remploy to demarcate certain trades according to gender, illustrates how pervasive such concepts were, existing in a company in which the traditional

[196] Sainsbury, 'Disabled People and the Personal Social Services', p. 188; Anderson, 'British Women, Disability and the Second World War', p. 50; Anderson, *War, Disability and Rehabilitation in Britain*, pp. 169–70; Hampton, *Disability and the Welfare State in Britain*, p. 119; Borsay, *Disability and Social Policy in Britain Since 1750*, p. 134; Thane, *Foundations of the Welfare State*, pp. 224–5.

assumption of male physical superiority in production did not apply. As this chapter has shown, however, this segregation was never absolute, even where it did exist, with cases of women taking on 'men's work' and men taking on 'women's work'. It has also been revealed that in many factories there was a very real 'gender mix', with little evidence of segregation on the factory floor. Here, male and female workers performed the same jobs side-by-side and socialised outside of work. In this way the peculiarities of Remploy and sheltered employment are demonstrated, with disability serving to overrule some of the traditional gender divisions common in open employment.[197] Once again we see variation at a factory level in terms of the gender mix and environment, further highlighting the lack of a typical Remploy experience. A Remploy worker in one factory might find themselves in an entirely male factory, and another in a factory with a genuine gender-mix, working alongside men and women and socialising with them outside of work.

That segregation was limited does not, of course, entail equality in status. This chapter has added the case of Remploy and the severely disabled to our understanding of inequality in women's employment in the period.[198] In terms of wages, Remploy followed the pattern of gender differentials until the establishment of equal pay in the 1970s. This was not due to a particular belief that this was justified in Remploy, but rather that it was important that Remploy emulate conditions in outside industry and not have wages in the government subsidised company exceed the norm elsewhere. While women were generally paid less with this principle in mind, this was mitigated in favour of women on a number of occasions and Remploy's position as a government company led to the establishment of equal pay in line with the 1970 Equal Pay Act, which was not the norm in outside industry. As a result, we see that in terms of wages,

[197] Bruley, *Women in Britain Since 1900*, pp. 99, 119; Thane, 'Towards Equal Opportunities?', p. 188; Glucksmann, *Women Assemble*, p. 281; Gladstone, *The Twentieth Century Welfare State*, pp. 119–22; Holloway, *Women and Work in Britain Since 1840*, p. 186.

[198] Lowe, *The Welfare State in Britain Since 1945*, pp. 42–3; Laybourn, *Unemployment and Employment Policies Concerning Women in Britain*, p. 187; Bruley, *Women in Britain Since 1900*, pp. 99–119; Summerfield, *Women Workers in the Second World War;* Glucksmann, *Women Assemble*, p. 281; Gladstone, *The Twentieth-Century Welfare State*, pp. 119–22; Holloway, *Women and Work in Britain Since 1840*, p. 186; Thane, 'Towards Equal Opportunities? Women in Britain Since 1945', pp. 183–208; Lewis, *Women in Britain Since 1945*, pp. 78–91.

while not providing equality until the end of the period, disabled women workers in Remploy did enjoy some comparative advantages owing to the particular nature of the company as the central government's sheltered employment scheme.

As to the extent of an existence of a 'glass ceiling' in promotion for female employees in Remploy, while supervisory positions upon the factory floor may have been attainable, more senior positions and certainly management were out of reach for all but a handful of women. Thus, women in Remploy appeared to have faced similar difficulties in advancement as those in open employment.[199] Similarly, in terms of representation at Board level, the maximum of one female member at any time left little support for issues concerning women workers. As a male-dominated environment, especially at senior levels, it was not until the very end of the period considered here that a fundamental re-think of the company in terms of operations and environments was beginning to be seriously considered. It is apparent, then, that Remploy did not cater equally for severely disabled men and women, leaving gender as a factor which would determine how one might access and experience sheltered employment.

[199] Laybourn, *Unemployment and Employment Policies Concerning Women in Britain*, p. 187; Bruley, *Women in Britain Since 1900*, p. 99; Summerfield, *Women Workers in the Second World War*; Holloway, *Women and Work in Britain Since 1840*, p. 209; Thane, 'Towards Equal Opportunities?', p. 184.

CHAPTER 6

The Mixed Economy and the Moving Frontier of the State

Introduction

Having focused upon Remploy as the central government scheme and as the chief provider during the period, this chapter will place the company within the broader field of sheltered employment. The traditional view of the postwar period was that the expansion of statutory welfare resulted in the curtailment of voluntary activity in those areas, until the sector experienced something of a resurgence in the mid-to-late 1960s.[1] This view has since been challenged with scholars such as Finlayson, Younghusband, Taylor, Prochaska, Kendall and Knapp illustrating the continued existence of voluntary welfare throughout the postwar period.[2] There is acceptance

[1] D. Gladstone, *The Twentieth-Century Welfare State* (Basingstoke, Palgrave Macmillan, 1999), p. 66; *The Future of Voluntary Organisations: Report of the Wolfenden Committee* (London, Croom Helm, 1978); B. Knight, *Voluntary Action (*London, Centris 1993); J. Hampton, *Disability and the Welfare State in Britain: Changes in Perception and Policy 1948–79* (Bristol, Policy Press, 2016); M. Bruce, *The Coming of the Welfare State* (London, Harper Collins, 1971); G Kitson-Clark, *An Expanding Society: Britain 1830–1900* (Cambridge, Cambridge University Press, 1967).

[2] G. Finlayson, *Citizen, State, and Social Welfare in Britain 1830–1990* (Oxford, Clarendon Press, 1994); E. Younghusband, *Social Work in Britain: 1950–1975* (London, Allen and Unwin, 1978); M. Taylor, 'Voluntary Action and the State', in D. Gladstone, (ed.) *British Social Welfare: Past, Present and Future* (London, UCL Press, 1995), p. 215; F. K. Prochaska, *The Voluntary Impulse: Philanthropy in Modern Britain*, (London, Faber,

© The Author(s), under exclusive license to Springer Nature Switzerland AG 2025

A. Holroyde, *Sheltered Employment and Disability in the British Welfare State*, New Directions in Welfare History,
https://doi.org/10.1007/978-3-031-87876-3_6

then, that there existed a 'mixed economy' of welfare, in which traditional voluntarism survived and acted as a 'junior partner' to expanding state provision.[3] The case of sheltered employment has not yet been considered in this area, though references to Remploy are often framed as though the company made previous schemes obsolete and became the only meaningful provider. While Anderson, for example, has hinted at the survival of voluntary workshops in the immediate postwar period, the extent of other sheltered employment provision has not been considered in any detail.[4] This chapter will therefore establish the existence and extent of a mixed economy in sheltered employment. This will serve both to clarify the place of Remploy within this wider field and to add the case of sheltered employment to this current understanding of welfare in the period.

As the statutory central government provider of sheltered employment, Remploy represented what is referred to in other areas of welfare as the 'frontier of the state'.[5] The mixed economy has not been seen as a static relationship between the state and voluntary provision, but rather one in which state involvement, represented by the 'frontier', has changed over time. The 'moving frontier' refers therefore to the changing relationship between central government, local government and the voluntary sector in delivering welfare provision.[6] Both Grier and Hampton have called for further examination of these complex interactions and this chapter seeks to do so for sheltered employment.[7] The exploration of the mixed economy in this chapter will therefore track the movement

1988); P. Thane, *Foundations of the Welfare State, 2nd Edition* (London, Longman, 1996), p. 277; J. Kendall and M. Knapp, *The Voluntary Sector in the United Kingdom* (Manchester, Manchester University Press, 1996), pp. 51–57.

[3] D. Owen, *English Philanthropy: 1660–1960* (London, Belknap Press, 1964), p. 527; Kendall and Knapp, *The Voluntary Sector in the United Kingdom*, pp. 51–7, 133–9; A. Digby, *British Welfare Policy: Workhouse to Workfare* (London, Faber and Faber, 1989), p. 89.

[4] J. Anderson, *War, Disability and Rehabilitation in Britain: 'Soul of a Nation'* (Manchester, Manchester University Press, 2011), p. 184.

[5] G. Finlayson, 'A Moving Frontier: Voluntarism and the State in British Social Welfare 1911–1949', *Twentieth Century British History*, vol. 1, no. 2 (1990), pp. 183–206.

[6] Finlayson, *Citizen, State and Social Welfare in Britain 1830–1990*, pp. 11–2; Kendall and Knapp, *The Voluntary Sector in the United Kingdom*, pp. 51–7.

[7] J. Grier, 'Voluntary Rights and Statutory Wrongs: The Case of Child Migration, 1948–67', *History of Education*, vol. 31 no. 3 (2002), pp. 263–4; Hampton, *Disability and the Welfare State in Britain*, p. 8.

of the company as the frontier of the state. In doing so it will examine the composition of the mixed economy, the changing place of Remploy within it, the complex relationships between the various providers and the degree to which it collectively delivered a cohesive sheltered employment system.

This chapter is structured according to three distinct periods which exemplify the movement of Remploy as the frontier of the state. The first section considers the period 1944–1951, with the initial creation of Remploy advancing the frontier dramatically. The following section begins with the halt to the expansion of Remploy explained in Chapter 3, and the resulting continuation of a mixed economy through to 1970. The final section concludes with the 1970s, when fundamental questions were raised about the effectiveness of the mixed economy and the potential of unification was explored.

The Frontier Advances, 1944–1951

As was shown in Chapter 2, there were a range of voluntary organisations offering sheltered employment before 1939. Prior to the creation of Remploy, sheltered employment for severely disabled people was solely provided by such organisations with some limited financial support from government under the MOL's 'scheme of grants'. The extent of this provision at the close of the Second World War was indicated by the newly formed Sheltered Employment Committee (SEC) of the NACED.[8] A report from May 1945 noted that the SEC had examined a list of 'those organisations at present included in the 'scheme of grants' which showed '16 organisations covering approximately 402 disabled persons'.[9] They also examined 'a further list of organisations providing sheltered employment but not having arrangements with the Ministry', which 'showed 22 organisations covering approximately 2744 disabled persons'.[10] The committee warned that this was only 'a general indication of the size of the field at present covered by any form of special provision'.[11] The

[8] The National Archives (TNA) LAB 20/173, SEC, 'Report to the National Advisory Council on the Employment of the Disabled, N.A.C. 9' (10.05.1945).

[9] Ibid.

[10] Ibid.

[11] TNA LAB 20/173, SEC, 'Minutes of the Second Meeting' (01.05.1945).

report also concluded that this provision was undoubtedly 'meagre and inadequate'.[12]

Details from this list of charitable sheltered employment examined by the SEC provide a useful illustration of the variations which existed in this field.[13] As well as some organisations providing dedicated sheltered workshops, there were also various forms of sheltered employment within wider welfare contexts, such as residential settlements, hospitals, TB sanatoria and training colleges. It is immediately apparent that the scale of such operations could vary widely, with several organisations providing employment for hundreds of disabled people, and some only very small numbers. For example, we see 600 disabled people reported as working at the Papworth Village Settlement, where they would live as well, and, by contrast, Cleethorpes Appliance Industries providing some form of sheltered employment to only 4.[14] Within these extremes it is apparent that, in general, such provision tended to cater for smaller numbers of disabled people. The list also reveals the various types of work undertaken in these voluntary workshops, with many continuing the traditional trades associated with sheltered employment, such as woodwork, upholstery and basket making.[15] Given the range of provision it is perhaps unsurprising that the wages paid to disabled workers were widely variable. In principle, charitable bodies were meant to approximate trade union rates and should have paid workers no less than the government's training allowances for severely disabled people.[16] In practice, there was

[12] TNA LAB 20/173, SEC, 'Report to the National Advisory Council on the Employment of the Disabled, N.A.C. 9' (10.05.1945).

[13] TNA LAB 20/173, SEC, 'Scheme of Grants to Undertakings Employing Severely Disabled Persons: Organisations at present included in the Scheme, S.E.C I' (1945); SEC, 'Undertakings Providing Employment for the Severely Disabled other than those at present included in the Ministry of Labour and National Service Scheme of Grants S.E.C 2' (1945).

[14] For more on village settlement schemes, see TNA PIN 15/34; 15/36; 15/37; D. Cohen, *The War Come Home: Disabled Veterans in Britain and Germany 1914–1939* (Los Angeles, University of California Press, 2001), p. 35.

[15] TNA LAB 20/173, SEC, 'Scheme of Grants to Undertakings Employing Severely Disabled Persons: Organisations at present included in the Scheme, S.E.C I' (1945); SEC, 'Undertakings Providing Employment for the Severely Disabled other than those at present included in the Ministry of Labour and National Service Scheme of Grants S.E.C 2' (1945).

[16] TNA LAB 20/173, MOL, 'Remuneration of Workers in Sheltered Employment' (1945).

wide variation with multiple formulas based on productivity or skill and a mix of time and piece rates.[17] A further notable variation existed in the explicit recruitment of particular groups of disabled people. In the most obvious example, sheltered employment in TB sanatoria, was, of course, available only for those with TB. Similarly, charities were largely set up to deal with particular 'causes' and their sheltered employment provision reflected this, often as just one aspect of wider welfare in which the charity was involved. Thus, sheltered workshops run by the British Legion provided only for ex-servicemen, while the workshop run by the Ayrshire Society for the Deaf, as its name suggests, provided sheltered employment only for deaf people. The list illustrates that most organisations did explicitly limit access by particular types of disability, gender, or grouping such as ex-servicemen at this time.

Initial discussions about postwar sheltered employment during the wartime Coalition Government presumed a continued role for the voluntary sector. The Tomlinson Report which informed the DPEA envisaged the continuation of the existing charitable undertakings which the new government scheme would serve to complement.[18] The wartime Minister of Labour, Ernest Bevin, highlighted in Chapter 2 as the individual chiefly responsible for establishing the scheme which would become Remploy, explained that in doing so 'it is not my intention to start competition with the institutions in existence'.[19] The terms of the DPEA itself did not specify what means of providing sheltered employment should be utilised, leaving such decisions to the MOL to decide.[20] This was again echoed in the initial plans for Remploy drawn up by the MOL towards the end of the war.[21] Consideration throughout wartime therefore consistently advocated and assumed that voluntary sheltered employment would continue. With such provision having proved inadequate to meet the scale of demand, necessitating the new government scheme, there was

[17] Ibid; TNA LAB 20/78, MOL, 'Note from Regional Controller, Training and Resettlement of Disabled Persons' (12.02.1945).

[18] *Report of Inter-departmental Committee on the Rehabilitation and Resettlement of Disabled Persons*, 6415 (1943), para. 90–1, pp. 34–5.

[19] Mr Ernest Bevin, *Hansard* (10.12.1943), vol. 395, cc. 1347; Mr Ernest Bevin, *Hansard* (24.03.1944), vol. 398, cc. 1215.

[20] DPEA.

[21] TNA LAB 20/108, MOL, 'Employment under Special Conditions: Outline of a Scheme under Section 15 of the Disabled Persons (Employment) Act, 1944' (June, 1944).

the presumption that Remploy would become the prime, but not sole, provider. A mixed economy in sheltered employment was therefore imagined by the Coalition Government for peacetime.

Under the Labour Government elected in 1945, however, the pendulum swung markedly towards the role of the state. With the rapid early expansion of the company, it was assumed Remploy would take over much, if not all, of the sheltered employment field.[22] This directive came from the Government itself, as the Remploy Board had expressed the wish to expand slowly and agreed in their first meeting that plans for the company should be adapted to prevent any overlap with existing organisations.[23] The Labour Government however, viewed Remploy as the desired agent for providing the envisaged comprehensive coverage, with the Minister of Labour, George Isaacs, explaining in the Commons that it was properly the role of the state to provide sheltered employment through Remploy.[24] As Marilyn Taylor has explained, Labour's general view of voluntarism at this time was that it was 'patronising and outdated', while Kendall and Knapp have suggested that many in the Labour Government, including Clement Attlee himself, 'expected and hoped' that the expansion of state welfare would see charitable services 'with their aura of middle-class patronage' made redundant.[25] Digby has further argued that the expansion of the role of the state became something of a common currency in almost all social policy discussion at this time.[26] For historians of disability such as Hampton, however, disabled people marked the exception to this rule, with a continuing reliance on non-statutory provision.[27] Remploy illustrates that this was not the case in all aspects, as in sheltered employment at least, the desire to see

[22] TNA BM 8/1, Disabled Persons Employment Corporation Limited, 'Minutes of the Twentieth Meeting of the Board of Directors' (25.03.1947).

[23] TNA BM 8/1, Disabled Persons Employment Corporation Limited, 'Minutes of the First meeting of the Board of Directors' (30.05.1945).

[24] Mr George Isaacs, *Hansard* (02.12.1947), vol. 445, cc. 186-8; TNA BM 8/ 1, Disabled Persons Employment Corporation Limited, 'Minutes of the Twentieth Meeting of the Board of Directors' (25.03.1947); TNA LAB 20/399, Disabled Persons Employment Corporation Limited, 'Executive Director Report No. 22' (21.07.1947).

[25] Taylor, 'Voluntary action and the state', p. 215; Kendall and Knapp, *The Voluntary Sector in the United Kingdom*, pp. 51–7.

[26] Digby, *British Welfare Policy*, p. 65.

[27] Hampton, *Disability and the Welfare State in Britain*, p. 57.

Remploy take over from charitable providers was entirely in keeping with the early-Attlee Government's expansion of the state and its wider attitude to welfare, social services, nationalisation and central planning.[28]

It is apparent that while voluntary organisations were not prohibited from offering sheltered employment, this became subject to them doing so 'efficiently' and providing 'co-operation' with the MOL's overall plan for Remploy.[29] Organisations would therefore have to demonstrate an ability to provide sheltered employment as effectively as Remploy, or face absorption into the company. This quickly became a reality as a number of voluntary workshops were taken over.[30] There is some evidence that this was based on the effectiveness of sheltered employment, with the MOL commenting on the poor quality of work provided through many charitable workshops in terms of the reliance on the traditional trades.[31] However, the chief measure and cause of absorption into Remploy was financial, with the postwar environment proving too challenging for many workshops, which had always been economically frail.

Such financial difficulty was partially due to the general postwar trading conditions which extended across industry, but this was undoubtedly

[28] D. Kavanagh and P. Morris, *Consensus Politics from Attlee to Major*, 2nd Edition (Oxford, Blackwell, 1994), pp. 24–5; J.E. Cronin, *The Politics of State Expansion: War, State and Society in Twentieth-Century Britain (*London, Routledge, 1991), pp. 153–7; K. Laybourn, *The Evolution of British Social Policy and the Welfare State, c.1800–1993* (Keele, Keele University Press, 1995), p. 231; K.O. Morgan, *Britain Since 1945: The People's Peace, 3rd Edition* (Oxford, Oxford University Press, 2001), p. 29; Taylor, 'Voluntary action and the state', p. 219.

[29] TNA LAB 20/173, MOL, 'Training and Employment of Blind Persons' (1945).

[30] TNA BM 8/1, Disabled Persons Employment Corporation Limited, 'Minutes of the Eighteenth Meeting of the Board of Directors' (28.01.1947); 'Minutes of the Eighteenth Meeting of the Board of Directors' (28.01.1947); 'Minutes of the Eighteenth Meeting of the Board of Directors' (28.01.1947); 'Minutes of the Nineteenth Meeting of the Board of Directors' (25.02.1947): 'Minutes of the Forty-First Meeting of the Board of Directors' (23.02.1949); Remploy Limited, 'Minutes of the Forty-Eighth Meeting of the Board of Directors' (26.10.1949); TNA BM 10/1, Remploy Limited, 'Review of the working of the Company during its first seven years' (March, 1953), p. 13.

[31] TNA LAB 20/78, MOL, 'Lord Roberts Memorial Workshops Fulham Factory' (February, 1951); MOL, 'Note of conversation' (09.09.1950); 'The Forces Help Society and Lord Roberts Workshops Gazette, Vol L, No. 1' (January, 1950); MOL, 'Note to Miss Acton' (24.12.1949); MOL, 'Note to Miss Acton' (11.08.1948); The Lord Roberts Memorial Workshops, 'Note from Miss Acton' (14.07.1948); MOL, 'Report on visit to the Lord Roberts Memorial Workshop Fulham' (01.04.1948); MOL, 'Note of Meeting' (23.06.1948).

exacerbated for these workshops by the creation of Remploy itself.[32] In announcing the formation of the company, Bevin stressed that he wished it to work in concert with voluntary organisations and the initial outline of Remploy produced in 1944 similarly stressed the need for close cooperation.[33] This did initially occur as Remploy began to be formed, with the Directors of the company seeking a great deal of advice from existing charitable workshops, particular the Lords Roberts Memorial Workshops, the largest provider at the time.[34] However, such cooperation soon vanished as the company began to operate, with Remploy and voluntary workshops left to compete for the scant work available in the immediate postwar climate. This was particularly the case for government contracts.[35] The awarding of these contracts to sheltered workshops had long been considered desirable, and in 1950 formal arrangements were introduced to give them a measure of priority.[36] This still left Remploy and the other providers in competition with each other.[37] Government contracts were not overly attractive financially, with both Remploy and the other workshops bemoaning the viability of what was offered, but they did provide a significant source of much-needed work and Remploy was awarded the majority of them.[38] Furthermore, the introduction of a state scheme in Remploy also reduced the impetus for public generosity through charitable donations to voluntary organisations, upon which they relied. Finlayson suggested that at this time the general public 'assumed

[32] Anderson, *War, Disability and Rehabilitation in Britain*, pp. 183–4.

[33] Mr Ernest Bevin, *Hansard* (10.12.1943), vol. 395, cc. 1347; Mr Ernest Bevin, *Hansard* (24.03.1944), vol. 398, cc. 1215; TNA LAB 20/108, MOL, 'Employment under Special Conditions: Outline of a Scheme under Section 15 of the Disabled Persons (Employment) Act, 1944' (June, 1944).

[34] See TNA LAB 20/187; 20/78, 'Note from Mr Isaacs' (12.12.1945).

[35] TNA BM 8/1, Disabled Persons Employment Corporation Limited, 'Minutes of the Thirty-First Meeting of the Board of Directors' (06.04.1948); TNA LAB 20/444, Disabled Persons Employment Corporation Limited, 'Executive Director Report No. 34' (21.10.1948).

[36] TNA LAB 20/1429, DE, 'Sheltered Employment: A Draft Consultative Document' (October, 1973), pp. 9, 27.

[37] Mr Llewellyn and Mr Isaacs, *Hansard* (07.11.1950), vol. 480, cv. 46.

[38] See Chapter 3 for Remploy and for Lord Roberts see TNA LAB 20/78, MOL, 'Note of conversation' (09.09.1950).

that the new welfare legislation rendered charities redundant or obsolete, and no longer felt obliged to support them'.[39] Prochaska similarly noted this as a common problem for many charitable organisations at this time.[40]

In the case of sheltered workshops several soon proved unviable, including the King's Roll War Disabled Men's Association Limited, which had recorded a loss of £4500 during 1948 and could no longer pay for its premises.[41] This was absorbed into Remploy, alongside others such as the Nursery School Equipment Centre in Edinburgh, Spero Industries Limited, Michael Works Limited and the Longton Disabled Soldiers' and Sailors' Cardboard Box Factory.[42] It is clear that the view of the MOL was that the best course of action was not to increase the grants awarded to help sustain the workshops, nor to see them close altogether, but instead to see them transferred to Remploy in the hope that the company could improve their fortunes. It is also important to consider that it was not simply a hope that ownership by Remploy would reduce losses, or would continue to provide sheltered employment despite a loss, that was expressed by the MOL. In this early period, it was still hoped, in common with the initial optimism which greeted the nationalisation of other parts of industry, that Remploy would prove able to contribute to the country's economy in a positive way and even run at a profit, which in turn could be reinvested to continue its expansion.[43]

Sheltered employment was also undertaken by LAs, which had been responsible for providing this service for blind people exclusively since

[39] Finlayson, *Citizen, State and Social Welfare in Britain 1830–1990*, p. 298.

[40] Prochaska, *The Voluntary Impulse*; Digby, *British Welfare Policy*, p. 89.

[41] TNA BM 8/1, Disabled Persons Employment Corporation Limited, 'Minutes of the Forty-First Meeting of the Board of Directors' (23.02.1949).

[42] TNA BM 8/1, Disabled Persons Employment Corporation Limited, 'Minutes of the Eighteenth Meeting of the Board of Directors' (28.01.1947); 'Minutes of the Nineteenth Meeting of the Board of Directors' (25.02.1947): 'Minutes of the Forty-First Meeting of the Board of Directors' (23.02.1949); Remploy Limited, 'Minutes of the Forty-Eighth Meeting of the Board of Directors' (26.10.1949); TNA BM 10/1, Remploy Limited, 'Review of the working of the Company during its first seven years' (March, 1953), p. 13.

[43] Mr Isaacs, *Hansard* (02.12.1947), vol. 445, cc. 186-8; P. Dorey, *British Politics Since 1945* (Oxford, Blackwell, 1995), pp. 7–9; T. Gourvish, 'The Rise (and Fall?) of State-Owned Enterprise', in T. Gourvish and A. O'Day (eds.), *Britain Since 1945* (Basingstoke, Macmillan, 1991), p. 111.

1920 as an element of welfare under the Blind Persons Act.[44] By the end of the Second World War most LAs had workshops in place with over 3000 blind persons employed overall.[45] The DPEA technically gave LAs 'permissive power' to provide sheltered workshops for 'sighted' severely disabled people as well, under direction from the MOL.[46] This was stated more explicitly in the National Assistance Act 1948. Designed to provide for those who slipped through the net of the contributory social insurance scheme which had been established by the National Insurance Act 1946, the National Assistance Act outlined a range of services LAs could offer for disabled people such as social centres, meals-on-wheels schemes and recreational outings.[47] As a result, LAs were empowered—though not obligated—to make arrangements for workshops as part of 'promoting the welfare' of those 'who are blind, deaf or dumb, and other persons who are substantially and permanently handicapped by illness, injury, or congenital deformity'.[48] Expectations here appear to have been considered somewhat ambiguous, however, and they focused instead on the clearer mandate of providing sheltered employment for blind people, with only the occasional inclusion of small numbers of sighted individuals within these existing workshops.[49]

Under the first postwar Labour governments the frontier of the state in sheltered employment thus advanced dramatically, with Remploy securing

[44] TNA LAB 13/1029, J. L. Edwards, 'Remploy: An Experiment in Sheltered Employment for the Severely Disabled in Great Britain', *International Labour Review*, Vol. LXXVII, No. 2 (February, 1958).

[45] TNA LAB 20/56, 'Memorandum by the Ministry of Health on the Welfare of the Blind together with a Note by the Board of Education on Training, R.D.5' (February, 1942); 'Interdepartmental Committee on the Rehabilitation of Disabled Persons: Extract from Minutes of Meeting held on 12th Feb 1942'; TNA LAB 20/173, SEC, 'Second Report to the National Advisory Council on the Employment of the Disabled: Appendix I' (1945).

[46] *Report of the Committee of Inquiry on The Rehabilitation Training and Resettlement of Disabled Persons*, 9883 (1956); DPEA, Section 15.

[47] D. Fraser, *The Evolution of the British Welfare State*, 4th Edition (Basingstoke, Palgrave Macmillan, 2009), p. 274; Hampton, *Disability and the Welfare State in Britain*, p. 58; Taylor, 'Voluntary Action and the State', p. 220.

[48] National Assistance Act 1948; TNA LAB 13/1029, Edwards, 'Remploy: An Experiment in Sheltered Employment for the Severely Disabled in Great Britain' (February, 1958).

[49] *Report of the Committee of Inquiry on The Rehabilitation Training and Resettlement of Disabled Persons*, 9883 (1956).

a large monopoly and being seen to set a new standard which would have to be met by other providers if they wished to continue. As Chapter 3 illustrated, however, the rapid expansion of Remploy caused both the Remploy Board of Directors and the Treasury to express concern at the financial cost and a 'slowdown' was adopted in order to allow the company a chance to consolidate its position. Had Remploy indeed operated at a profit as was hoped, and not called itself for a period of consolidation, it is possible that its role would have continued to increase and advanced the frontier of the state further still.

The Frontier Halts, 1951–1970

As shown in Chapter 3, the slowdown of the expansion of Remploy became a permanent halt under the Conservative Government elected in 1951 and the scope of Remploy was to be limited in terms of economic performance throughout the remainder of the period. With the company not expanding as was initially intended there remained a greater demand for sheltered employment than Remploy itself was placed to deliver. As a result, alternative providers of sheltered employment continued to operate and by 1956 the MOL recorded that there remained some 30 charitable organisations offering work for 858 disabled people.[50] Financial pressures remained high and as such, there were mixed fortunes experienced by these workshops into the 1960s. Some organisations, such as the British Legion Cambrian Factory and the Manton Association, had no choice but to either cede control of workshops or close down altogether.[51] At the same time there were also several new workshops established, with a new Camphill Village Trust Workshop, a laundry unit run by the Scottish Council for the Care of Spastics, and a workshop created by the Industrial Therapy Organisation operating in 1962.[52] By 1965 therefore, the numbers of disabled employees in charitable workshops remained steady at some 863 people.[53]

[50] TNA LAB 43/268, MOL, 'Note on letter dated 17th May 1956 from Mr Willey, MP' (1956).

[51] TNA LAB 20/1073, SEC, 'Provision of Sheltered Employment by Local Authorities and Voluntary Bodies' (November, 1962).

[52] Ibid.

[53] TNA LAB 20/1073, NACED, 'Sheltered Employment Committee Reports'.

Greater expansion in alternative sheltered employment occurred as a result of an increasing role for LAs. In 1956, the Piercy Report noted that excluding those for the blind, 'no workshops have yet been provided by local authorities', with the extent of progress limited to plans for one such workshop having been 'approved'.[54] This was to change as the 1958 amendment to the original DPEA made it clear that LAs had the power to provide sheltered employment and, under direction of the MOL, 'a duty to exercise their powers'.[55] As a result, by 1962 the MOL could note that 85% of LAs had by then taken powers to provide sheltered employment in some form.[56] These figures also included existing provision for blind persons but it is clear that in terms of sighted disabled people, LAs had begun to take on the task as well. This involved the increasing incorporation of sighted disabled people into existing workshops as well as the creation of dedicated new ones. Not all of these workshops were under the direct control of the LA, however, as it became increasingly common for them to utilise voluntary organisations as delivery agencies.[57] This arrangement had been set out in the National Assistance Act as one of the ways in which LAs could provide welfare services for the disabled.[58] With both LAs and charitable workshops under funding pressures this was an attractive option to jointly deliver sheltered employment provision, and has been identified as a common occurrence across other forms of welfare in the period as well.[59] In 1960, the number of disabled people in these 'agency' workshops was 90 and by 1965 this had increased to 296.[60]

[54] *Report of the Committee of Inquiry on The Rehabilitation Training and Resettlement of Disabled Persons*, 9883 (1956).

[55] Disabled Persons (Employment) Act (Amendment) 1958.

[56] TNA LAB 20/1073, SEC, 'Provision of Sheltered Employment by Local Authorities and Voluntary Bodies' (November, 1962); SEC, 'Provision of Sheltered Employment by Local Authorities and Voluntary Bodies, S.E.C.107' (September, 1964).

[57] TNA LAB 20/1073, SEC, 'Provision of Sheltered Employment by Local Authorities and Voluntary Bodies' (November, 1962); NACED, 'Sheltered Employment Committee Reports'.

[58] National Assistance Act 1948.

[59] J. Hampton, 'Disabled People and the Classic Welfare State, 1948–1975: Changes in Perception, Developments in Policy', unpublished PhD Thesis, University of Bristol (2012), p. 10; M. Brenton, *The Voluntary Sector in British Social Services* (Harlow, Prentice Hall Press, 1985), p. 27.

[60] TNA LAB 20/1073, NACED, 'Sheltered Employment Committee Reports'.

Table 6.1 Number of sighted disabled workers in sheltered employment, 1958–1970

Year	*Section II disabled people in Workshops*		*Section II disabled people (sighted) in Blind workshops*	*Total*	*Section II registered unemployed*[61]
	Remploy	*LA & Voluntary*			
1958	6185	867	42	7,094	–
1959	6,156	1,073	59	7,288	4,199
1960	6,303	1,089	78	7,470	4,313
1961	6,203	1,055	126	7,384	4,543
1962	6,359	1,121	198	7,678	4,864
1963	6,291	1,240	220	7,751	5,511
1964	6,519	1,520	272	8,311	5,978
1965	6,823	1,650	372	8,845	6,141
1966	6,817	1,686	337	8,840	6,382
1967	6,817	1,827	381	9,057	7,533
1968	7,179	1,999	409	9,605	8,630
1969	7,447	1,978	466	9,891	9,602
1970	7,505	2,132	493	10,130	10,013

Sources TNA BM 10/48, Remploy Limited, 'Objectives and Criteria of Success: Appendix 5' (1980), p. 73; TNA LAB 20/1071, MOL, 'Unemployed Registered Disabled Persons by Age Groups'; Mr. Green, *Hansard*, (16.04.1962), vol. 658, cc. 12-3w; TNA LAB 20/1429, DE, 'Sheltered Employment: A Draft Consultative Document: Table VIII Section II Register 1963–73' (October, 1973). For unemployed see additional footnote

Table 6.1 indicates the overall growth in sheltered employment provision delivered by LA and voluntary providers, illustrating that although they remained a 'junior partner', there was nevertheless a genuine 'mixed economy' in operation.

The survival and expansion of alternative provision was the result of a number of factors. Political ideology was clearly important. The continuation of a role for a mixed economy in sheltered employment was consistent with the political discourse and wider context of welfare in this period. As Taylor noted, the importance of the voluntary sector as a valuable 'junior partner' in welfare had become increasingly recognised.[62]

[61] For 1959–1961, TNA LAB 20/1071, MOL, 'Unemployed Registered Disabled Persons by Age Groups'. For 1962, Mr. Green, *Hansard*, (16.04.1962), vol. 658, cc. 12-3w. For 1963–70, TNA LAB 20/1429, DE, 'Sheltered Employment: A Draft Consultative Document: Table VIII Section II Register 1963–73' (October, 1973).

[62] Taylor, 'Voluntary Action and the State', p. 223.

Furthermore, while there is no clear demarcation between the attitudes of the Attlee and subsequent Conservative Governments towards Remploy, as the Board themselves felt that continued expansion was unsustainable, the perpetuating of this standstill and hence continuation of sheltered employment provision through charitable services during the 1950s was consistent with the general Conservative outlook on limiting the role of the state, utilising private funding and its sympathy with voluntary enterprise.[63]

Similarly, it has been noted in Chapter 3 that the return of a Labour Government in 1964 did not see a return to a major expansion of Remploy. A continuation of a mixed economy was again consistent with the views of the Labour Party at this time, with voluntary enterprise no longer considered objectionable. While in opposition the Party had curbed its expectations for further widespread nationalisation and the shock of the rediscovery of poverty, highlighted by the publication in 1965 of Brian Abel-Smith and Peter Townsend's *The Poor and the Poorest*, had shown that the central welfare state had failed to eradicate all social problems.[64] This was also the time which saw the resurgence of non-statutory groups, primarily in the new form of campaigning groups drawing inspiration from civil rights movements in the United States, with some well-known examples including the Child Poverty Action Group, Shelter and DIG.[65] Such organisations were more openly critical of government and better able to foster public pressure for policy change.[66] This new form of voluntarism was inherently more acceptable to Labour, contrasting with the aura of middle-class philanthropy which

[63] Kavanagh and Morris, *Consensus Politics*, pp. 25–6; Taylor, 'Voluntary Action and the State', p. 223; Kendall and Knapp, *The Voluntary Sector in the United Kingdom*, pp. 133–9.

[64] Kendall and Knapp, *The Voluntary Sector in the United Kingdom*, pp. 51–7; Digby, *British Welfare Policy*, pp. 65, 89; Kavanagh and Morris, *Consensus Politics*, pp. 27–8; Fraser, *The Evolution of the Welfare State*, p. 300.

[65] Gladstone, *The Twentieth-Century Welfare State*, pp. 66–9; R. Page, *Revisiting the Welfare State* (Maidenhead, Open University Press, 2007), pp. 49–54; R. Lowe, *The Welfare State in Britain Since 1945* (Basingstoke, Palgrave Macmillan, 2005), p. 286.

[66] G. Millward, 'Invalid Definitions, Invalid Responses: Disability and the Welfare State, 1965–1995', unpublished PhD Thesis, London School of Hygiene and Tropical Medicine (2013), pp. 29–33.

had previously been typical of charitable organisations.[67] Though sheltered workshops remained a traditional form of charitable enterprise, the overall image of the voluntary sector was more acceptable to Labour and its potential benefits in delivering welfare more accepted.

Funding was also an important factor in the continuation of a mixed economy. As Chapter 3 illustrated, the hoped-for profit from Remploy was not to occur. Remploy was not unique in this regard but it was far more costly in direct terms for the Government than the other providers, with the financial responsibility for Remploy held entirely by the Exchequer.[68] For LA and approved charitable undertakings, governments offered grants, the largest of which was a 'deficiency grant' which covered 75% of the financial loss for a workshop for the year but was limited to a maximum amount.[69] This limit was £100 per disabled worker in 1956, which increased to £240 in 1961, and reached £430 the following decade.[70] The rest of the costs were borne by either the LA, as part of their overall welfare budget, or through the fundraising activities of the particular charity. In the case of those voluntary workshops operating on behalf of an LA, central government contributed 50% of the funding and the LA and charity 25% each.[71] Central government therefore made only a contribution, alongside contributions from the charitable organisations or from LA budgets. There were also occasions

[67] Kendall and Knapp, *The Voluntary Sector in the United Kingdom*, pp. 51–7.

[68] TNA LAB 20/1429, DE, 'Sheltered Employment: A Draft Consultative Document' (October, 1973), pp. 28–9.

[69] TNA LAB 43/268, MOL, 'Note on letter dated 17th May 1956' (1956); TNA LAB 20/1038, MOL, 'Employment in Sheltered Workshops: Conditions for the payment of grants and allowances to Voluntary Undertakings employment severely disabled persons' (November, 1961).

[70] TNA LAB 43/268, MOL, 'Note on letter dated 17th May 1956' (1956); TNA LAB 20/1038, MOL, 'Employment in Sheltered Workshops: Conditions for the payment of grants and allowances to Voluntary Undertakings employment severely disabled persons' (November, 1961); TNA LAB 20/1073, SEC, 'Provision of Sheltered Employment by Local Authorities and Voluntary Bodies' (November, 1962); TNA LAB 20/1429, DE, 'Sheltered Employment: A Draft Consultative Document' (October, 1973), pp. 28–9; TNA LAB 20/1478, DE, 'Sheltered Employment: Dealings with Local Authorities' (1975).

[71] TNA LAB 20/1478, DE, 'Sheltered Employment: Dealings with Local Authorities' (1975).

where, owing to fundraising successes, charitable workshops required no grant at all.[72]

The direct cost of Remploy to government was much greater. It is not possible to provide direct comparative information for the entire period, but there are a number of useful examples. The Piercy Report noted that for the financial year 1954/55, the MOL had provided financial support for LA workshops for blind persons totalling 'approximately £367,000' and for charitable workshops totalling 'about £94,000'.[73] These workshops provided employment for almost 5000 workers.[74] The cost of Remploy for the same period totalled £2,903,000, in support of 6500 workers.[75] When calculated on a crude per-worker basis, we can see that the MOL was contributing £92 per worker for the year to LA and charitable workshops, compared to £447 per worker in Remploy. Given this, it is perhaps easy to see why the mixed economy, with additional funding available from charitable donations or LA budgets, continued to prove an attractive option for successive governments.[76]

It is also possible to detect a loss of faith in the ability of Remploy to provide sheltered employment in a superior way to the other providers. While this was chiefly reflected in financial results, the key test for any company, there were also concerns about its operations. Remploy's management had first been subject to serious criticism in the Fourth Report of the Select Committee on Estimates in 1952, which was widely publicised and which was deemed by Remploy to have been 'disastrous' for the company's reputation.[77] As well as this bad publicity, and despite the MOL officially noting its support for Remploy, it is clear in some of

[72] See reports in TNA LAB 20/78.

[73] *Report of the Committee of Inquiry on The Rehabilitation Training and Resettlement of Disabled Persons*, 9883 (1956).

[74] Ibid.

[75] TNA LAB 13/1029, Edwards, 'Remploy: An Experiment in Sheltered Employment for the Severely Disabled in Great Britain', (February, 1958), p. 13.

[76] TNA LAB 13/1029, Edwards, 'Remploy: An Experiment in Sheltered Employment for the Severely Disabled in Great Britain', (February, 1958), p. 13.

[77] *Fourth Report from the Select Committee on Estimates*, 162 (1952); TNA LAB 20/653, 'Note of a Meeting between the Minister and the Board of Remploy Limited on 16th May' (16.05.1952); TNA BM 10/2, Remploy Limited, 'A Brief Outline of the Birth and Early Development of Remploy Limited' (May, 1979), p. 8. See also TNA LAB 20/929.

the correspondence among MOL officials that doubts lingered about the capability of its management.[78]

The growing role for LA's following the 1958 amendment to the DPEA was also consistent with the delivery of welfare services more generally.[79] This has recently been highlighted in the case of disabled people by Hampton, who described the increasing, though varying, efforts of LAs to deliver welfare provision across the 1950s and 1960s.[80] Similarly, the system of LA and central government funding to voluntary organisations was not limited to sheltered employment, but was a common relationship, with a considerable number of charitable welfare organisations at least part-funded by national or local government.[81] As Gladstone noted, this increasing reliance on state funding 'raised the issue of the independence' of the voluntary sector.[82] In the case of sheltered employment, there was a concurrent increase in regulation as this closer relationship developed. This was a softer frontier of the state, but an important one which saw the infringement, albeit within limits, of central government on the independence of the charitable sector. The Piercy Report in 1956, while commending the role of voluntary workshops, maintained that the continued support of the MOL should be dependent on the ability of the workshops to provide 'a service of good standard', and that they remained open to inspection from MOL officials.[83] The standard was codified further and inspections formalised in a guide for sheltered workshops circulated in 1962.[84] This noted that grants were only available to those workshops approved by the MOL and that this

[78] See Chapter 3 and TNA LAB 20/929.

[79] Millward, 'Invalid Definitions, Invalid Responses', pp. 29–33.

[80] Hampton, *Disability and the Welfare State in Britain*, pp. 59–65.

[81] Brenton, *The Voluntary Sector in British Social Services*, p. 27; Gladstone, *The Twentieth-Century Welfare State*, pp. 66–9; Kendall and Knapp, *The Voluntary Sector in the United Kingdom*, pp. 51–7, 133–9.

[82] Kendall and Knapp, *The Voluntary Sector in the United Kingdom*, pp. 51–7, 133–9; Gladstone, *The Twentieth-Century Welfare State*, pp. 66–9.

[83] *Report of the Committee of Inquiry on The Rehabilitation Training and Resettlement of Disabled Persons*, 9883 (1956).

[84] TNA LAB 20/1038, MOL, 'Employment in Sheltered Workshops: Conditions for the payment of grants and allowances to Voluntary Undertakings employment severely disabled persons' (November, 1961); TNA LAB 20/1429, DE, 'Sheltered Employment: A Draft Consultative Document' (October, 1973), p. 14.

approval was based on a number of conditions, such as providing 'genuine employment', paying wages and providing a 'normal' 40 hour week.[85] The organisation itself had to run the workshop 'efficiently', not take any profits, and prove able to provide sufficient funding to meets its proportion of the costs.[86] As before, it was noted that the workshop 'must be open to inspection by duly authorised officers of the Ministry of Labour', and that approval was subject to review 'from time to time'.[87] LA and charitable workshops were therefore subject to an assessment of standards if they were in receipt of government support and did not escape from pressure to improve workshop performance.[88] This should not be overstated however, as beyond inspection and general monitoring, there is no evidence of punitive action being taken against any workshop. The DE noted that in practice its control over LA and voluntary workshops had always been 'limited' and this was to remain the case throughout this period and beyond.[89]

The form voluntary sheltered employment provision took continued to be varied. In the majority of cases both charitable and LA workshops tended to cater for smaller numbers of workers than was typical in Remploy factories. In 1958, J. L. Edwards, an MOL official, claimed in his article on the development of Remploy, that as the company had focused its initial expansion on areas with high numbers of severely disabled people, there were by then few areas where 'the concentration of suitable disabled unemployed is large enough' to warrant large factories.[90] He noted that those workshops run by LAs or charities tended therefore, to focus on the remaining 'relatively small local concentrations

[85] TNA LAB 20/1038, MOL, 'Employment in Sheltered Workshops: Conditions for the payment of grants and allowances to Voluntary Undertakings employment severely disabled persons' (November, 1961).

[86] Ibid.

[87] Ibid.

[88] TNA LAB 20/1429, DE, 'Sheltered Employment: A Draft Consultative Document' (October, 1973), p. 53.

[89] Ibid., p. 63; TNA BM 3/54, Remploy Limited, 'Co-operation in Sheltered Employment: Notes of a Meeting between Remploy and ESA' (26.07.1976); TNA ET 2/32, MSC, 'Sheltered Workshops: Guidelines for local authorities' (1978); C. Barnes, *Disabled People in Britain and Discrimination* (London, C. Hurst & Co., 2000), p. 71.

[90] TNA LAB 13/1029, Edwards, 'Remploy: An Experiment in Sheltered Employment for the Severely Disabled in Great Britain' (February, 1958), pp. 14–15.

of disabled people'.[91] Though not absolute, this suggests something of a demarcation therefore, with Remploy's initial expansion providing large-scale factories where there was shown to be large numbers of eligible employees, and LAs and charities then providing smaller scale workshops.[92] This presents a tangible example of the non-statutory sector being a 'junior partner' in the mixed economy. According to the DE, by the 1970s, LA and charitable workshops usually involved catering for '30–40' workers 'in less predominantly industrial areas'.[93] Where demand was even smaller in rural or remote areas, sheltered employment was 'almost entirely' composed of charitable provision.[94] It is also apparent that no other sheltered employment scheme ever approached Remploy's overall scale. Whereas Remploy operated a network of factories, the vast majority of LA and voluntary workshops were uncoordinated individual units.[95] The largest network outside Remploy belonged to Lord Roberts Memorial Workshops with five workshops at the start of the period, and two more in operation by 1965.[96]

A further key difference was that charities continued to focus upon particular groups of disabled people. Chapter 4 has illustrated the reality of recruitment into Remploy as based upon potential productivity rather than by groupings of disability or by ex-service status. Chapter 5 indicated that while Remploy was male-dominated, women were not excluded from the company explicitly in terms of central policy. Independent charitable workshops could limit recruitment however they wished to focus on their particular 'causes', and a list of these workshops presented to the SEC shows that this continued to be the case into the 1960s.[97] Thus, for example, the Scottish Council for Care of Spastics workshop provided

[91] Ibid.

[92] TNA LAB 20/1429, DE, 'Sheltered Employment: A Draft Consultative Document' (October, 1973), pp. 20, 30, 63.

[93] Ibid., p. 24.

[94] Ibid., pp. 24, 30.

[95] TNA LAB 20/1478, Remploy Limited, 'Managing Director to Department of Employment' (09.04.1975).

[96] See TNA LAB 20/173, SEC, 'Scheme of Grants to Undertakings Employing Severely Disabled Persons: Organisations at present included in the Scheme, S.E.C I' (1945); TNA LAB 20/1073, SEC, 'Approved arrangements made by Local Authorities for providing sheltered employment for severely disabled sighted persons' (1965).

[97] Ibid.

solely for those with cerebral palsy, while the Yateley Industries for Disabled Girls catered only for women. There is also evidence to suggest that this continued into the following decade as well, as the DE noted that while some organisations catered 'for all or most categories of disabled people', charitable provision 'typically' involved catering for a specific group, again based around gender, disability or ex-service status.[98] Such establishments could also, like Remploy, employ non-Section II workers. Unlike Remploy however, they were not subject to a limit, and how many Section I or non-disabled people were employed was ultimately down to the organisation itself.[99] Financial assistance from governments in this period however, was limited to a 'per employee' deficiency grant available only to Section II employees, meaning the organisation would have to fund such cases itself.[100]

As to whether employees within these workshops were then selected on a similar basis to Remploy, in terms of maximising productivity, there is something of a mixed picture. Anderson suggested that charitable sheltered workshops 'were not willing to accept lower standards of production from their workers'.[101] It is possible that a remark from the Lord Roberts Memorial Workshop in Fulham in 1951 that they were having difficult in 'finding suitable disabled men' for light assembly woodwork, indicates that they were indeed looking for a certain level of ability or productivity, though it is also possible this referred to ex-service personnel for whom the charity catered.[102] Certainly, the Piercy Report of 1956 had recommended that sheltered employment should be reserved for those that were capable of productive employment, and this applied to sheltered employment generally. However, contrary to this, the DE noted that there had long been a widespread belief that LA and charitable workshops tended

[98] TNA LAB 20/1429, DE, 'Sheltered Employment: A Draft Consultative Document' (October, 1973), p. 21.

[99] TNA LAB 20/1038, MOL, 'Employment in Sheltered Workshops: Conditions for the payment of grants and allowances to Voluntary Undertakings employment severely disabled persons' (November, 1961).

[100] Ibid.

[101] Anderson, *War, Disability and Rehabilitation in Britain*, pp. 183–4.

[102] TNA LAB 20/78, MOL, 'Lord Roberts Memorial Workshops Fulham Factory' (February, 1951).

to employ those with a lower production capacity than did Remploy.[103] Similarly a Remploy Group Director, who worked closely with voluntary and LA workshops, suggested that those disabled people considered unable to meet Remploy's productivity level were sometimes accepted by other workshops owing to their greater willingness 'to accept additional low output personnel into their workshops'.[104] This indicates that while productivity was a factor in recruitment, this was generally considered to be to a lesser extent that was the case for Remploy.

In terms of the types of work undertaken, LA workshops, having developed in the early 1960s, had adapted quickly to providing the so-called 'new trades', focusing primarily upon light engineering and carpentry.[105] While many charitable workshops also pursued these areas, a significant number continued to rely on the traditional sheltered employment trades.[106] For both LA and voluntary workshops, the work undertaken was largely determined by the perceived ability of the workers to carry out certain tasks, and the local and independent nature of the workshops which prevented capital investment, marketing and large-scale orders.[107] In some respects this was different to Remploy, which attempted to focus upon national markets with standard product lines and was not, in principle, overly interested in local orders.[108] An example of the kind of production which Remploy was aiming for was the securing of sole manufacturing and sales rights for the Swedish *Lundia* shelving range, which remained a key product for decades.[109] This sort of deal could only occur because of Remploy's size which allowed it 'to bear the risks and sustain

[103] TNA LAB 20/1429, DE, 'Sheltered Employment: A Draft Consultative Document' (October, 1973), pp. 61–2.

[104] TNA BM 3/47, Remploy Limited, 'Group Director B.A.S: Entry Standard for Employment in Remploy' (31.01.1975); Remploy Limited, 'Note from Group Director BAS to Remploy MD: Entry Standard for Employment in Remploy' (18.02.1975).

[105] TNA LAB 20/1429, DE, 'Sheltered Employment: A Draft Consultative Document: Table IV' (October, 1973), p. 25.

[106] Ibid.

[107] TNA LAB 20/1429, DE, 'Sheltered Employment: A Draft Consultative Document' (October, 1973), p. 25; LAB 20/78, MOL, 'Note of conversation' (09.09.1950); LAB 20/1144, MOL, 'Borough of Swindon Enterprise Work Inspection Report' (July, 1966).

[108] TNA BM 10/1, Remploy Limited, 'A Review of the working of the Company during its first seven years' (March, 1953), pp. 7–8.

[109] TNA BM10/2, Remploy Limited, 'A Brief Outline of the Birth and Early Development of Remploy Limited' (May, 1979), p. 21.

the overheads involved in a national marketing operation'.[110] However, as has been noted in Chapter 3, this attempt to focus on a national market was not always successful, especially in Remploy's early days, and with work scarce, many factories engaged in whatever could be found, with numerous reports of factory managers sourcing local work in the same way as other workshops continued to do.[111] Even when Remploy was organised into trade groupings with standard product lines from the 1950s onwards, there remained continued variation in the precise type of trade in factories. Work was never very secure and, given the nature of the company, was always in demand. Therefore we see some of the traditional trades, such as the 'brush and broom trade' undertaken by charitable workshops continue in Remploy factories as well, either because of a lack of alternatives or because it was considered more suitable for the employees.[112] It is not clear therefore how much of a difference between a national operation like Remploy and the smaller local contracts undertaken in other workshops was felt on the production floor itself.

It is also apparent that other providers, in common with Remploy, faced certain commercial pressures. Though charities and LAs provided sheltered employment more explicitly as a form of welfare than was the case with Remploy, the need to be as productive as possible within this remit still held some importance. The Lord Roberts Workshop's records reveal struggles with similar issues to Remploy, such as the securing of work and productivity issues which required further deficiency grants from the MOL.[113] The financial situation of all workshops was monitored by the Ministry and its successors and there were concerns raised on a number of occasions about their economic sustainability.[114] As the DE noted, such commercial difficulties were largely 'inherent in the concept

[110] TNA LAB 20/1429, DE, 'Sheltered Employment: A Draft Consultative Document' (October, 1973), p. 25.

[111] See Chapter 3; TNA BM 10/2, Remploy Limited, 'A Brief Outline of the Birth and Early Development of Remploy Limited' (May, 1979).

[112] TNA BM 3/54, Remploy Limited, 'Remploy in the Long-Term: Appendix 10' (28.02.1977).

[113] TNA LAB 20/78, MOL, 'Note of conversation' (09.09.1950).

[114] *Report of the Committee of Inquiry on The Rehabilitation Training and Resettlement of Disabled Persons*, 9883 (1956); TNA LAB 20/1429, DE, 'Sheltered Employment: A Draft Consultative Document' (October, 1973), pp. 53–5; TNA LAB 20/1462, NACED, 'Sheltered Employment Annual Report' (1975).

of sheltered employment'.[115] Though not under the same pressure as Remploy, LA and charitable workshops in receipt of government funds were not immune from calls to increase commercial efficiency.[116]

With the full expansion of Remploy having been abandoned, alternative provision in sheltered employment increased and remained throughout the period, irrespective of changes in government. Such provision proved cost-effective for central government and conformed to the pattern for support for a mixed economy in welfare more generally. This included voluntary organisations, some new, some continued from before the war, and an increasing role for undertakings operated by LAs both independently and in partnership. The result was the existence of a diverse 'tripartite mixed economy' in sheltered employment.

The National Consultation and Question of Unification, 1970–1979

The effectiveness of this tripartite mixed economy came under question in the 1970s during a process of national consultation. This was instigated by the Conservative Government elected in 1970 under Edward Heath, as part of a wider reorganisation of central and local government designed to modernise and 'make public administration more dynamic'.[117] This included the restructuring of the employment service, with the formation of two new agencies to implement policy, the Employment Services Agency (ESA) and the Training Services Agency, alongside the creation in 1973 of the Manpower Services Commission (MSC) which was given responsibility for manpower policy.[118] The Local Authority Social Services Act of 1970, the Social Work (Scotland) Act 1968 and the Chronically Sick and Disabled Persons Act 1970 further increased the role of LAs with regards to disabled people across a range of provision such as 'social workers, occupational therapists, residential and day centre facilities, holidays, meals on wheels, respite services and disability aids

[115] TNA LAB 20/1429, DE, 'Sheltered Employment: A Draft Consultative Document' (October, 1973), pp. 53–5.

[116] Ibid., p. 53.

[117] Dorey, *British Politics Since 1945*, p. 85; M. Hill, *The Welfare State in Britain: A Political History since 1945* (Aldershot, Edward Elgar Publishing, 1993), p. 103.

[118] Ibid.

and adaptations'.[119] Local government itself was extensively reorganised following the passing of the Local Government Act 1972.[120] During this process, the Executive Council of the County Councils Association asked for clarity as to its role in providing sheltered employment.[121] As a result, the DE published and distributed a 'Consultative Document' in 1973 on the future of sheltered employment, which was followed by a period of discussion over the following two years—during which time a Labour Government replaced Heath's in 1974. With Labour having moved to the Left following its defeat in 1970, touting an agenda of further nationalisation and a promise of a comprehensive employment service for disabled people, the possibility was raised for a fundamental change in sheltered employment provision.[122]

The DE's Consultative Document, outlined the 'increasing difficulty' in operating the current tripartite system and the various options for sheltered employment going forward.[123] Contrary to the image portrayed by Edwards in his article, of Remploy and the other providers together forming a cohesive overall system, the Consultative Document revealed the various problems which had developed in the mixed economy over the preceding years which had prevented this from happening.[124] Chiefly this was the result of a lack of cooperation among the various providers. With difficult trading conditions a common problem since the Second World War, the competition for work between the providers had remained constant. This was still most keenly felt in terms of government contracts, which Remploy had continued to dominate, much to the chagrin of

[119] A. Roulstone and S. Prideaux, *Understanding Disability Policy* (Bristol, Policy Press, 2012), p. 37.

[120] Younghusband, *Social Work in Britain*, pp. 247–8.

[121] TNA BM 3/47, Remploy Limited, 'Group Director B.A.S: Entry Standard for Employment in Remploy: Appendix A' (31.01.1975); TNA LAB 20/1429, DE, 'Sheltered Employment: A Draft Consultative Document' (October, 1973), p. 2; Kendall and Knapp, *The Voluntary Sector in the United Kingdom*, pp. 51–7; J. A. Chandler, *Explaining Local Government: Local Government in Britain since 1800* (Manchester, Manchester University Press, 2007), pp. 201–5.

[122] Hampton, *Disability and the Welfare State in Britain*, p. 145; Kavanagh and Morris, *Consensus Politics*, pp. 28–9.

[123] TNA LAB 20/1429, DE, 'Sheltered Employment: A Draft Consultative Document' (October, 1973), pp. 69–70.

[124] TNA LAB 13/1029, Edwards, 'Remploy: An Experiment in Sheltered Employment for the Severely Disabled in Great Britain' (February, 1958), p. 14.

other workshops.[125] Competition appears to have developed into mutual antipathy and even hostility between Remploy and the charitable and LA workshops. The Consultative Document noted an example of a case where an LA had flatly refused a proposal to share workshop space with the company.[126] Such conflict was most acute in relations between Remploy and the other providers, but there were also problems between LAs and voluntary bodies, since the former had a duty to provide sheltered employment for disabled people generally, whereas the latter usually existed to support a particular group, which could lead to disagreement when they ran workshops together.[127]

The initial discussions during the formation of Remploy had warned against the duplication of service between Remploy and other workshops resulting from a lack of coordination.[128] However, this was highlighted as a key problem in the Consultative Document, which noted no less than 38 instances of duplications of service, with a Remploy factory and another workshop located in the same locality.[129] As well as being uneconomic, this also created an uneven system with some areas having multiple workshops, and others none at all, highlighting the limitation of the kind of demarcation suggested by Edwards.[130] To a degree this was unavoidable in the case of independent charitable provision which varied greatly based on the resources, aims and whims of the bodies directing them.[131] Indeed, this problem of 'unequal geographical coverage' has

[125] TNA LAB 20/1429, DE, 'Sheltered Employment: A Draft Consultative Document' (October, 1973), p. 27.

[126] Ibid., p. 63.

[127] Ibid., pp. 62–3.

[128] TNA LAB 20/108, MOL, 'Employment under Special Conditions: Outline of a Scheme under Section 15 of the Disabled Persons (Employment) Act, 1944' (June, 1944).

[129] TNA LAB 20/1429, DE, 'Sheltered Employment: A Draft Consultative Document' (October, 1973), pp. 85–6; TNA BM 3/54, Remploy Limited, 'Remploy in the Long-Term, Appendix 2: Remploy in Sheltered Employment in the U.K.' (22.04.1977); TNA BM 8/79, Remploy Limited, 'Minutes of the Three Hundred and Thirty-Third Meeting of the Board of Directors' (13.09.1975).

[130] TNA BM 8/79, Remploy Limited, 'Minutes of the Three Hundred and Thirty-Third Meeting of the Board of Directors' (13.09.1975); TNA LAB 13/1029, Edwards, 'Remploy: An Experiment in Sheltered Employment for the Severely Disabled in Great Britain' (February, 1958), pp. 14–5.

[131] TNA LAB 20/1429, DE, 'Sheltered Employment: A Draft Consultative Document' (October, 1973), p. 24.

been noted as a common critique of charitable organisations in the period generally.[132] More coordination might be expected from Remploy and LAs in terms of how they positioned themselves.[133] However, with mutual distrust, such coordination was virtually non-existent, leaving no collective approach to achieving effective coverage.[134]

This also highlighted the lack of a uniform experience of sheltered employment, as two disabled people in the same area could experience vastly different working conditions depending on the kind of workshop they joined.[135] Thus the DE noted that disabled workers in one workshop 'cannot help but wonder whether they are not perhaps being inequitably dealt with'.[136] Remploy in particular advocated the benefits of disabled workers having 'the same general conditions' regardless of location, which of course they felt uniquely placed to provide.[137] It has already been demonstrated that Remploy factories were, in reality, far from uniform, but they were undoubtedly more so than was the case with the other disparate providers. A particular concern expressed by the DE in this regard was the variation and levels of wages in many workshops. As was illustrated in the previous chapter, Remploy's wages were initially negotiated with the unions of the various trades undertaken, with a reduction to reflect the decreased productivity of the disabled workers, which was then replaced with a standard Remploy rate. Despite repeated calls from the DE and Remploy for a unified wage structure, and concerns expressed by the former at some examples of 'extremely low'

[132] Digby, *British Welfare Policy*, p. 89; Thane, *Foundations of the Welfare State*, p. 277.

[133] TNA LAB 20/1429, DE, 'Sheltered Employment: A Draft Consultative Document' (October, 1973), pp. 20, 30.

[134] Ibid., pp. 63, 70–1.

[135] TNA BM 8/79, Remploy Limited, 'Minutes of the Three Hundred and Thirty-Third Meeting of the Board of Directors' (13.09.1975); TNA BM 3/54, Remploy Limited, 'Remploy in the Long-Term, Appendix 2: Remploy in Sheltered Employment in the U.K.' (22.04.1977).

[136] TNA LAB 20/1429, DE, 'Sheltered Employment: A Draft Consultative Document' (October, 1973), p. 62.

[137] TNA BM 3/54, Remploy Limited, 'Remploy in the Long-Term, Appendix 2: Remploy in Sheltered Employment in the U.K.' (22.04.1977); TNA LAB 20/1478, Remploy Limited, 'Managing Director to Department of Employment' (09.04.1975).

pay, wages paid to disabled employees in charitable and LA workshops varied considerably.[138]

The Consultative Document concluded that the tripartite structure was dysfunctional, and had resulted in the uneven distribution of workshops, confusion over financing, differing wages for workers and protracted negotiations, discussions and compromises in planning.[139] Having outlined such problems, it then made clear that the view of the DE was that the unification of sheltered employment under a single authority was necessary.[140] To this end, the Department proposed two possible systems, one involved the devolution of responsibility for sheltered employment to local government, and the other would bring all provision under central government control.[141] The first option would see workshops and factories operated by LAs. Remploy would become a National Agency, funded entirely by the LAs, providing management consultancy, marketing, product development and sales.[142] All charitable workshops would have to act as agents of the LAs to continue to receive funding.[143] The benefits of this proposal, outlined by the DE, related to the current welfare responsibilities of LAs, the fundamentally local nature of sheltered workshops and the potential for comprehensive integration with other welfare services.[144] The second option would see central government control of all aspects of sheltered employment, with the expansion of Remploy to perform the role.[145] Under this system Remploy would take over all other workshops, with independent charitable workshops who wished to continue being funded, working as agents of the company.[146] The benefits of such a national scheme to

[138] TNA LAB 20/1429, DE, 'Sheltered Employment: A Draft Consultative Document, Table VII' (October, 1973); BM 3/54, Remploy Limited, 'Remploy in the Long-Term' (22.04.1977), p. 9.

[139] TNA LAB 20/1429, DE, 'Sheltered Employment: A Draft Consultative Document' (October, 1973), pp. 63, 70–2.

[140] Ibid., pp. 69–72.

[141] Ibid., p. 72.

[142] Ibid., pp. 75–6.

[143] Ibid., p. 78.

[144] Ibid., pp. 85–6.

[145] Ibid., p. 79.

[146] Ibid.

streamlined planning, uniform employment conditions and wages and a cohesive industrial strategy were noted, with Remploy's position as the only example of such an operation highlighted.[147] Both options involved the placing of voluntary workshops under the remit of either local or central government.

Protracted discussions ensued, involving Remploy, LAs, government ministers, the NACED, the MSC, the TUC, the Confederation of British Industry, the National Association of Industries for the Blind and Disabled (NAIBD) and the National League of the Blind and Disabled (NLBD)—with the DE attempting to balance the various viewpoints.[148] It is important to note that these deliberations did include a voice for disabled people themselves, though this was limited to only two organisations, the NAIBD and the NLBD. The move away from the traditional paternalistic advocacy for disabled people by 'well-meaning' non-disabled people has been noted as a key development in the period.[149] This engagement with the relevant communities targeted by welfare appears to be a common feature across services and was intended to provide a 'counterweight to the "top-down" nature of the statutory welfare state'.[150] That only two such organisations were consulted illustrates that adequate representation still had some way to go, but it does represent an initial step in this direction.

[147] Ibid., p. 89.

[148] TNA LAB 20/1478, 'Note, DE "The Future of Sheltered Employment"' (26.03.1975); MSC, 'Sheltered Employment: Paper by the Secretariat'.

[149] Millward, 'Invalid Definitions, Invalid Responses', pp. 29–33.

[150] Gladstone, *The Twentieth-Century Welfare State*, pp. 66–9.

While broad agreement was reached on the desirability to unify sheltered employment, there was deep disagreement over how this should be achieved.[151] Predictably, Remploy favoured unification under central government, and LAs unification under themselves, and each strongly opposed the other scheme.[152] It is impossible to ignore the sense of mutual distrust and enmity between Remploy and the representatives of the other providers.[153] The justifications used by each side as to why they should take over a unified system reveal some of the opinions they had of each other. Remploy's criticism of LA control centred around the lack of focus on sheltered employment when compared to their other welfare responsibilities; a lack of expertise among social work officials, particularly in terms of the commercial necessities of operating a large scheme; and a lack of unity among the LAs that would result in a 'chaotic and fragmented system'.[154] Under LA control, Remploy felt that sheltered employment would be reduced 'to a shambles, operated...by a large number of independent and unskilled local authorities'.[155] The LAs chief criticism of Remploy was its focus on commercial efficiency and tendency

[151] TNA LAB 20/1478, MSC, 'Sheltered Employment: Paper by the Secretariat'; Confederation of British Industry, 'Note "Sheltered Employment for Disabled People"' (28.05.1974); TUC, 'Note "Sheltered Employment for Disabled People"' (15.08.1974); DE, 'Sheltered Employment: Note of a meeting with Representatives of The National League of the Blind and Disabled' (24.03.1975); Association of Metropolitan Authorities, 'Note to Department of Employment "Sheltered Employment"' (06.03.1975); Association of County Councils, 'Note to Department of Employment "The Future of Sheltered Employment"' (27.02.1975).

[152] TNA LAB 20/1478, Remploy Limited, 'Managing Director to Department of Employment' (09.04.1975); TNA LAB 20/1478, MSC, 'Sheltered Employment: Paper by the Secretariat'; Confederation of British Industry, 'Note "Sheltered Employment for Disabled People"' (28.05.1974); TUC, 'Note "Sheltered Employment for Disabled People"' (15.08.1974); DE, 'Sheltered Employment: Note of a meeting with Representatives of The National League of the Blind and Disabled' (24.03.1975); Association of Metropolitan Authorities, 'Note to Department of Employment "Sheltered Employment"' (06.03.1975); Association of County Councils, 'Note to Department of Employment "The Future of Sheltered Employment"' (27.02.1975).

[153] See TNA LAB 20/1478.

[154] TNA LAB 20/1478, Remploy Limited, 'Managing Director to Department of Employment' (09.04.1975).

[155] TNA BM 3/54, Remploy Limited, 'The Remploy View' (February, 1974), p. 25.

to demand maximum productivity from workers, rejecting those unable to meet a high 'industrial tempo', rather than focusing on welfare.[156]

Remploy outlined their own argument for control in a document called 'The Remploy View', emphasising their experience of largely performing such a role already.[157] However, according to the DE, this proposal 'had virtually no support outside Remploy', and indeed was 'strongly opposed in some important quarters'.[158] What these 'important quarters' were, was not mentioned. The Remploy reply to the DE assessment questioned the reasoning behind this opposition, 'and if these reasons are based on the up-to-date situation'.[159] That there was something of a loss of faith in Remploy's management has already been noted and this perception appears to have influenced these discussions. The result was that even while it remained technically an option under discussion, a DE official revealed in correspondence that 'at official level in the Department we no longer regard this as a serious contender'.[160]

Proposals for LA control were also put forward, stressing their current responsibilities for social services and the local flexibility such a scheme would afford.[161] As with Remploy, the DE noted that the proposals had 'no support outside local authorities'.[162] With both initial options considered unworkable, the Department was left with the option of either maintaining the status quo, or to follow the suggestion made by the NACED that responsibility should be given to the MSC to

[156] See for example, TNA LAB 20/1478, Association of Metropolitan Authorities & Association of County Councils, 'Sheltered Employment – Local Government and the Future of Remploy' (February, 1975).

[157] TNA LAB 20/1478, Remploy Limited, 'Managing Director to Department of Employment' (09.04.1975); TNA BM 3/54, Remploy Limited, 'Remploy in the Long-Term, Appendix 2: Remploy in Sheltered Employment in the U.K.' (22.04.1977).

[158] TNA LAB 20/1478, DE, 'Note, "Sheltered Employment"' (12.03.1975); DE, 'Note, "The Future of Sheltered Employment"' (26.03.1975).

[159] TNA LAB 20/1478, Remploy Limited, 'Managing Director to Department of Employment' (09.04.1975).

[160] TNA LAB 20/1478, DE, 'Note, "The Future of Sheltered Employment"' (26.03.1975).

[161] TNA LAB 20/1478, Association of County Councils, 'Secretary to Department of Employment "The Future of Sheltered Employment"' (27.02.1975); DE, 'Note, "The Future of Sheltered Employment"' (26.03.1975).

[162] TNA LAB 20/1478, DE, 'Note, "Sheltered Employment"' (12.03.1975); DE, 'Note, "The Future of Sheltered Employment"' (26.03.1975).

oversee the different providers.[163] Thus the existing mixed economy would continue, but with a body providing a measure of overview. This proposal was accepted by the DE, and the final decision was announced in the Commons in December 1975 by Labour's Joint Parliamentary Under-Secretary of State for Employment, Harold Walker.[164] Noting the agreement that a unified system would be advantageous, but that 'no form of unification...would command sufficiently widespread support', it was decided that the present tripartite system would remain.[165] This continuation of a mixed economy under Labour was also consistent with wider welfare. Once in power, Labour had curbed its expectations for further state expansion, and with the climate of economic crisis which pervaded much of its term removing the economic growth upon which expansion was predicated, the mixed economy more generally remained largely untouched.[166] The end result of the process was thus the transfer of administration of sheltered employment under the tripartite system to the MSC with an aim to engender closer cooperation between the various providers.[167]

By the mid-1970s therefore, there continued to be a diverse mix of sheltered employment other than Remploy, as can be seen in Table 6.2. There were similar numbers of workshops run independently by LAs and voluntary organisations, employing similar numbers of people, as well as a number of agency relationships and the inclusion of a significant number of sighted people in blind workshops.[168] Although there

[163] TNA LAB 20/1478, DE, 'Note, "The Future of Sheltered Employment"' (26.03.1975); DE, 'Note, "Sheltered Employment"' (12.03.1975); DE, 'Review of Policies and Services for Disabled People' (09.06.1975), pp. 1–3.

[164] TNA BM 3/54, Remploy Limited, 'Remploy in the Long-Term, Appendix 3: Managing Director's Bulletin' (11.12.1975).

[165] Ibid.

[166] Kavanagh and Morris, *Consensus Politics*, pp. 28–9; Digby, *British Welfare Policy*, p. 65.

[167] TNA BM 3/54, Remploy Limited, 'Remploy in the Long-Term, Appendix 3: Managing Director's Bulletin' (11.12.1975).

[168] TNA LAB 20/1073, NACED, 'Sheltered Employment Committee Reports'; TNA LAB 20/1462, NACED, 'Sheltered Employment Annual Report' (1975).

Table 6.2 Sheltered workshops excluding Remploy, 1975

Provider	*No. of Factories/Units*	*Number in Employment (Sighted)*
LA (Sighted)	28	1014
LA (Blind)	29	400
Charity acting as agents for LA's (Sighted)	7	272
Charity acting as agents for LA's (Blind)	27	275
Independent Charity (Sighted)	26	1123
TOTAL	117	3,084

Source TNA LAB 20/1462, NACED, 'Sheltered Employment Annual Report' (1975)

were isolated reports of some workshops having to reduce their workforce 'owing to lack of work', the overall trend was growth.[169] LAs in particular expanded their role, with many increasing capacity or creating new workshops.[170] A mixed economy in sheltered employment continued therefore, with Remploy remaining, as the MSC noted, only a 'part' of this overall provision.[171] Table 6.3 reveals, however, that while provision among other providers continued to grow, as with other forms of welfare, the voluntary sector still remained the 'junior partner' in the postwar mixed economy.[172] The majority of sheltered employment continued to be provided through central government in the form of Remploy.

Though the unification of sheltered employment failed, attempts were made to foster closer cooperation between the providers.[173] This had begun during the consultative process itself, with Remploy's senior management expressing a wish to develop 'closer and closer relations'

[169] TNA LAB 20/1462, NACED, 'Sheltered Employment Annual Report' (1975).

[170] Ibid.

[171] TNA BM 8/79, Remploy Limited, 'Minutes of the Three Hundred and Forty-Seventh Meeting of the Board of Directors' (16.12.1976); 'Minutes of the Three Hundred and Twenty-Eighth Meeting of the Board of Directors' (20.03.1975); TNA BM 10/48, DE, 'Finding Employment for Handicapped Young People' (1979).

[172] Digby, *British Welfare Policy*, p. 89.

[173] TNA BM 3/54, Remploy Limited, 'Remploy in the Long-Term, Appendix 3: Managing Director's Bulletin' (11.12.1975).

Table 6.3 Number of sighted disabled workers in sheltered employment, 1970–1978

Year	*Section II disabled people in Workshops*		*Section II disabled people (sighted) in Blind workshops*	*Total*	*Section II registered unemployed*[174]
	Remploy	*LA & Voluntary*			
1970	7,505	2,132	493	10,130	10,013
1971	7,518	2,193	555	10,266	11,120
1972	7,746	2,303	577	10,626	12,105
1973	7,959	2,505	660	11,124	11,164
1974	8,077	2,638	639	11,354	10,989
1975	8,308	2,495	675	11,478	11,101
1976	8,514	2,538	690	11,742	11,457
1977	7,972	2,682	728	11,382	10,901
1978	7,894	2,800	777	11,471	9,719

Source TNA BM 10/48, Remploy Limited, 'Objectives and Criteria of Success: Appendix 5 and Appendix 6' (July, 1980); TNA LAB 20/1429, DE, 'Sheltered Employment: A Draft Consultative Document: Table VIII Section II Register 1963–73' (October, 1973); Mr. Harold Walker, *Hansard* (20.03.1975), vol. 888, cc. 536-42w; TNA BM 10/34, Remploy Limited, 'Report of the Working Party on the Mix of Disabilities Employed by Remploy, Table II' (June, 1981), p. 13. For unemployed see additional footnote

with LA and charitable bodies.[175] In an effort to help 'break the ice', Remploy carried out 'Operation Information' during 1974 and 1975, inviting LA Directors of Social Services to Remploy factories and providing information about the company.[176] Some LAs responded to this, with 73 Directors and their colleagues taking up the invitation to visit in 1974, and '17 County Authorities, 6 Metropolitan County Authorities and 15 Voluntary Societies' requesting information.[177] Following the

[174] For 1970–73, TNA LAB 20/1429, DE, 'Sheltered Employment: A Draft Consultative Document: Table VIII Section II Register 1963–73' (October, 1973). For 1974, Mr. Harold Walker, *Hansard* (20.03.1975), vol. 888, cc. 536-42w. For 1975–76, TNA BM 10/48, Remploy Limited, 'Objectives and Criteria of Success: Appendix 6' (July, 1980). For 1977–78, TNA BM 10/34, Remploy Limited, 'Report of the Working Party on the Mix of Disabilities Employed by Remploy, Table II' (June, 1981), p. 13.

[175] TNA LAB 20/1478, Remploy Limited, 'Managing Director to Department of Employment' (09.04.1975).

[176] TNA BM 3/54, Remploy Limited, 'Remploy in the Long-Term, Appendix 2: Remploy in Sheltered Employment in the U.K.' (22.04.1977).

[177] Ibid.

consultative process, the Remploy Managing Director again reiterated the company's willingness to foster 'the closest cooperation between all those concerned with sheltered employment'.[178] LAs and charitable organisations also showed some willingness, liaising with the ESA to establish a discussion group with the same aim.[179]

Such efforts appear, however, to have generated little tangible result. The ESA noted the difficulty in getting the various providers of sheltered employment to take real action to cooperate and remove themselves from 'entrenched positions'.[180] The LA and voluntary bodies feared the loss of their autonomy, and many remained reticent of working with Remploy.[181] There was a 'continued existence of suspicion' among the other providers that any cooperation would see Remploy take a preferential place.[182] The result was that calls for closer cooperation continued for the remainder of the period, but with virtually nothing constructively achieved.[183] By the end of the decade, Remploy noted that the company continue to be damned as being 'too professional' by other organisations, who 'almost without exception' held it in 'low esteem'.[184] As a result, the uneven

[178] TNA LAB 20/1478, Remploy Limited, 'Managing Director to Department of Employment' (09.04.1975); TNA BM 3/54, Remploy Limited, 'Remploy in the Long-Term, Appendix 3: Managing Director's Bulletin' (11.12.1975).

[179] TNA BM 3/54, Remploy Limited, 'Co-operation in Sheltered Employment: Notes of a Meeting between Remploy and ESA' (26.07.1976); Remploy Limited, 'Remploy in the Long-Term, Appendix 2: Remploy in Sheltered Employment in the U.K.' (22.04.1977).

[180] TNA BM 3/54, Remploy Limited, 'Co-operation in Sheltered Employment: Notes of a Meeting between Remploy and ESA' (26.07.1976).

[181] Ibid.

[182] Ibid.

[183] TNA LAB 20/1478, DE, 'Review of Policies and Services for Disabled People' (09.06.1975), p. 7; TNA BM 3/54, Remploy Limited, 'Remploy in the Long-Term' (22.04.1977), p. 2; TNA BM 10/48, Remploy Limited, 'Company Objectives and Criteria of Financial Success' (July, 1980), p. 57; TNA BM 8/80, Remploy Limited, 'Minutes of the Three Hundred and Eightieth Meeting of the Board of Directors' (20.12.1979).

[184] TNA BM 10/48, Remploy Limited, 'Objectives and Criteria of Success' (July, 1980), pp. 56–7; TNA BM 8/80, Remploy Limited, 'Minutes of the Three Hundred and Eightieth Meeting of the Board of Directors' (20.12.1979).

distribution of sheltered employment throughout the country, and the wide variability in conditions, continued as before.[185]

Conclusions

It has been demonstrated that sheltered employment, as with other areas of welfare provision identified by scholars, operated throughout the period of the classic welfare state as a mixed economy. Remploy was not the sole meaningful provider of sheltered employment, operating instead as the 'senior' partner in a tripartite mixed economy, alongside workshops provided by voluntary organisations and LAs, both independently and in concert. The voluntary sector in sheltered employment survived the Second World War and the increase in statutory welfare which followed, to become a 'junior partner', while LAs took on an increasing role. Examination of this mixed economy reveals some of the common aspects among providers, as well as areas where Remploy operated, or attempted to operate, differently. In this way the case of sheltered employment supports the current understanding of a complex mixed economy of welfare across the period.[186]

In examining Remploy as the 'moving frontier of the state', it is clear that the understanding of how sheltered employment should be provided did not remain static, but changed over time. Upon its creation, the company was positioned as *the* sheltered employment provider which would take over much, if not all, of the field and set a new standard in efficiency and efficacy. The case of Remploy illustrates that, contrary to the view of Hampton, some aspects of disability provision did reflect the expansion of the state into areas of welfare undertaken by the initial Attlee Government.[187] This expansion of the frontier proved to be short lived, however, as over the course of subsequent governments, a truly mixed economy was established and maintained. In part this was due to ideology, with recognition of the limits of the state to solve all social problems and

[185] TNA BM 3/54, Remploy Limited, 'Remploy in the Long-Term, Appendix 2: Remploy in Sheltered Employment in the U.K.' (22.04.1977).

[186] Kendall and Knapp, *The Voluntary Sector in the United Kingdom*, pp. 51–7, 133–9; Finlayson, *Citizen, State and Social Welfare in Britain 1830–1990*; Younghusband, *Social Work in Britain;* Taylor, 'Voluntary Action and the State', p. 215; Prochaska, *The Voluntary Impulse*; Thane, *Foundations of the Welfare State*, p. 277.

[187] Hampton, *Disability and the Welfare State in Britain*, p. 57.

the merits of voluntarism, sincerely believed in by Conservative governments, also becoming accepted by Labour when in power. As a result, the continuation of a mixed economy became somewhat common ground for both major parties in government, and this is evident in the case of sheltered employment as in welfare more generally. It is also apparent that the economic benefits to the Treasury of moving some of the burden to LAs and charitable organisations was a further important factor when weighed against the costs of supporting Remploy.

Despite this support for the mixed economy, there were clearly a number of problems in its application which by the 1970s could no longer be ignored. This was coupled with a political climate open to further provision for disabled people and a reorganisation of local and central government. The result was that the unification of sheltered employment under a single authority was raised as a serious idea with real support. This failed however, in large part due to mistrust and disagreement about how it should be achieved. No providers wished to relinquish control of sheltered employment to the other, and thus unification ultimately failed and the tripartite mixed economy endured.

In his article published in 1958, Edwards, an MOL official, suggested that Remploy operated seamlessly alongside the other providers to deliver a cohesive and comprehensive scheme of sheltered employment for the severely disabled.[188] Despite employing an increasing number of severely disabled people during the period, Chapter 4 has already indicated that neither Remploy itself, nor the mixed economy of sheltered employment as a whole, succeeded in providing 'full employment' for all those eligible. The deep divisions among the providers of sheltered employment highlight that the mixed economy did not combine to deliver a cohesive sheltered employment service. Wide variations existed across providers with workshops differing in terms of size, scope and working conditions. With no meaningful cooperation, it is apparent that a disabled person's experience of sheltered employment would similarly vary widely. This study has already shown that Remploy was not a cohesive catch-all scheme, and here it is evident that this was also the case for the overall field of sheltered employment, which was characterised instead by competition, and variations in coverage and conditions.

[188] TNA LAB 13/1029, Edwards, 'Remploy: An Experiment in Sheltered Employment for the Severely Disabled in Great Britain' (February, 1958), p. 14.

CHAPTER 7

Conclusions

Through detailed examination of Remploy, this book has sought to clarify fundamental aspects of how the company functioned, and use this as a new lens through which to explore corresponding aspects of the British welfare state, shedding further light on the history of disability in the postwar period.

Importantly, Remploy was clearly not created simply as a means of segregating unproductive workers in order to placate industry and thereby ease the acceptance of the other measures of the DPEA.[1] A scheme of state-run sheltered employment was a point of campaign for a number of groups representing disabled people in the interwar period, and the records examined here attest to a seemingly genuine belief in those most involved in its creation, that a national sheltered employment scheme was in the best interest of, and desired by, the disabled people it was designed to serve. In the context of this period, it is therefore a mistake to see

[1] H. Bolderson, *Social Security, Disability and Rehabilitation: Conflicts in the Development of Social Policy 1914–1946* (London, Jessica Kingsley Publishers, 1991), pp. 109–110; A. Borsay, *Disability and Social Policy in Britain Since 1750: A History of Exclusion* (Basingstoke, Palgrave Macmillan, 2005). See also S. Humphries and P. Gordon, *Out of Sight: The Experience of Disability 1900–1950* (Plymouth, Northcote House, 1992), p. 138; S. Wheatcroft, *Worth Saving: Disabled Children During the Second World War* (Manchester, Manchester University Press, 2013), pp. 168–70.

© The Author(s), under exclusive license to Springer Nature Switzerland AG 2025

A. Holroyde, *Sheltered Employment and Disability in the British Welfare State*, New Directions in Welfare History,
https://doi.org/10.1007/978-3-031-87876-3_7

Remploy as part of a narrative of deliberate discrimination. At a time when the realistic alternative, based upon the lessons learned in the aftermath of the First World War, appeared to be large-scale unemployment for these severely disabled people, sheltered employment was considered a valid and beneficial service to provide, which fulfilled a real need.

Furthermore, it is clear that Remploy was not a spontaneous reaction to the Second World War. Instead, longer term developments, alongside the war itself, were among the factors which played a part in its creation, with the key contribution coming from the individual drive of Bevin to see the scheme first into the DPEA, and then into implementation. In terms of the wider debate over the factors which led to the creation of the welfare state, the case of Remploy has thus been shown not to sit at the extreme end of the scale in supporting Titmuss' view of the primacy of the Second World War, but rather to support the acceptance of a range of influencing factors, including, but not limited to, the war, as important in establishing the postwar settlement.[2] Beyond clarifying the origins of Remploy, this conclusion also highlights the importance of looking beyond the timeframes of wars, and the two World Wars of the twentieth century in particular, in considering developments in disability policy.

It is also evident that Remploy was not created with a predetermined purpose fully established, beyond a general conception of providing a national scheme of sheltered employment. With nothing comparable in existence, it was not until the Remploy Board of Directors held their first meeting in 1945 that the many issues in attempting to establish such a scheme were really considered. The first issue of *Remploy News* explained that the company 'was something entirely new to the industrial world and we had, therefore, to learn by experience. There were no precedents to follow; no textbooks to guide us. It was a completely new field of endeavour that had to be probed and explored before the right answers could be found'.[3] Such a comment was certainly justified, as it was in postwar Britain, through Remploy, that the realities of operating a national sheltered employment scheme were first confronted.

[2] K. Laybourn, *The Evolution of British Social Policy and the Welfare State, c.1800–1993* (Keele, Keele University Press, 1995), pp. 217–8; T.H. Marshall, *Social Policy in the Twentieth-Century* (London, Hutchinson, 1975), pp. 84, 99; R. Lowe, *The Welfare State in Britain Since 1945* (Basingstoke, Palgrave Macmillan, 2005) pp. 16–7; D. Gladstone, *The Twentieth-Century Welfare State* (Basingstoke, Palgrave Macmillan, 1999), p. 51.

[3] *Remploy News*, 1 (December, 1952).

Given this, the early conflicts examined in Chapter 3 are perhaps unsurprising. The key element revealed here has been the development in the understanding of what sheltered employment should mean, based upon a notion of 'genuine employment' which was first articulated by the Remploy Board itself, and then adopted by ministers and officials as the guiding principle to determine policy. Though this was initially resisted by the early Attlee Government, and sometimes later contested by politicians, this became the approach taken by successive governments for the remainder of the period. This conception of sheltered employment envisioned the factories not as places to simply keep disabled people occupied, segregated, or rehabilitated, but rather as places that tolerated reduced productivity—as long as this was within acceptable limits—and did consider the welfare of disabled employees, but which also sought to emulate commercial, productive and 'genuine' working environments as far as was possible. Such places were therefore only partially 'sheltered' from the realities of competitive, commercial mainstream employment, and this was understood to be necessary in order for the disabled employees to receive the perceived benefits of this kind of provision. While this was considered the ideal for all sheltered employment, it was particularly stressed for Remploy. The benefits of employment, encompassing a range of aspects for both the individual and wider society such as health, wellbeing and economic security, have continued to be evoked by policy-makers, and debated by academics, across various contexts and populations into the modern day. In this case, with 'genuine employment' becoming the key element, either out of genuine belief in that being the virtue of sheltered employment, or as a means of justifying the focus on commercial efficiency in controlling public expenditure, it is clear that there was no sudden change from a humanitarian focus in the period examined here to economic imperatives in the 1980s.[4] In Remploy, commercial efficiency was always important as a policy, both in terms of operating within the limits set by government for expenditure, and in terms of fulfilling what was understood as its role.

Contrary to the notion that disability was not 'discovered' as a political issue until the 1960s, this was certainly not the case in terms of

[4] C. Barnes, *Disabled People in Britain and Discrimination* (London, C. Hurst & Co., 2000), p. 73; G. Millward, 'Invalid Definitions, Invalid Responses: Disability and the Welfare State, 1965–1995', unpublished PhD Thesis, London School of Hygiene and Tropical Medicine (2013), pp. 184–5.

Remploy.[5] Rather, the scope of the company was discussed, and indeed contested, at a political level from the earliest days of its operation. This occurred initially within Labour under Attlee, and then most notably during the subsequent years of Conservative government. The 1950s saw Remploy referenced frequently by Labour MPs in opposition and, in the middle of the decade, evoked as a serious attack on the Government. Sheltered employment, and more specifically Remploy itself, therefore represents an area of disability policy which was always 'visible' and politically relevant prior to the 1960s. In terms of the wider debate around the existence of a postwar consensus, therefore, Remploy represented an area of initial contest between the two major parties. However, both parties in government ultimately responded to Remploy in broadly the same way—expressing a desire to expand provision, but only within the limits of what was considered possible based upon the commercial strength of the company and the economic conditions which dictated collective public expenditure priorities. As such, something of the 'consensus in action', described by Millward and Hampton in their studies of disability, can be seen to apply to Remploy as well.[6]

This consensus extended to an acceptance of the benefits of a mixed economy. Remploy was not the only provider of sheltered employment during the postwar period, with voluntary provision surviving the Second World War, and, later joined by LAs, operating within a genuine tripartite mixed economy. The case of sheltered employment can therefore be included as a further element in our understanding of a mixed economy of welfare existing across the period, in which the new statutory provision became the 'senior partner'.[7] A moving frontier of the state within this

[5] J. Hampton, 'Discovering Disability: The General Classes of Disabled People and the Classic Welfare State, 1948–1964', *The Historian*, vol. 75, no. 1 (2013), pp. 70–1; J. Hampton, *Disability and the Welfare State in Britain: Changes in Perception and Policy 1948–79* (Bristol, Policy Press, 2016), pp. 8, 50; S. Sainsbury, 'Disabled People and the Personal Social Services', in D. Gladstone, (ed.) *British Social Welfare: Past, Present and Future* (London, UCL Press, 1995), pp. 183–8; E. Younghusband, *Social Work in Britain: 1950–1975* (London, Allen and Unwin, 1978), pp. 210–11.

[6] Millward, 'Invalid Definitions, Invalid Responses', pp. 165, 284; Hampton, *Disability and the Welfare State in Britain*, p. 244.

[7] G. Finlayson, *Citizen, State, and Social Welfare in Britain 1830–1990* (Oxford, Clarendon Press, 1994); Younghusband, *Social Work in Britain*; M. Taylor, 'Voluntary Action and the State', in D. Gladstone, (ed.) *British Social Welfare: Past, Present and Future* (London, UCL Press, 1995), p. 215; F. K. Prochaska, *The Voluntary Impulse:*

mixed economy, in the form of Remploy, is also apparent, with changes in the perception of how sheltered employment provision should be delivered and administered over time. That the tripartite approach did not equate to a coherent overall system, highlights the need to examine the interactions between providers in any mixed economy, as in the case here, it is clear that a fractious relationship developed, particularly between Remploy and other workshops, which directly impacted how sheltered employment was delivered.[8] Whatever the intentions of ministers and officials in outlining multi-layered systems to deliver public services, it is useful to have such examples as a reminder that personalities and perceptions among delivery providers can ultimate play a key role in determining the efficacy of implementation.

The aspect of Remploy which has perhaps generated the most misconception is the composition of its workforce. Most importantly, it is evident that Remploy was not a 'catch-all' scheme for severely disabled people. Throughout the period, access to Remploy was restricted, by a range of barriers and in the form of medical and bureaucratic gatekeepers, to a select number of severely disabled people. Contrary to the popular notion, this selection was not based upon ex-service status, as even the notion of a preference for this group was soon to disappear. It is apparent therefore that the privileges held by this group in welfare and employment ceased to be universal after the Second World War, and in the case of Remploy at least, Bevin succeeded in removing the origin of a person's disability as the primary determiner in the award of such provision.[9] Thus

Philanthropy in Modern Britain, (London, Faber, 1988); P. Thane, *Foundations of the Welfare State, 2nd Edition* (London, Longman, 1996), p. 277; D. Owen, *English Philanthropy: 1660–1960* (London, Belknap Press, 1964), p. 527; J. Kendall and M. Knapp, *The Voluntary Sector in the United Kingdom* (Manchester, Manchester University Press, 1996), pp. 51–7, 133–9; A. Digby, *British Welfare Policy: Workhouse to Workfare* (London, Faber and Faber, 1989), p. 89.

[8] The National Archives (TNA) LAB 13/1029, J. L. Edwards, 'Remploy: An Experiment in Sheltered Employment for the Severely Disabled in Great Britain', *International Labour Review*, vol. LXXVII, No. 2 (February, 1958), p. 14.

[9] W. J. Gagen, 'Remastering the Body, Renegotiating Gender: Physical Disability and Masculinity during the First World War, the case of J.B. Middlebrook', *European Review of History*, vol. 14, no. 4 (2007), pp. 536–7; J. Bourke, *Dismembering the Male: Men's Bodies, Britain and the Great War* (London, Reaktion Books, 1996), pp. 37–9; Hampton, *Disability and the Welfare State in Britain*, pp. 53–4; J. Anderson, "Turned into Taxpayers': Paraplegia, Rehabilitation and Sport at Stoke Mandeville, 1944–56', *Journal of Contemporary History*, vol. 38, no. 3 (2003), pp. 469–70; J. Anderson, *War, Disability*

the 'general classes' identified by Hampton as remaining under-served by the welfare state, were on an equal footing in accessing sheltered employment as those disabled by war or industrial accident.[10] It has also been demonstrated that bar certain specific exceptions, selection was not based upon a person's disability itself.[11] The case of gender in selection is not as clear-cut, however this appears again to not have been the primary deciding factor. While alternative sheltered employment providers did in many cases still focus on these 'groups', this book has demonstrated that as a corollary of the importance of commercial efficiency, the chief focus on selection for Remploy was on individual productivity. It was this measure as 'potential' which guided recruitment, and this measure in 'practice' which governed retention.

The common feature of the Remploy workforce was therefore an ability to meet and maintain the productivity requirements of their local factory. In terms of the current understanding of the exclusion of disabled people from the benefits of the 'golden age' of welfare and employment in the period, this study has offered a more nuanced picture in examining a previously unexplored group in those 'severely disabled people' eligible for sheltered employment.[12] On one level, it is has been illustrated that the achievement of 'full employment' was not extended to the Section II population.[13] Neither Remploy, nor the field of sheltered employment as a whole, was ever able to provide for all those made eligible for such provision under the DPEA. The possibility of meeting this need was only briefly expressed and was swiftly abandoned. In part this was due to practical issues concerning reach, and the emerging reality of the costs involved, but this was also due to the adoption of 'genuine employment' as the guiding policy which condoned an additional benchmark

and Rehabilitation in Britain: 'Soul of a Nation' (Manchester, Manchester University Press, 2011), p. 211.

[10] Hampton, *Disability and the Welfare State in Britain.*

[11] Anderson, *War, Disability and Rehabilitation in Britain,* p. 183.

[12] Borsay, *Disability and Social Policy in Britain Since 1750*, p. 168; Hampton, *Disability and the Welfare State in Britain.*

[13] Lowe, *The Welfare State in Britain Since 1945*, pp. 80–1, 115–9; R. Page, *Revisiting the Welfare State* (Maidenhead, Open University Press, 2007), p. 38; D. Fraser, *The Evolution of the British Welfare State*, 4th Edition (Basingstoke, Palgrave Macmillan, 2009), pp. 267–8; H. Glennerster, *British Social Policy: 1945 to the Present*, 3rd Edition (Oxford, Blackwell Publishing, 2007), p. 5; Laybourn, *The Evolution of British Social Policy and the Welfare State*, p. 241.

of productivity for disabled workers. It was therefore quickly established that in practice there were not two employment categories of disabled people as defined by the DPEA, but rather three. Thus, despite being eligible under the legislation in place, a significant number of Section II disabled people were considered not productive enough to warrant a place in sheltered employment. In this way, it is possible to say that sheltered employment can be added to the other measures of the DPEA in terms of them failing to live up to their initial promise, with a significant number excluded from this provision.[14] At the same time, it is important to recognise that this was in large part due to this change in conception of how sheltered employment should function which occurred in this period. It must also be considered that while it is understandable to focus on where provision failed to match original intention, Remploy did succeed in providing sheltered employment, including a wide range of social and welfare activities, for many thousands of disabled people under both the financial constraints of government's welfare expenditure and the challenges of the manufacturing industry. Furthermore, it cannot be ignored that for some employees the emphasis on productivity may have proven to be beneficial as a stepping-stone to mainstream employment and career advancement. This did, however, undoubtedly leave a large proportion of severely disabled people 'left behind' as they proved unable to meet the productivity requirements.

In considering these issues of recruitment and retention, it is apparent that the case of Remploy further demonstrates a continued paternalism evident in the measures of the welfare state. Severely disabled recruits were, at every stage of the recruitment process and once employed, continuously subject to assessment as to their capabilities and suitability for a place in a factory. This assessment was carried out by medical professionals, civil servants and Remploy officials. It was these parties who were the determiners of a person's capability for work, and importantly in the case of Remploy, whether they were meeting it during their employment. While there was some evidence of individual MPs advocating on behalf of employees, and some initial examples of the involvement of organisations representing disabled people in the consultative process in the

[14] Borsay, *Disability and Social Policy in Britain Since 1750*, pp. 135–9, 168; Hampton, *Disability and the Welfare State in Britain;* H. Bolderson, 'The Origins of the Disabled Persons Employment Quota and its Symbolic Significance', *Journal of Social Policy*, vol. 9, no. 2 (1980), pp. 171, 184.

1970s, the case of Remploy suggests that the challenges to the paternalistic state identified by Glennerster as appearing in the 1960s were slow to extend to the severely disabled.[15] This approach continued unabated throughout the period of the classic welfare state, and the broader aspects of medical and functional assessment to determine eligibility for statutory provision in benefits and services has endured into the present day. Given the promised plans for reform in these areas at the time of writing, it is useful to understand that this approach to determine disabled people's access to support has a long history.

In exploring the case of severely disabled women, this book has responded to the call for historians to consider the different experiences of women in employment.[16] It has been shown that sheltered employment was part of the welfare state's provision that was indeed, as Sainsbury and others have suggested, allocated primarily to men, thereby offering support to the notion that disabled women suffered something of a 'double disability'.[17] Similarly, it is apparent that the prevailing view of women's employment in general having involved segregation, lower pay, inferior status and limited advancement, was also reflected in sheltered employment through Remploy.[18] However, it is also the

[15] Glennerster, *British Social Policy*, p. 99.

[16] S. Bruley, *Women in Britain Since 1900* (Basingstoke, Palgrave, 1999), p. 93.

[17] M. Oliver, *The Politics of Disablement* (Basingstoke, Macmillan, 1990), p. 70; Anderson, *War, Disability and Rehabilitation in Britain*, p. 168; J. Anderson, 'British Women, Disability and the Second World War', *Contemporary British History*, vol. 20, no. 1 (2006); Hampton, *Disability and the Welfare State in Britain*, p. 119; G. Millward, 'Social Security Policy and the Early Disability Movement—Expertise, Disability, and the Government, 1965–77', *Twentieth Century British History*, vol. 26, no. 2 (2015), pp. 281–2; Thane, *Foundations of the Welfare State*, pp. 224–5; Sainsbury, 'Disabled People and the Personal Social Services', p. 188.

[18] Lowe, *The Welfare State in Britain Since 1945*, pp. 42–3; K. Laybourn, *Unemployment and Employment Policies Concerning Women in Britain, 1900–1951* (Lampeter, Edwin Mellen Press, 2002), p. 187; Bruley, *Women in Britain Since 1900*, pp. 99–119; P. Summerfield, *Women Workers in the Second World War: Production and Patriarchy in Conflict* (London, Routledge, 1984); M. Glucksmann, *Women Assemble: Women Workers and the New Industries in Inter-War Britain* (London, Routledge, 1990), p. 281; Gladstone, *The Twentieth-Century Welfare State*, pp. 119–22; G. Holloway, *Women and Work in Britain Since 1840* (London, Routledge, 2005), p. 186; P. Thane, 'Towards Equal Opportunities? Women in Britain since 1945', in T. Gourvish and A. O'Day (eds.), *Britain Since 1945* (Basingstoke, Macmillan, 1991), pp. 183–208; J. Lewis, *Women in Britain Since 1945: Women, Family, Work and the State in the Post-War Years* (Oxford, Blackwell, 1992), pp. 78–91; J. Lewis, *Women in England 1870–1950: Sexual Divisions*

case that 'gender' was mitigated to a degree by 'disability', as segregation in Remploy was neither absolute nor typical for many factories, and while wages for women were less than those for men, they were occasionally adapted in ways which proved comparatively beneficial for female employees. Collectively, this highlights the importance of considering intersectionality, as it is apparent that severely disabled women had a specific experience of employment within Remploy.

Remploy itself was clearly not a coherent monolithic scheme, and any notion of a 'single Remploy experience' is a mirage. Central policy did not reflect a uniform reality in the factory, with wide variation in working environments, conditions and personnel. One employee might find themselves working in a pristine and custom-built factory within easy-commuting distance from home, working on a long-term production order which proved stimulating and rewarding, under a factory manager keen to promote the welfare of his workforce, while enjoying the benefits of socialising with colleagues with the potential of meeting a future husband or wife. Another person might equally find themselves struggling to travel to a dilapidated converted building, mixing periods of uninteresting and monotonous busy work with long stretches of idleness, under a manager desperate to improve their commercial performance and in a factory with few social activities. Though Remploy did become more standardised as the period progressed, differences across factories clearly remained the norm. When this is considered alongside the further variations outlined in Chapter 6 among the other providers of sheltered employment, it is apparent that, for the severely disabled, sheltered employment was something of a lottery based upon location. A criticism of sheltered employment at the start of the twentieth century was that it was 'decentralised and inconsistent', with opportunities varying widely depending on location.[19] By the end of the period considered here, despite the creation of Remploy and attempts to improve coordination of the various providers, this was still largely the case.

Finally, this book has demonstrated that any image of the period of the classic welfare state as a 'golden age' for sheltered employment is

and Social Change (Brighton, Wheatsheaf Books Ltd, 1984); H. Bradley, *Men's Work, Women's Work* (Cambridge, Polity Press, 1989), p. 116.

19 M. Kowalsky, "This Honourable Obligation": The King's National Roll Scheme for Disabled Ex-servicemen, 1915–1944', *European Review of History*, vol. 14, no. 4 (2007), pp. 576–7.

an illusion. The conclusions here build upon those of John Carrier and Ian Kendall, who examined the NHS in the period, and similarly challenged the notion of any 'golden age' prior to Thatcherism.[20] There was no clear demarcation in policy towards Remploy and sheltered employment following the election of the Thatcher Government in 1979. As had been the case prior to this point, under the premise of providing 'genuine employment', sheltered employment continued to have the support of government, and with commercial efficiency reflecting continuity rather than revolution, Remploy continued much as before with employee numbers steadily increasing to reach 9,000 by the end of the 1980s.[21] It was at this same time that fundamental change occurred, and the first signs of the end of sheltered employment began to appear, with the launch of the 'Interwork' scheme in 1988, whereby the transition of employees from sheltered employment into the mainstream labour market turned from being an approved side effect, to a central aim.[22] Though the continually escalating cost of Remploy, against the backdrop of a declining manufacturing sector, was clearly a factor, this adjustment was also part of a wider agenda in Britain focused on 'inclusion' which increasingly viewed sheltered employment as inherently discriminatory and archaic. While governments across the postwar period had applied pressure to reduce the costs of Remploy, none had questioned the fundamental desirability of providing sheltered employment. It was this questioning of its inherent nature which was to ultimately mark the beginning of the end for Remploy as a sheltered employment provider, as it adapted over the following two decades to become an employment services provider supporting disabled people and those with barriers to work into mainstream employment.

[20] J. Carrier and I. Kendall, *Health and the National Health Service* (London, Athlone Press, 1998), pp. 192–8.

[21] See Board of Director Meeting Minutes in TNA BM 8/80.

[22] Mr Lee, *Hansard* (29.06.1989), vol. 155, cc. 559w; TNA BM 3/67, Remploy Limited, 'Report on Employment of Disabled People in Remploy-1979: Analysis of length of service of severely disabled persons employed in all Remploy factories' (1979); TNA BM 3/54, Remploy Limited, 'Sheltered Employment for Disabled People, A Consultative Document: The Remploy View' (February, 1974), p. 20.

Bibliography

TNA—The National Archives, Kew, London

Welsh Office

BD 40, Economic Planning Division (1951–1998).

Remploy Limited

BM 3/7, Correspondence with Ministry of Labour (1948–59).
BM 3/32, Premises correspondence (1964–72).
BM 3/47, Employment Policy (1975–76).
BM 3/54, Remploy in the long term: report and correspondence (1977).
BM 3/55, Meetings between Remploy and Manpower Services Commission: minutes (1976–78).
BM 3/67, Report on employment of disabled people in Remploy (1980).
BM 3/70, Report of the Working Party on the Mix of Disabilities Employed by Remploy (1981).
BM 3/71, Hailey Working Party on Objectives and Criteria of Success: working papers (1979).
BM 3/72, Hailey Working Party on Objectives and Criteria of Success: working papers (1979–80).

© The Editor(s) (if applicable) and The Author(s), under exclusive license to Springer Nature Switzerland AG 2025

A. Holroyde, *Sheltered Employment and Disability in the British Welfare State*, New Directions in Welfare History,
https://doi.org/10.1007/978-3-031-87876-3

BM 3/74, Hailey Working Party on Objectives and Criteria of Success: final report (1979).
BM 4/1, Memorandum and Articles of Association of Remploy (1945).
BM 5/1, Personnel Department Circulars (1967–75).
BM 5/9, Circulars and Standing Instructions: Factory Manager's Guide (1949).
BM 6/2, Remploy News 30–33 (1956).
BM 6/3, Remploy News 34–36 (1957).
BM 6/4, Remploy News 37–40 (1958).
BM 6/5, Remploy News 41–44 (1959).
BM 6/6, Remploy News 45–48 (1960).
BM 6/7, Remploy News 49–52 (1961).
BM 6/8, Remploy News 53–56 (1962).
BM 6/9, Remploy News 57–60 (1963).
BM 6/10, Remploy News 61–64 (1964).
BM 6/11, Remploy News 65–68 (1965).
BM 6/12, Remploy News 69–71 (1966).
BM 6/13, Remploy News 72–75 (1967).
BM 6/14, Remploy News 76–79 (1968).
BM 6/15, Remploy News 80–83 (1969).
BM 6/16, Remploy News 84–85 (1970).
BM 6/17, Remploy News 86–87 (1971).
BM 6/18, Remploy News 88–91 (1972).
BM 6/19, Remploy News 92–94 (1973).
BM 6/20, Remploy News 95–100 (1974).
BM 8/1, Minutes of Board Meetings (1945–50)/General Meetings (1945–49).
BM 8/2, Minutes of Board Meetings (1950–61)/General Meetings (1950–60).
BM 8/3, Minutes of Board Meetings (1961–68)/General Meetings (1961–67).
BM 8/4, Board Papers: miscellaneous (1952–53).
BM 8/5, Board Papers: miscellaneous (1955–55).
BM 8/6, Board Papers: miscellaneous (1954–55).
BM 8/7, Board Papers: miscellaneous (1955–57).
BM 8/8, Board Papers: miscellaneous (1957–58).
BM 8/9, Board Papers: miscellaneous (1958–59).
BM 8/10, Board Papers: miscellaneous (1959–60).
BM 8/11, Board Papers: miscellaneous (1960–62).

BM 8/12, Board Papers: miscellaneous (1962–64).
BM 8/13, Executive Director reports 67–77 (1951–52).
BM 8/14, Executive Director reports 85–92 (1953–54).
BM 8/15, Executive Director reports 93–101 (1954).
BM 8/16, Executive Director reports 102–108 (1955).
BM 8/17, Executive Director reports 109–115 (1955–56).
BM 8/18, Executive Director reports 116–120 (1956).
BM 8/19, Executive Director reports 121–122 (1956).
BM 8/20, Managing Director reports 1–11 (1952–53).
BM 8/21, Managing Director reports 12–18 (1953–54).
BM 8/22, Managing Director reports 19–27 (1954).
BM 8/23, Managing Director reports 28–34 (1954–55).
BM 8/32, Managing Director reports 84–89 (1960).
BM 8/43, Managing Director reports 178–187 (1968–69).
BM 8/49, Minutes of Board Meetings / General Meetings (1968–74).
BM 8/50, Miscellaneous Board Papers and Correspondence (1968–74).
BM 8/51, Managing Director reports 188–198 (1969–70).
BM 8/53, Managing Director reports 211–221 (1971–72).
BM 8/79, Minutes of Board Meetings (1975–78).
BM 8/80, Minutes of Board Meetings (1978–82).
BM 8/81, Managing Director Reports 248–254 (1975).
BM 8/82, Managing Director Reports 255–261 (1975–76).
BM 8/83, Managing Director Reports 262–269 (1976).
BM 8/84, Board Papers and Miscellaneous Correspondence (1975–77).
BM 8/85, Board Papers and Miscellaneous Correspondence (1978–79).
BM 10/1, Review of first 7 years of Remploy by Executive Director (1953).
BM 10/2, Outline of birth and early Remploy by R.E. Benjamin (1979).
BM 10/7, Model factory Plans (1946–48).
BM 10/12, Survey of Remploy undertaken by Organisation and Methods Division of the Treasury: Report with Directors' Comments (1955).
BM 10/19, Fact-finding survey of typical Remploy factories prepared by Messrs. Parry and Critchley of Ministry of Labour, with Working Directors' observations (1955).
BM 10/26, Standard Factory Plan (1975).
BM 10/34, Report of the Working Party on the Mix of Disabilities Employed by Remploy (1981).
BM 10/48, Remploy: Company Objectives and Criteria of Financial Success (Hailey Report) (1979–80).

BM10/53, Remploy Facts (1986).

War Cabinet and Cabinet

CAB 24/73/30, The Labour Situation. Report from the Ministry of Labour (1919).

CAB 24/80/62, The Labour Situation. Report from the Ministry of Labour (1919).

CAB 24/84/92, The Labour Situation. Report from the Ministry of Labour (1919).

CAB 24/87/60, The Labour Situation. Report from the Ministry of Labour (1919).

CAB 24/88/84, The Labour Situation. Report from the Ministry of Labour (1919).

CAB 24/106/55, The Labour Situation. Report from the Ministry of Labour (1920).

CAB 24/121/7, Ministry of Labour Weekly Report (1921).

CAB 24/123/79, The Employment of Severely Disabled Men (1921).

CAB 24/125/13, The Employment of Severely Disabled Ex-Servicemen (1921).

CAB 27/49, Miscellaneous Committees: Demobilisation (1919).

CAB 67/9/160, Rehabilitation, Training and Employment of Disabled Persons (1941).

CAB 71/5, Lord President's Committees: Minutes and Papers: Papers 159–226 (1941).

Manpower Services Commission

ET 2/32, Publicity and Information: The Disabled Persons Register: an employment service for disabled people (1977).

MOL and Successors

LAB 13/1029, International Labour Division and Overseas Department: Article on Remploy for the International Labour Review (1957–59).

LAB 14/429, Factory and Welfare Advisory Board minutes 35–37 (1943).

LAB 20/2, Report of Glen Committee (1940–41).

LAB 20/3, Formation of Glen Committee (1940).

LAB 20/35, Remploy Executive Director's Report (1949).
LAB 20/43, Remploy: Executive Director's Reports (1951).
LAB 20/48, Rehabilitation Board of War Casualties: memorandum (1940).
LAB 20/56, Inter-departmental committee on rehab and resettlement (1942).
LAB 20/78, Lord Roberts Workshops (1943–51).
LAB 20/84, Ince Committee papers (1934–45).
LAB 20/85, Ince Committee papers (1934–48).
LAB 20/87, Ince Committee agenda and minutes (1943–45).
LAB 20/91, Tomlinson Report, Amendments to quota scheme (1943–44).
LAB 20/108, Sheltered employment scheme (1944–45).
LAB 20/109, Registration of disabled persons: policy and procedure with regard to conditions and disqualifications (1944–45).
LAB 20/113, Remploy appointment of chairman and directors (1944–45).
LAB 20/120, Remploy appointment of chairman and directors (1944–48).
LAB 20/127, Guide for use in the placing of disabled persons and survey of Disabled Persons Resettlement Officer's placing work (1944–57).
LAB 20/173, Sheltered employment scheme committee of National Advisory Council on the employment of the disabled (1945–46).
LAB 20/187, Remploy Executive Director reports (1945–46).
LAB 20/189, Revised programme of basic training for Disablement Resettlement Officers (1945–47).
LAB 20/200, Remploy, remuneration of workers (1945–52).
LAB 20/201, Remploy, procedure for submitting disabled persons for work (1945–53).
LAB 20/215, Section 15: instruction to Regional Offices on eligibility; Ministry of Labour circular 139/198 (1945–58).
LAB 20/241, Guide for the use of local offices in the placing of disabled persons, additions, amendments etc ED738 (1946–51).
LAB 20/253, Remploy, minutes of Regional Executive Officer's conference (1945–48).
LAB 20/328, Disablement resettlement officer handbook (1946–47).
LAB 20/350, Statistical form, numbers of unemployed registered disabled persons, position of non-registered disabled persons (1946–57).
LAB 20/381, Analysis of unemployed disabled (1947–49).

LAB 20/399, Reports by executive director (1946–47).
LAB 20/416, Proposed extension of the Roll to cover disabled men of WW2: meetings and solicitor's opinion (1938–60).
LAB 20/444, Report by executive director (1948).
LAB20/453, Suggestion for slowing down Remploy programme by the chairman, Minister's agreement (1949).
LAB 20/584, Solicitor's ruling on section 15 of 1944 Act relating to sheltered employment (1945–47).
LAB 20/591, National Advisory Council, trend of unemployment among registered disabled men and women (1951–52).
LAB 20/653, Criticism of Remploy in report of Select committee on estimates, reply of Ministry of Labour (1952).
LAB 20/707, Remploy, factory programme (1946–66).
LAB 20/929, Remploy: Ministerial decisions and policy questions (1954–62).
LAB 20/1035, Numbers of severely disabled persons in Remploy factories (1961–62).
LAB 20/1038, Employment in sheltered workshops: Leaflet (DP/L11) (1959–62).
LAB 20/1052, Analysis of the severely disabled unemployed (1960–61).
LAB 20/1054, Remuneration of severely disabled workers in factories (1961).
LAB 20/1071, Enquiry into the cause of the persistent increase in the numbers of Section II unemployed (1962–65).
LAB 20/1073, Sheltered employment for severely disabled persons in approved undertakings: papers prepared for the Sheltered Employment Committee (1962–65).
LAB 20/1100, National Advisory Council for the Employment of the Disabled (NACED): Minutes of meetings (1945–1947).
LAB 20/1140, Training of disablement resettlement officers: policy (1963–66).
LAB 20/1144, Swindon Borough Council sheltered workshop: enterprise works (1963–67).
LAB 20/1173, Wages of disabled workers (1963–68)
LAB 20/1429, Sheltered Employment, A Draft Consultative Document issued by the Department of Employment (1973).
LAB 20/1462, Annual reports to the NAC on Employment of disabled in sheltered workshops and Remploy factories (1975).

LAB 20/1478, Review of policies and services for the disabled; sheltered employment; general policy (1974–75).
LAB 43/204, Private Office Paper: Selected Case Files: Mrs E H Braddock MP: query on output increase of disabled persons at Remploy factory (1954).
LAB 43/268, Private Office Paper: Selected Case Files: Remploy and the employment of handicapped persons: meetings with a group of Labour MPs (1956).

Ministry of Pensions

PIN 15/33, Disabled men unemployable on account of their disability: proposed examination by Commissioners of Medical Services (1920–39).
PIN 15/34, Inter-Departmental Committee on Unemployables (1920).
PIN 15/35, Inter-Departmental Committee on Unemployables (1920).
PIN 15/36, Inter-Departmental Committee on Unemployables (1920).
PIN 15/37, Inter-Departmental Committee on Unemployables (1920–21).
PIN 15/38, Disabled men unemployable on account of their disability: correspondence and resolutions from outside organisations (1921–37).

Treasury

T222/1085, Organisation and Methods Division: Remploy review (1953–56).
T224/1891, Agriculture, Transport and Trade Division: Financial assistance to Remploy (1964–69).
T227/1106, Social Services Division Files: Remploy (1959–60).

Newspapers and Periodicals

Daily Dispatch.

Daily Herald.

Daily Mail.

Daily Telegraph.

Exeter and Plymouth Gazette.

Financial Times.

International Labour Review.

News Chronicle.

Sunday Dispatch.

The Dundee Advertiser.

The Guardian.

The Lancet.

The Manchester Guardian.

The Nottingham Journal.

The Telegraph.

The Times.

Westminster Gazette.

House of Commons Papers and Government Documents

Report of the Committee appointed by the President of the Local Government Board upon the Provision and Employment of Sailors and Soldiers Disabled in the War, 7915 (1915).

Report from the Select Committee on Pensions, 185 (1920).

Ministry of Labour, Committee on Re-Employment of Ex-Servicemen, Interim Report, 951 (1920).

Social Insurance and Allied Services, 6404 (1942).

Report of Inter-departmental Committee on the Rehabilitation and Resettlement of Disabled Persons, 6415 (1943).

Fourth Report from the Select Committee on Estimates, 162 (1952).

Report of the Committee of Inquiry on The Rehabilitation Training and Resettlement of Disabled Persons, 9883 (1956).

The Future of Voluntary Organisations: Report of the Wolfenden Committee (London, Croom Helm, 1978).

Department of Employment, The Net Exchequer Costs of Sheltered Employment, (Research Paper No. 69, 1989).

The Government Statistical Service, Unemployment statistics from 1881 to the present day (1996).

Legislation

Blind Persons Act 1920.

Disabled Persons (Employment) Act 1944.

Education Act 1944.

National Insurance Act 1946.

National Assistance Act 1948.

Disabled Persons (Employment) Act (Amendment) 1958.

Mental Health Act 1959.

Social Work (Scotland) Act 1968.

Chronically Sick and Disabled Persons Act 1970.

Equal Pay Act 1970.

Local Authority Social Services Act 1970.

Local Government Act 1972.

Remploy Material

Remploy News 1–29 (1952–1955); 101–131 (1975–1979).
Remploy News: We Have a Part to Play (1988).
Remploy News: Golden Jubilee Special (1995).

Websites

Historic Hansard / Hansard, Contains Parliamentary information licensed under the Open Parliament Licence v3.0. Open Parliament Licence–UK Parliament

Office for National Statistics.
Oxford Dictionary of National Biography.
UK Parliamentary Papers.

Secondary Sources

Addison, P., *The Road to 1945: British Politics and the Second World War*, (London, Cape, 1975).
Addison, P., *The Road to 1945: British Politics and the Second World War* (London, Pimlico, 1994).
Addison, P., *No Turning Back: The Peacetime Revolutions of Post-War Britain* (Oxford, Oxford University Press, 2010).
Addison, P., and Jones, H., (eds.) *A Companion to Contemporary Britain, 1939–2000* (Oxford, Blackwell, 2005).
Alborn, T., 'Senses of Belonging: The Politics of Working-class Insurance in Britain, 1880–1914', *Journal of Modern History*, vol. 73, no.3 (2001), pp. 561–602.
Anderson, J., "Turned into Taxpayers': Paraplegia, Rehabilitation and Sport at Stoke Mandeville, 1944–56', *Journal of Contemporary History*, vol. 38, No. 3 (2003), pp. 461–475.
Anderson, J., 'British Women, Disability and the Second World War', *Contemporary British History*, vol. 20, no. 1 (2006), pp. 37–53.
Anderson, J., 'Review Article: Voices in the Dark: Representations of Disability in Historical Research', *Journal of Contemporary History*, vol. 44, no. 1 (2009), pp. 107–116.
Anderson, J., *War, Disability and Rehabilitation in Britain: 'Soul of a Nation'* (Manchester, Manchester University Press, 2011).
Anderson, J., "Jumpy Stump': Amputation and Trauma in the First World War', *First World War Studies*, vol. 6, no. 1, (2015), pp. 9–19.

© The Editor(s) (if applicable) and The Author(s), under exclusive license to Springer Nature Switzerland AG 2025

A. Holroyde, *Sheltered Employment and Disability in the British Welfare State*, New Directions in Welfare History,
https://doi.org/10.1007/978-3-031-87876-3

Anderson, J., and Carden-Coyne, A., 'Enabling the Past: New Perspectives in the History of Disability', *European Review of History*, vol. 14, no. 4 (2007), pp. 447–457.

Anderson, J., and Pemberton, N., 'Walking Alone: Aiding the War and Civilian Blind in the Inter-war Period', *European Review of History*, vol. 14, no. 4 (2007), pp. 459–79.

Ashford, D.E., 'The Whig Interpretation of the Welfare State', *Journal of Policy History*, vol. 1, no. 1 (1989), pp. 24–43.

Barnes, C., *Disabled People in Britain and Discrimination* (London, C.Hurst & Co., 2000).

Barnes, C., Oliver, M., and Barton, L., (eds.) *Disability Studies Today* (Cambridge, Polity Press, 2002).

Barnett, C., *The Audit of War: The Illusion and Reality of Britain as a Great Nation* (London, Macmillan, 1986).

BBC News 'What are Remploy workers doing now?', (31.11.2014). http://www.bbc.co.uk/news/uk-29843567 . Accessed 16 August 2024.

Béland, D., et al., 'Introduction', in Béland, D., et al., (eds.) *The Oxford Handbook of the Welfare State: Second Edition* (Oxford, Oxford University Press, 2021), pp. 1–19.

Bell, D., *The End of Ideology: On the Exhaustion of Political Ideas in the Fifties*, (London, Collier-Macmillan, 1962).

Bellamy, J.M., and Saville, J., (eds.), *Dictionary of Labour Biography, Vol. 9* (Palgrave Macmillan: Basingstoke, 1993).

Bernstein, F.L., 'Rehabilitation Staged: How Soviet Doctors "Cured" Disability in the Second World War', in Burch, S., and Rembis, M., (eds.) *Disability History* (Urbana, University of Illinois Press, 2014), pp. 218–236.

Bickenbach, J., *Physical Disability and Social Policy* (Toronto, University of Toronto Press, 1993).

Bohata, K., et al., *Disability in Industrial Britain: A Cultural and Literary History of Impairment in the Coal Industry, 1880–1948* (Manchester, Manchester University Press, 2020).

Bolderson, H., 'The Origins of the Disabled Persons Employment Quota and its Symbolic Significance', *Journal of Social Policy*, vol. 9, no. 2 (1980), pp. 169–186.

Bolderson, H., *Social Security, Disability and Rehabilitation: Conflicts in the Development of Social Policy 1914–1946* (London, Jessica Kingsley Publishers, 1991).

Borsay, A., *Disability and Social Policy in Britain Since 1750: A History of Exclusion* (Basingstoke, Palgrave Macmillan, 2005).

Borsay, A., 'Disability in British Poetry of the First World War', *Disability & Society*, vol. 30, no. 4 (2015), pp. 499–512.

Bourke, J., *Dismembering the Male: Men's Bodies, Britain and the Great War* (London, Reaktion Books, 1996).
Bradley, H., *Men's Work, Women's Work* (Cambridge, Polity Press, 1989).
Braybon, G., and Summerfield, P., *Out of the Cage: Women's Experiences in Two World Wars* (London, Routledge, 2013).
Brenton, M., *The Voluntary Sector in British Social Services* (Harlow, Prentice Hall Press, 1985).
Bridgen, P., and Lowe, R., *Welfare Policy Under the Conservatives 1951–1964* (London, PRO, 1998).
Briggs, A., 'The Welfare State in Historical Perspective', *European Journal of Sociology*, vol. 2, no. 2, (1961), pp. 221–258.
Brown, J., *The British Welfare State: A Critical History* (Oxford, Blackwell, 1995).
Bruce, M., *The Coming of the Welfare State* (London, Harper Collins, 1971).
Bruley, S., *Women in Britain Since 1900* (Basingstoke, Palgrave, 1999).
Bryder, L., *Below the Magic Mountain: A Social History of Tuberculosis in Twentieth-Century Britain* (Oxford, Clarendon Press, 1988).
Bullock, A., *The Life & Times of Ernest Bevin: Volume Two, Minister of Labour 1940–1945* (London, Heinemann, 1967).
Burch, S., 'Disability History: Suggested Readings – An Annotated Bibliography', *The Public Historian*, vol. 27, no. 2 (2005), pp. 63–74.
Burch, S., and Rembis, M., *Disability Histories* (Urbana, University of Illinois Press, 2014).
Butler, R., and Parr, H., (eds.) *Mind and Body Space: Geographies of illness, impairment and disability* (Abingdon, Routledge, 1999).
Calder, A., *The People's War: Britain 1939–1945* (London, Pimlico, 1969).
Calder, A., *The Myth of the Blitz* (London, Pimlico, 1991).
Campbell, J., and Oliver, M., *Disability Politics: Understanding Our Past, Changing Our Future* (London, Routledge, 1996).
Carden-Coyne, A., 'Ungrateful Bodies: Rehabilitation, Resistance and Disabled American Veterans of the First World War', *European Review of History*, vol. 14, no. 4 (2007), pp. 543–565.
Carden-Coyne, A., *Reconstructing the Body: Classicism, Modernism, and the First World War* (Oxford, Oxford University Press, 2009).
Carnevali, F., and Strange, J., (eds.) *20th Century Britain: Economic, Cultural and Social Change*, 2nd Edition (Harlow, Pearson, 2007).
Carrier, J., and Kendall, I., *Health and the National Health Service* (London, Athlone Press, 1998).
Carter, E.W., Bendetson, S., and Guiden, C.H., 'Family Perspectives on the Appeals of and Alternatives to Sheltered Employment for Individuals with Severe Disabilities', *Research and Practice for Persons with Severe Disabilities*, 43(3), (2018), pp. 145–164.

Chandler, J.A., *Explaining Local Government: Local Government in Britain since 1800* (Manchester, Manchester University Press, 2007).

Childs, D., *Britain Since 1945: A Political History*, 5th Edition (London, Routledge, 2001).

Cohen, D., *The War Come Home: Disabled Veterans in Britain and Germany, 1914–1939* (Los Angeles, University of California Press, 2001).

Cohen, D., 'Will to Work: Disabled Veterans in Britain and Germany after the First World War', in D. A. Gerber (ed.) *Disabled Veterans in History* (Ann Arbor, University of Michigan Press, 2012), pp. 295–321.

Coxall, B., and Robins, L., *British Politics Since the War* (Basingstoke, Macmillan, 1998).

Crompton, R., and Sanderson, K., *Gendered Jobs & Social Change* (London, Unwin Hyman, 1990).

Cronin, J.E., *The Politics of State Expansion: War, State and Society in Twentieth-Century Britain* (London, Routledge, 1991).

Curtis, B., and Thompson, S., "A plentiful crop of cripples made by all this progress': Disability, Artificial Limbs and Working-Class Mutualism in the South Wales Coalfield, 1890–1948', *Social History of Medicine,* vol. 27, no. 4 (2014), pp. 708–727

Curtis, B., and Thompson, S., 'Disability and the Family in South Wales Coalfield Society, c.1920–1939', *Family and Community History,* vol. 20, no. 1, (2017), pp. 25–44.

Dale, P., and Melling, J., (eds.) *Mental Illness and Learning Disability since 1850: Finding a Place for Mental Disorder in the United Kingdom* (Oxon, Routledge, 2006).

Deacon, A., 'Spending More to Achieve less? Social Security Since 1945' in D. Gladstone, (ed.) *British Social Welfare: Past, Present and Future* (London, UCL Press, 1995), pp. 71–97.

Deakin, N., *The Politics of Welfare: Continuities and Change* (London, Harvester Wheatsheaf, 1994).

Digby, A., *British Welfare Policy: Workhouse to Workfare* (London, Faber and Faber, 1989).

Dorey, P., *British Politics since 1945* (Oxford, Blackwell, 1995).

Dudink, S., Hagemann, K., and Tosh, J., (eds.) *Masculinities in Politics and War: Gendering Modern History* (Manchester, Manchester University Press, 2004).

Dunleavy, P., and Husbands, C.T., *British Democracy at the Crossroads: Voting and Party Competition in the 1980s* (London, Allen & Unwin, 1985).

Dunleavy, P., and O'Leary, B., *Theories of the State: The Politics of Liberal Democracy,* (Basingstoke, Macmillan, 1987).

Dutton, D., *British Politics Since 1945*, 2nd Edition (Oxford, Blackwell, 1997).

Eastwood, G.G., *George Isaacs: Printer, Trade-union Leader, Cabinet Minister* (London, Odhams Press, 1952).

Edwards, J.L., 'Remploy: An Experiment in Sheltered Employment for the Severely Disabled in Great Britain', *International Labour Review*, vol. LXXVII, no. 2 (1958).
Ellison, N., and Pierson, C., (eds.) *Developments in British Social Policy* (Basingstoke, Macmillan, 1998).
Ellison, N., and Pierson, C., (eds.) *Developments in British Social Policy 2* (Basingstoke, Palgrave Macmillan, 2003).
Elsey, E., 'The Rehabilitation and Employment of Disabled Ex-Servicemen after the Two World Wars'. Unpublished PhD Thesis, University of Teesside (1994).
Elsey, E., 'Disabled Ex-servicemen's Experiences of Rehabilitation and Employment After the First World War', *Oral History*, vol. 25, no. 2 (1997), pp. 49–58.
Ernst, W., (ed.) *Histories of the Normal and the Abnormal* (Abingdon, Routledge, 2006).
Esping-Anderson, G., *The Three Worlds of Welfare Capitalism* (Princeton, Princeton University Press, 1990).
Fawcett, H., and Lowe, R., (eds.) *Welfare Policy in Britain: The Road From 1945* (Basingstoke, Macmillan, 1999).
Finlayson, G., 'A Moving Frontier: Voluntarism and the State in British Social Welfare 1911–1949', *Twentieth Century British History*, vol. 1, no. 2 (1990), pp. 183–206.
Finlayson, G., *Citizen, State, and Social Welfare in Britain 1830–1990* (Oxford, Clarendon Press, 1994).
Fleischer, D.Z., and Zames, F., *The Disability Rights Movement: From Charity to Confrontation* (Philadelphia, Temple University Press, 2011).
Francis, M., 'The Domestication of the Male? Recent Research on Nineteenth- and Twentieth-Century British Masculinity', *The Historical Journal*, vol. 45, no. 3 (2002), pp. 637–52.
Francis, M., 'Leisure and Popular Culture', in Zweiniger-Bargielowska, I., (ed.), *Women in Twentieth-Century Britain* (London, Routledge, 2014), pp229–243.
Fraser, Duncan., 'The Postwar Consensus: A Debate Not Long Enough?', *Parliamentary Affairs*, vol. 53, no. 2 (2000), pp. 347–362.
Fraser, D., *The Welfare State* (Stroud, Sutton, 2000).
Fraser, D., *The Evolution of the British Welfare State*, 4th Edition (Basingstoke, Palgrave Macmillan, 2009).
Gagen, W.J., 'Disabling Masculinity: Ex-servicemen, Disability, and Gender-identity, 1914–1930'. Unpublished PhD Thesis, University of Essex (2004).
Gagen, W.J., 'Remastering the Body, Renegotiating Gender: Physical Disability and Masculinity during the First World War, the case of J.B. Middlebrook', *European Review of History*, vol. 14, no. 4 (2007), pp. 525–41.

Garland-Thomson, R., (ed.) *Freakery: Cultural Spectacles of the Extraordinary Body* (New York, New York University Press, 1996).

Gerber, D.A., 'Disabled Veterans, the State, and the Experience of Disability in Western Societies, 1914–1950', *Journal of Social History*, vol. 36, no. 4 (2003), pp. 899–916.

Gerber, D.A., 'Introduction: Finding Disabled Veterans in History', in D.A. Gerber (ed.) *Disabled Veterans in History* (Ann Arbor, University of Michigan Press, 2012), pp. 1–51.

Gerber, D.A., (ed.) *Disabled Veterans in History* (Ann Arbor, University of Michigan Press, 2012).

Gladstone, D., 'The Welfare State and the State of Welfare', in D. Gladstone, (ed.) *British Social Welfare: Past, Present and Future* (London, UCL Press, 1995), pp. 1–27.

Gladstone, D., *The Twentieth-Century Welfare State* (Basingstoke, Palgrave Macmillan, 1999).

Gleeson, B., 'Disability Studies: A Historical Materialist View', *Disability & Society*, vol. 12, no. 2 (1997), pp. 179–202.

Gleeson, B., *Geographies of Disability* (London, Routledge, 1999).

Glennerster, H., *British Social Policy: 1945 to the Present*, 3rd Edition (Oxford, Blackwell Publishing, 2007).

Glucksmann, M., *Women Assemble: Women Workers and the New Industries in Inter-War Britain* (London, Routledge, 1990).

Gorsky, M., *Patterns of Philanthropy: Charity and Society in Nineteenth-century Bristol* (London, Boydell Press, 1999).

Gough, I., *The Political Economy of the Welfare State, Critical Texts in Social Work and the Welfare State* (London, Palgrave Macmillan, 1979).

Gourvish, T., 'The Rise (and Fall?) of State-Owned Enterprise', in Gourvish, T., and O'Day, A., (eds.), *Britain Since 1945* (Basingstoke, Macmillan, 1991), pp. 111–133.

Grier, J., 'Voluntary Rights and Statutory Wrongs: The Case of Child Migration, 1948–67', *History of Education*, vol. 31 no. 3 (2002), pp. 263–80.

Gulland, J., *Gender, Work and Social Control: A Century of Disability Benefits* (Palgrave Macmillan, 2019).

Hall, E., 'Workspaces: Refiguring the Disability—Employment Debate', in Butler, R., and Parr, H., (eds.) *Mind and Body Space: Geographies of Illness, Impairment and Disability* (Abingdon, Routledge, 1999), pp. 138–154.

Hampton, J., 'Disabled People and the Classic Welfare State, 1948–1975: Changes in Perception, Developments in Policy'. Unpublished PhD Thesis, University of Bristol (2012).

Hampton, J., 'Discovering Disability: The General Classes of Disabled People and the Classic Welfare State, 1948–1964', *The Historian*, vol. 75, no. 1 (2013), pp. 69–93.

Hampton, J., *Disability and the Welfare State in Britain: Changes in perception and policy 1948–79* (Bristol, Policy Press, 2016).
Harris, B., *The Origins of the British Welfare State* (Basingstoke, Palgrave Macmillan, 2004).
Harris, J., 'Political Thought and the Welfare State 1870–1914: An Intellectual Framework for British Social Policy', *Past and Present*, vol. 135 (1992), pp. 116–141.
Harris, J., and Roulstone, A., *Disability, Policy and Professional Practice* (London, Sage, 2011).
Harrison, B., 'The Rise, Fall and Rise of Political Consensus in Britain since 1940', *History: Journal of the Historical Association*, vol. 84, no. 274 (1999), pp. 301–24.
Hay, R., 'Employers and Social Policy in Britain: the Evolution of Welfare Legislation, 1905–14', *Social History*, vol. 2, no. 4 (1977), pp. 435–55.
Hemphill, E., and Kulik, C.T., 'The Tyranny of Fit: Yet another Barrier to Mainstream Employment for Disabled People in Sheltered Employment', *Social Policy & Administration*, 51:7, (Dec 2017), pp. 1119–34;
Hill, M., *The Welfare State in Britain: A Political History since 1945* (Aldershot, Edward Elgar Publishing, 1993).
Holloway, G., *Women and Work in Britain Since 1840* (Abingdon, Routledge, 2005).
Holroyde, A., 'Sheltered Employment and Mental Health in Britain: Remploy c.1945–81', in S.J. Taylor and A. Brumby (eds.), *Healthy Minds in the Twentieth Century: In and Beyond the Asylum* (Palgrave Macmillan, 2020), pp. 113–35.
Holt, R., 'Sport and Recreation', in P. Addison and H. Jones (eds.) *A Companion to Contemporary Britain 1939–2000* (Oxford, Blackwell, 2005), pp. 110–26.
Holt, R., and Mason, T., *Sport in Britain 1945–2000* (Oxford, Blackwell, 2000).
Hudson, G.L., 'Disabled Veterans and the State in Early Modern England', in Gerber, D.A., (ed.) *Disabled Veterans in History* (Ann Arbor, University of Michigan Press, 2012), pp. 117–44.
Humphries, S., and Gordon, P., *Out of Sight: The Experience of Disability 1900–1950* (Plymouth, Northcote House, 1992).
Hutchinson, I., Atherton, M., & Virdi, J., (eds.) *Disability and the Victorians: Attitudes, Interventions, Legacies* (Manchester, Manchester University Press, 2022).
Hyde, M., 'Sheltered and Supported Employment in the 1990s: The Experiences of Disabled Workers in the UK', *Disability & Society*, vol. 13, no. 2 (1998), pp. 199–215
Jefferys, K., *The Churchill Coalition and Wartime Politics, 1940–1945* (Manchester, Manchester University Press, 1991).

Jefferys, K., *Retreat from the New Jerusalem, British Politics 1951–64*, (London, Palgrave, 1997).

Jeffries, J., 'The Remploy Resource', *Industrial Management & Data Systems*, vol. 86, no. 1/2, (1986), pp. 7–9.

Johnson, N., *The Welfare State in Transition: The Theory and Practice of Welfare Pluralism* (Amherst, The University of Massachusetts Press, 1987).

Jones, C., and Porter, R., (eds.) *Reassessing Foucault: Power, Medicine and the Body* (London, Routledge, 1994).

Jones, H., 'Introduction', in Jones, H., and Kandiah, M., (eds.), *The Myth of Consensus: New Views on British History, 1945–64* (Basingstoke, 1996), pp. xiii–xvii.

Jones, H., and Kandiah, M., (eds.) *The Myth of Consensus* (Basingstoke, Macmillan, 1996).

Jones, H., 'The State and Social Policy', in Zweiniger-Bargielowska, I., (ed.), *Women in Twentieth-Century Britain* (London, Routledge, 2014), pp. 321–335.

Jones, K., *The Making of Social Policy in Britain 1830–1990*, 2nd Edition (London, Athlone Press, 1996).

Jones, M., and Lowe, R., *From Beveridge to Blair: The First Fifty Years of Britain's Welfare State, 1948–98* (Manchester, Manchester University Press, 2002).

Kavanagh, D., and Morris, P., *Consensus Politics from Attlee to Major*, 2nd Edition (Oxford, Blackwell, 1994).

Kelly, S., *The Myth of Mr. Butskell: The Politics of British Economic Policy, 1950–55* (Aldershot, Ashgate, 2002).

Kendall, J., and Knapp, M., *The Voluntary Sector in the United Kingdom* (Manchester, Manchester University Press, 1996).

Kinder, J.M., "Lest We Forget': Disabled Veterans and the Politics of War Remembrance in the United States' in Burch, S., and Rembis, M., (eds.) *Disability History* (Urbana, University of Illinois Press, 2014), pp. 163–182.

King, L., *Family Men: Fatherhood and Masculinity in Britain, 1914–1960* (Oxford, Oxford University Press, 2015).

King, L., 'How Men Valued Women's Work: Labour In and Outside the Home in Post-War Britain', *Contemporary European History*, 28 (2019), pp. 454–468.

Kitson-Clark, G., *An Expanding Society: Britain 1830–1900* (Cambridge, Cambridge University Press, 1967).

Knight, B., *Voluntary Action* (London, Centris 1993).

Kochan, A., 'Remploy: Disabled and Thriving', *Assembly Automation*, vol. 16, no. 1 (1996), pp. 40–41.

Koven, S., 'Remembering and Dismemberment: Crippled Children, Wounded Soldiers and the Great War in Great Britain', *American Historical Review*, vol. 99, no. 4, (1994), pp. 1167–202.

Koven, S., and Michel, S., 'Womanly Duties: Maternalist Politics and the Origins of Welfare States in France, Germany, Great Britain and the United States, 1880–1920', *American Historical Review*, vol. 95, no. 4 (1990), pp. 1076–1108.

Koven, S., and Michel, S., (eds.), *Mothers of a New World: Maternalist Politics and the Origins of Welfare States* (London, Routledge, 1993).

Kowalsky, M., 'Enabling the Great War: Ex-servicemen, the Mixed Economy of Welfare and the Social Construction of Disability, 1899–1930'. Unpublished PhD Thesis, University of Leeds (2007).

Kowalsky, M., "This Honourable Obligation": The King's National Roll Scheme for Disabled Ex-servicemen, 1915–1944', *European Review of History*, vol. 14, no. 4 (2007), pp. 567–84.

Kudlick, C., 'Disability History: Why We Need Another "Other', *The American Historical Review*, vol. 108, no. 3 (2003), pp. 763–793.

Land, A., Lowe, R., and Whiteside, N., *The Development of the Welfare State 1939–1951: A Guide to Documents in the Public Record Office* (London, HMSO, 1992).

Laybourn, K., *A History of British Trade Unionism, c.1770–1990* (Stroud, Alan Sutton, 1992).

Laybourn, K., *The Evolution of British Social Policy and the Welfare State, c.1800–1993* (Keele, Keele University Press, 1995).

Laybourn, K., (ed.) *Modern Britain since 1906: A Reader* (London, I.B. Tauris and Co., 1999).

Laybourn, K., *Unemployment and Employment Policies Concerning Women in Britain, 1900–1951* (Lampeter, Edwin Mellen Press, 2002)

Lewis, J., *Women in England 1870–1950: Sexual Divisions and Social Change* (Brighton, Wheatsheaf Books Ltd, 1984).

Lewis, J., *Women in Britain Since 1945: Women, Family, Work and the State in the Post-War Years* (Oxford, Blackwell, 1992).

Lewis, J., 'Gender, the Family and Women's Agency in the Building of States: the British Case', *Social History*, vol. 19, no. 1 (1994), pp 37–55.

Linker, B., 'On the Borderlands of Medical and Disability History: A Survey of the Fields', *Bulletin of the History of Medicine*, vol. 87, no. 4 (2013), pp. 499–535.

Lipset, S.M., *Political Man*, (London, Mercury Books, 1963).

Lonsdale, S., *Work and Inequality* (Harlow, Longman, 1985).

Lonsdale, S., *Women and Disability: The Experience of Physical Disability Among Women* (Basingstoke, Macmillan, 1990).

Long, V., *The Rise and Fall of the Healthy Factory: The Politics of Industrial Health in Britain, 1914–60* (Basingstoke, Palgrave Macmillan, 2011).

Longmate, N., *How We Lived Then: A History of Everyday Life during the Second World War* (London, Pimlico, 2002).

Longmore, P.K., and Umansky, L., 'Disability History: From the Margins to the Mainstream', in Longmore, P.K., and Umansky, L., (eds.) *The New Disability History: American Perspectives* (New York, New York University Press, 2001), pp. 1–29.

Lowe, R., 'The Second World War, Consensus, and the Foundation of the Welfare State', *Twentieth Century British History*, vol. 1, no. 2 (1990), pp. 152–82.

Lowe, R., 'Introduction: The Road from 1945', in H. Fawcett and R. Lowe (eds.) *Welfare Policy in Britain: The Road from 1945* (Basingstoke, Macmillan, 1999), pp. 1–17.

Lowe, R., *The Welfare State in Britain Since 1945* (Basingstoke, Palgrave Macmillan, 2005).

Lubenow, W.C., *The Politics of Government Growth: Early Victorian Attitudes Towards State Intervention 1833–1848*, (Newton Abbot, David & Charles, 1971).

MacDonagh, O., 'The Nineteenth Century Revolution in Government- A Reappraisal', *Historical Journal*, vol. 1, no. 1 (1958), pp. 52–67.

MacDonagh, O., *Early Victorian Government* (London, Weidenfeld and Nicolson, 1977).

Malisoff, H., 'The British Disabled Persons (Employment) Act', *Industrial and Labor Relations Review*, vol. 5, no. 2 (1952), pp. 249–57.

Mantin, M., 'Educational Experiences of Deaf Children in Wales: The Cambrian Institution for the Deaf and Dumb, 1847–1914'. Unpublished PhD Thesis, Swansea University (2010).

Mantin, M., 'Coalmining and the National Scheme for Disabled Ex-Servicemen after the First World War', *Social History*, vol. 41, no. 2 (2016), pp. 155–170.

Marshall, T.H., *Social Policy in the Twentieth Century* (London, Hutchinson, 1975).

Martin, K.C., *Hard and Unreal Advice: Mothers, Social Science and the Victorian Poverty Experts* (Basingstoke, Palgrave Macmillan, 2008).

Marwick, A., 'Middle Opinion in the Thirties: Planning, Progress and Political 'Agreement'', *English Historical Review*, vol. 79, no. 311 (1964), pp. 285–98.

Marwick, A., *Britain in the Century of Total War: War, Peace and Social Change 1900–1967* (Middlesex, Penguin, 1970).

Marwick, A., *War and Social Change in the Twentieth Century: a Comparative study of Britain, France, Germany, Russia and the US* (London, Macmillan, 1974).

Marwick, A., *A History of the Modern British Isles, 1914–1999* (Oxford, Blackwell, 2000).
Marwick, A., *British Society Since 1945*, 4th Edition (London, Penguin, 2003).
McCarthy, H., *Double Lives: A History of Working Motherhood* (London, Bloomsbury, 2020).
McCloskey, D., 'Paid Work' in Zweiniger-Bargielowska, I., (ed.), *Women in Twentieth-Century Britain* (London, Routledge, 2014), pp. 165–79.
Meyer, J., "Not Septimus Now': Wives of Disabled Veterans and Cultural Memory of the First World War in Britain', *Women's History Review*, vol. 13, no. 1 (2004), pp. 117–138.
Miliband, R., *Parliamentary Socialism: A study in the politics of labour* (London, Merlin Press, 1972).
Millward, G., 'Invalid Definitions, Invalid Responses: Disability and the Welfare State, 1965–1995'. Unpublished PhD Thesis, London School of Hygiene and Tropical Medicine (2013).
Millward, G., 'Social Security Policy and the Early Disability Movement – Expertise, Disability, and the Government, 1965–77', *Twentieth Century British History*, vol. 26, no. 2 (2015), pp. 274–97.
Millward, G., 'A Disability Act? The Vaccine Damage Payments Act 1979 and the British Government's Response to the Pertussis Vaccine Scare', *Social History of Medicine*, vol. 30, no. 2 (2017), pp. 429–447.
Misra, J., and Akins, F., 'The Welfare State and Women: Structure, Agency, and Diversity', *Social Politics*, vol. 5, no. 3 (1998), pp. 260–78.
Morgan, K.O., *Labour in Power 1945–51* (Oxford, Oxford University Press, 1984).
Morgan, K.O., *Britain Since 1945: The People's Peace, 3rd Edition* (Oxford, Oxford University Press, 2001).
Morris, J., *Pride Against Prejudice: A Personal Politics of Disability* (London, The Women's Press, 1991).
Moreton, T., 'Sheltered Employment: Gateway or "Road Block"?', *Personnel Review*, vol. 21, no. 6 (1992), pp. 37–54.
Mounsey, C., (ed.), *The Idea of Disability in the Eighteenth Century* (Lewisburg, Bucknell University Press, 2014).
Muir, K., "That bastard's following me!' Mentally Ill Australian Veterans Struggling to Maintain Control', in Turner, D.M., and Stagg, K., (eds.) *Social Histories of Disability and Deformity* (Abingdon, Routledge, 2006), pp. 161–174.
Myer-Kelly, M., 'The Child Poverty Action Group, 1965–1974: the Origins and Effectiveness of a Single Issue Pressure Group'. Unpublished PhD Thesis, University of Bristol (2001).
Oakley, A., and Williams, A.S., (eds.) *The Politics of the Welfare State* (London, UCL Press, 1994).

Oliver, M., *The Politics of Disablement* (Basingstoke, Macmillan, 1990).
Oliver, M., and Barnes, C., *Disabled People and Social Policy: From Exclusion to Inclusion* (London, Longman, 1998).
Ott, K., Serlin, D., and Mihm, S., (eds.) *Artificial Parts, Practical Lives: Modern Histories of Prosthetics* (New York, New York University Press, 2002).
Owen, D., *English Philanthropy: 1660–1960* (London, Belknap Press, 1964).
Page, R., *Revisiting the Welfare State* (Maidenhead, Open University Press, 2007).
Page, R., and Silburn, R., (eds.) *British Social Welfare in the Twentieth Century* (Basingstoke, Macmillan, 1998).
Paul, E.A., Millar, F.D., and Paul, J., (eds.) *The Welfare State* (Cambridge, Cambridge University Press, 1997).
Peacock, A.T & Wiseman, J., *The Growth of Public Expenditure in the United Kingdom* (Unwin University Books, 1967).
Pelling, H., *Britain and the Second World War* (London, Collins, 1970).
Pelling, H., *A History of British Trade Unionism*, 3rd Edition (Harmondsworth, Penguin, 1977).
Pemberton, H., 'The Transformation of the Economy', in P. Addison and H. Jones (eds.) *A Companion to Contemporary Britain 1939–2000* (Oxford, Blackwell, 2005), pp. 180–202.
Pemberton, N., 'Enabling the Past: New Perspectives in the History of Disability', *History Workshop Journal*, no. 61 (2006), pp. 292–295.
Pierson, C., *Beyond the Welfare State? The New Political Economy of Welfare* (Cambridge, Polity Press, 1991).
Pierson, C., 'Theory in British Social Policy', in N. Ellison & C. Pierson (eds.) *Developments in British Social Policy* (London, Macmillan, 1998), pp. 17–30.
Pimlott, B., 'The Myth of Consensus', in Smith, L.M., (ed.), *The Making of Britain: Echoes of Greatness,* (Basingstoke, Macmillan, 1988), pp. 129–141.
Pimlott, B., *Frustrate Their Knavish Tricks: Writings on Biography, History and Politics* (London, Harper Collins, 1994).
Prochaska, F., *The Voluntary Impulse: Philanthropy in Modern Britain* (London, Faber and Faber, 1988).
Pugh, M., *Women and the Women's Movement in Britain, 1914–59* (London, Macmillan, 1992).
Quayson, A., *Aesthetic Nervousness: Disability and the Crisis of Representation* (New York, Columbia University Press, 2007).
Reiss, M., *Blind Workers Against Charity: The National League of the Blind of Great Britain and Ireland, 1893–1970* (London, Palgrave Macmillan, 2015).
Reznick, J., *Healing the Nation: Soldiers and the Culture of Caregiving in Britain During the Great War* (Manchester, Manchester University Press, 2005).
Reznick, J., 'Work-Therapy and the Disabled British Soldier in Great Britain in the First World War: The Case of Shepherd's Bush Military Hospital,

London', in D. A. Gerber (ed.) *Disabled Veterans in History* (Ann Arbor, University of Michigan Press, 2012), pp. 185–203.
Robinson, M., *Shell-shocked British Army Veterans in Ireland, 1918–39: A Difficult Homecoming (*Manchester, Manchester University Press, 2022).
Rollings, N., 'Poor Mr Butskell: A Short Life, Wrecked by Schizophrenia"? *Twentieth Century British History*, vol. 5, no. 2 (1994), pp. 183–205.
Roper, M., and Tosh, J., (eds.) *Manful Assertions: Masculinities in Britain since 1800* (London, Routledge, 1991).
Rose, S.O., *Which People's War? National Identity and Citizenship in Wartime Britain 1939–1945* (Oxford, Oxford University Press, 2003).
Rosen, G., (ed.) *Dictionary of Labour Biography* (London, Policio's Publishing, 2001).
Roulstone, A., and Barnes, C., (eds.) *Working Futures? Disabled People, Policy and Social Inclusion* (Bristol, Policy Press, 2005).
Roulstone, A., and Prideaux, S., *Understanding Disability Policy* (Bristol, Policy Press, 2012).
Ryde, P., *Out on a Limb* (British Limbless Ex-Service Men's Association, 1982).
Sainsbury, S., 'Disabled People and the Personal Social Services', in D. Gladstone, (ed.) *British Social Welfare: Past, Present and Future* (London, UCL Press, 1995), pp. 183–195.
Sandell, R., Dodd, J., and Garland-Thomson, R., *Re-presenting Disability: Activism and Agency in the Museum* (Abingdon, Routledge, 2010).
Seaman, L.C.B., *Post-Victorian Britain, 1902–1951* (London, Methuen and Co., 1966).
Seldon, A., 'Consensus: A Debate Too Long?', *Parliamentary Affairs,* vol. 47, no. 4 (1994), pp. 501–514.
Shah, S., and Priestley, M., *Disability and Social Change: Private Lives and Public Policies* (Bristol, Policy Press, 2011).
Shakespeare, T., 'The Social Model of Disability', in Davies, L.J., (ed.) *The Disability Studies Reader*, 4th Edition (Abingdon, Routledge, 2013), pp. 214–221.
Skocpol, T., and Ritter, G., 'Gender and the Origins of Modern Social Policies in Britain and the United States', *Studies in American Political Development,* vol. 5, no. 1 (1991), pp. 36–93.
Slorach, R., *A Very Capitalist Condition: A History and Politics of Disability* (London, Bookmarks, 2016).
Smith, H.L., (ed.), *War and Social Change: British Society in the Second World War,* New Edition (Manchester, Manchester University Press, 1990).
Smith, L.M., (ed.) T*he Making of Britain: Echoes of Greatness* (Basingstoke, Macmillan, 1988).

Soeker, M.S., et al., 'The Experiences and Perceptions of Persons with Disabilities Regarding Work Skills Development in Sheltered and Protective Workshops', *Work*, 59:2 (2018), pp. 303–14.

Stephens, M., *Ernest Bevin: Unskilled Labourer and World Statesman 1881–1951* (London, TGWU, 1981).

Stevenson, J., *British Society 1914–45* (London, Penguin, 1984).

Stewart, J., 'The Twentieth Century: an Overview', in R. Page and R. Silburn (eds.) *British Social Welfare in the Twentieth Century* (London, Macmillan, 1999), pp. 15–32.

Stiker, H., *A History of Disability* (Ann Arbor, University of Michigan Press, 1999).

Stone, D., *The Disabled State* (Philadelphia, Temple University Press, 1984).

Storch, R.D., "The Plague of Blue Locusts': Police Reform and Popular Resistance in Northern England 1840–1857', *International Review of Social History*, vol. 20, no. 1 (1975), pp. 61–90.

Storch, R.D., 'The Policeman as Domestic Missionary: Urban Discipline and Popular Culture in Northern England, 1850–1880', *Journal of Social History*, vol. 9, no. 4 (1976), pp. 481–509.

Summerfield, P., *Women Workers in the Second World War: Production and Patriarchy in Conflict* (London, Routledge, 1984).

Taylor, M., 'Voluntary Action and the State', in D. Gladstone, (ed.) *British Social Welfare: Past, Present and Future* (London, UCL Press, 1995), pp. 214–204.

Thane, P., 'The Working Class and State "Welfare" in Britain 1880–1914', *Historical Journal*, vol. 27, no. 4 (1984), pp. 877–900.

Thane, P., 'Government and Society in England and Wales, 1750–1914', in F.M.L. Thompson (ed.), *The Cambridge Social History of Britain 1750–1950, vol. 3, Social Agencies and Institutions* (Cambridge, Cambridge University Press, 1990), pp. 1–62.

Thane, P., 'Visions of Gender in the Making of the British Welfare State' in G. Bock and P. Thane (eds.), *Maternity and Gender Policies: Women and the Rise of the European Welfare States, 1880s–1950s* (London, Routledge, 1991).

Thane, P., 'Towards Equal Opportunities? Women in Britain since 1945', in Gourvish, T., and O'Day, A., (eds.), *Britain Since 1945* (Basingstoke, Macmillan, 1991), pp. 183–208.

Thane, P., 'Women in the British Labour Party and the Construction of State Welfare, 1906–39' in S. Koven and S. Michel (eds.), *Mothers of a New World: Maternalist Politics and the Origins of Welfare States* (London, Routledge, 1993), pp. 343–77.

Thane, P., *Foundations of the Welfare State*, 2nd Edition (London, Longman, 1996).

Thane, P., 'Voluntary Action in Britain since Beveridge', in Oppenheimer, M., and Deakin, N., (eds.) *Beveridge and Voluntary Action in Britain and the Wider British World* (Manchester: Manchester University Press, 2011), pp. 121–34.

Thompson, P., *The Voice of the Past: Oral History*, 3rd edition (Oxford: Oxford University Press, 2000).

Thorpe, A., 'Myth and Counter-myth in Second World War British Politics', in Williams, C., and Edwards, A., (eds.) *The Art of the Possible: Politics and Governance in Modern British History, 1885–1997* (Manchester, Manchester University Press, 2015), pp. 121–142.

Timmins, N., *The Five Giants: A Biography of the Welfare State*, New Edition (London, Harper Collins, 2001).

Titmuss, R.M. *Problems of Social Policy* (London, HMSO and Longmans, 1950).

Topliss, E., *Provision for the Disabled* (Oxford, Basil Blackwell, 1979).

Toye, R., 'From "Consensus" to "Common Ground": The Rhetoric of the Postwar Settlement and its Collapse', *Journal of Contemporary History*, vol. 48, no. 1, (2012), pp. 3–23.

Tremain, S., (ed.) *Foucault and the Government of Disability* (Ann Arbor, University of Michigan Press, 2005)

Turner, A., and McIvor, A., "Bottom Dog Men': Disability, Social Welfare and Advocacy in the Scottish Coalfields in the Interwar Years, 1918–1939', *Scottish Historical Review*, 96:2 (2017), pp. 187–213.

Turner, D.M., 'Disability History: Looking Forward to a Better Past?', *History Workshop Journal*, no. 71 (2011), pp. 283–287.

Turner, D.M., and Blackie, D., *Disability in the Industrial Revolution: Physical impairment in British coalmining, 1780–1880* (Manchester, Manchester University Press, 2018).

Turner, D.M., and Stagg, K., (eds.) *Social Histories of Disability and Deformity* (Abingdon, Routledge, 2006).

Van Der Torre, L. and Fenger, M., 'Policy Innovations for Including Disabled People in the Labour Market: A study of Innovative Practices of Dutch Sheltered Work Companies', *International Social Security Review*, 67:2 (2014), pp. 67–84.

Visier, L., 'Sheltered Employment for Persons with Disabilities', *International Labour Review*, 137:3 (1998), pp. 347–65.

Weiler, P., *Ernest Bevin* (Manchester, Manchester University Press, 1993).

Welshman, J., 'Inside the Walls of the Hostel, 1940–74' in P. Dale and J. Melling, *Mental Illness and Learning Disability Since 1850* (Abingdon, Routledge, 2006), pp. 200–223.

Wheatcroft, S., *Worth Saving: Disabled children during the Second World War* (Manchester, Manchester University Press, 2013)

Wightman, C., *More than Munitions: Women, Work and the Engineering Industries 1900–1950* (Harlow, Longman, 1999).

Wilson, D.S., 'Gender: Change and Continuity', in P. Addison and H. Jones (eds.) *A Companion to Contemporary Britain 1939–2000* (Oxford, Blackwell, 2005), pp. 245–62.

Wilson, D.S., 'A New Look at the Affluent Worker: The Good Working Mother in Post-War Britain', *Twentieth Century British History*, Vol. 17, no. 2 (2006), pp. 206–29.

Wilson, D.S., 'Gender, Race and Ideal Labour Force' in L. Ryan and W. Webster (eds.), *Gendering Migration: Masculinity, Femininity and Ethnicity in Post-War Britain* (Aldershot, Ashgate, 2008), pp. 89–103.

Wilson, E., *Women and the Welfare State* (London, Tavistock Publications, 1977).

Wootton, G., *The Politics of Influence: British Ex-servicemen, Cabinet Decisions and Cultural Change, 1917–57* (London, Routledge and Kegan Paul, 1963).

Wright, G., *The Ordeal of Total War, 1939–1945* (London, Harper & Row, 1968).

Younghusband, E., *Social Work in Britain: 1950–1975* (London, Allen and Unwin, 1978).

Zweiniger-Bargielowska, I., (ed.) *Women in Twentieth-Century Britain* (London, Routledge, 2014).

Index

© The Editor(s) (if applicable) and The Author(s), under exclusive license to Springer Nature Switzerland AG 2025

A. Holroyde, *Sheltered Employment and Disability in the British Welfare State*, New Directions in Welfare History,
https://doi.org/10.1007/978-3-031-87876-3

The manufacturer's authorised representative in the EU is Springer Nature Customer Service Centre GmbH, Europaplatz 3, 69115 Heidelberg, Germany. If you have any concerns regarding our products, please contact ProductSafety@springernature.com

Printed and bound by CPI Group (UK) Ltd, Croydon, CR0 4YY

05/10/2026

02228125-0010